Monoclonal Antibodies and Functional Cell Lines

Progress and Applications

Monoclonal Antibodies and Functional Cell Lines

Progress and Applications

Edited by

Roger H. Kennett

University of Pennsylvania School of Medicine
Philadelphia, Pennsylvania

Kathleen B. Bechtol

The Wistar Institute of Anatomy and Biology
Philadelphia, Pennsylvania

and

Thomas J. McKearn

Cytogen Corporation
Princeton, New Jersey

Plenum Press • New York and London

Library of Congress Cataloging in Publication Data

Main entry under title:

Monoclonal antibodies and functional cell lines.

Bibliography: p.
Includes index.
1. Antibodies, Monoclonal. 2. Cell lines. I. Kennett, Roger H. II. Bechtol,
Kathleen B. III. McKearn, Thomas J. [DNLM: 1. Monoclonal antibodies. 2. Cell
line. W1 BI918P v.1 / QW 575 M475]
QR186.85.M657   1984   616.07'93   84-4847
ISBN 0-306-41567-4

© 1984 Plenum Press, New York
A Division of Plenum Publishing Corporation
233 Spring Street, New York, N.Y. 10013

Printed in the United States of America

Contributors

KATHLEEN B. BECHTOL, The Wistar Institute of Anatomy and Biology, Philadelphia, Pennsylvania 19104

FRANK BERTHOLD, Department of Human Genetics, University of Pennsylvania School of Medicine, Philadelphia, Pennsylvania 19104, and Universitätskinderklinik, D 6300 Giessen, Federal Republic of Germany

S. H. BLOSE, Cold Spring Harbor Laboratory, Cold Spring Harbor, New York 11724

CLAYTON A. BUCK, The Wistar Institute of Anatomy and Biology, Philadelphia, Pennsylvania 19104

DAVID W. BUCK, Cetus Immune Research Laboratories, Palo Alto, California 94303. Present address: Becton Dickinson Monoclonal Center, Inc., Mountain View, California 94043

ROBERTO L. CERIANI, Children's Hospital Medical Center, Bruce Lyons Memorial Research Laboratory, Oakland, California 94609

CHRISTINE CLARK, Bethesda Research Laboratories, Gaithersburg, Maryland 20877

CAROLINE H. DAMSKY, The Wistar Institute of Anatomy and Biology, Philadelphia, Pennsylvania 19104

CINDI DECKER, Department of Biochemistry and Biophysics, University of Pennsylvania School of Medicine, Philadelphia, Pennsylvania 19104

BRADLEY J. DYER, Cetus Immune Research Laboratories, Palo Alto, California 94303

J. R. FERAMISCO, Cold Spring Harbor Laboratory, Cold Spring Harbor, New York 11724

CHERYL A. FISHER, Department of Anatomy, University of Pennsylvania School of Medicine, Philadelphia, Pennsylvania 19104

FRANK W. FITCH, Committee on Immunology, Department of Pathology, University of Chicago, Chicago, Illinois 60637

ANDREW L. GLASEBROOK, Department of Immunology, Swiss Institute for Experimental Cancer Research, Epalinges S./Lausanne, Switzerland CH 1006. Current address: The Salk Institute, San Diego, California 92138

SEN-ITIROH HAKOMORI, Division of Biochemical Oncology, Fred Hutchinson Cancer Research Center, and University of Washington, Seattle, Washington 98104

HARRY HARRIS, Department of Human Genetics, University of Pennsylvania School of Medicine, Philadelphia, Pennsylvania 19104

MARY KATE HART, Department of Pathology, Divisions of Research Immunology and Laboratory Medicine, University of Pennsylvania School of Medicine, Philadelphia, Pennsylvania 19104

ALAN F. HORWITZ, Department of Biochemistry and Biophysics, University of Pennsylvania School of Medicine, Philadelphia, Pennsylvania 19104

NAOHIKO IKEGAKI, Department of Human Genetics, University of Pennsylvania School of Medicine, Philadelphia, Pennsylvania 19104

ZDENKA L. JONAK, Department of Human Genetics, University of Pennsylvania School of Medicine, Philadelphia, Pennsylvania 19104

ROGER H. KENNETT, Department of Human Genetics, University of Pennsylvania School of Medicine, Philadelphia, Pennsylvania 19104

KAREN A. KNUDSEN, The Wistar Institute of Anatomy and Biology, Philadelphia, Pennsylvania 19104

LOIS ALTERMAN LAMPSON, Department of Anatomy, University of Pennsylvania School of Medicine, Philadelphia, Pennsylvania 19104

JAMES W. LARRICK, Cetus Immune Research Laboratories, Palo Alto, California 94303

CAROL J. LAWTON, Department of Anatomy, University of Pennsylvania School of Medicine, Philadelphia, Pennsylvania 19104

RONALD LEVY, Department of Medicine, Stanford University, Stanford, California 94305

J. J. C. LIN, Cold Spring Harbor Laboratory, Cold Spring Harbor, New York 11724. Present address: Department of Zoology, University of Iowa, Iowa City, Iowa 52242

MICHAEL LINK, Department of Pediatrics, Stanford University, Stanford, California 94305

ELLIOTT K. MAIN, Department of Pathology, Divisions of Research Immunology and Laboratory Medicine and of Obstetrics and Gynecology, University of Pennsylvania School of Medicine, Philadelphia, Pennsylvania 19104

DAVID G. MALONEY, Department of Medicine, Stanford University, Stanford, California 94305

F. MATSUMURA, Cold Spring Harbor Laboratory, Cold Spring Harbor, New York 11724

GERD G. MAUL, The Wistar Institute of Anatomy and Biology, Philadelphia, Pennsylvania 19104

THOMAS J. MCKEARN, Cytogen Corporation, Princeton-Forrestal Center, Princeton, New Jersey 08540

RICHARD A. MILLER, Department of Medicine, Stanford University, Stanford, California 94305

NICOLA T. NEFF, Department of Biochemistry and Biophysics, University of Pennsylvania School of Medicine, Philadelphia, Pennsylvania 19104

ALAN OSEROFF, Department of Medicine, Stanford University, Stanford, California 94305

ANSELMO OTERO, National Cancer Center for Scientific Research, Havana, Cuba

S. MICHAEL PHILLIPS, Allergy and Immunology Section, University of Pennsylvania School of Medicine, Philadelphia, Pennsylvania 19104

ANDREW RAUBITSCHEK, Cetus Immune Research Laboratories, Palo Alto, California 94303

DAVID P. RICHMAN, Department of Neurology, Division of the Biological Sciences, University of Chicago, and Pritzker School of Medicine, Chicago, Illinois 60637

G. SENYK, Cetus Immune Research Laboratories, Palo Alto, California 94303

PAUL STRATTE, Department of Medicine, Stanford University, Stanford, California 94305

KENNETH E. TRUITT, Cetus Immune Research Laboratories, Palo Alto, California 94303

ROSEMARY J. VERSTEEGEN, Bethesda Research Laboratories, Gaithersburg, Maryland 20877

J. WANG, Cetus Immune Research Laboratories, Palo Alto, California 94303

DARCY B. WILSON, Department of Pathology, Divisions of Research Immunology and Laboratory Medicine, University of Pennsylvania School of Medicine, Philadelphia, Pennsylvania 19104

JAMES P. WHELAN, Department of Anatomy, University of Pennsylvania School of Medicine, Philadelphia, Pennsylvania 19104

DENI M. ZODDA, SmithKline Diagnostics, Sunnyvale, California 90486

Preface

This volume serves as a follow-up to our previous book, *Monoclonal Antibodies—Hybridomas: A New Dimension in Biological Analyses.* We continue the theme of monoclonal antibodies and their applications, attempting to cover some of the areas not covered in the previous volume. We again include an appendix describing methods useful to those who are beginning to apply these techniques in their own laboratories.

This volume will be followed by another concentrating on the combination of monoclonal antibody techniques with molecular genetic techniques to study structure/function relationships at the level of both the gene and gene product.

Roger H. Kennett
Kathleen B. Bechtol

Philadelphia, Pennsylvania

Thomas J. McKearn

Princeton, New Jersey

Acknowledgments

Roger Kennett acknowledges the patience and support of his wife, Carol, and his family, friends, and colleagues during the work on this volume, and again thanks, above all, the Lord, Jesus Christ.

Kathleen Bechtol wishes to thank colleagues and friends for their support and understanding during the months of preparation of this volume.

Tom McKearn acknowledges and thanks his wife, Pat, and his family for their support and encouragement.

Contents

Part V Developing Areas of Biotechnology

11 Production of Human Monoclonal Antibodies   275

David W. Buck, James W. Larrick, Andrew Raubitschek,
Kenneth E. Truitt, G. Senyk, J. Wang, and Bradley J. Dyer

12 Monoclonal Antibodies and Molecular Genetics: Oncogenes
    and Oncogene Products   311

Roger H. Kennett, Zdenka L. Jonak, and Naohiko Ikegaki

13 Functional Murine T-Cell Clones   341

Frank W. Fitch and Andrew L. Glasebrook

Appendix Additional Methods for Production and
    Characterization of Monoclonal Antibodies
    and Continuous Cell Lines

PART I
INTRODUCTION

1
Introduction

Reflections on Nine Years of Monoclonal Antibodies from Hybridomas

ROGER H. KENNETT, KATHLEEN B. BECHTOL, AND THOMAS J. MCKEARN

I. Biotechnology's "Coming of Age"

It has been 9 years since Kohler and Milstein (1975) first reported the production of monoclonal antibodies with predefined specificity. During the intervening time, these reagents have become valuable tools in biomedical research, some have been given FDA approval, and they have been used on patients for therapy; moreover, recent biotechnology newsletters indicate that the first "over-the-counter" monoclonal antibody kit is now available.

Monoclonal antibody technology grew very rapidly after its introduction, as indicated by Figure 1, showing the citations of Kohler and Milstein's original article. The "log phase" of growth lasted for several years, and the number of citations per year continues to grow even through the seventh year after the original report. The "genealogy" of hybridoma production is pictured in Figure 2. Although somewhat simplified, it represents the two major technical advances that made hybridoma production possible—the derivation of mouse plasmacytoma cell lines (Potter, 1972) and the techniques of somatic cell hybridization (Ephrussi, 1972; Kennett, 1979). A similar wedding of enzymology and molecular biology contributed to the development of recombinant DNA techniques, and there are already signs that these two new offspring, which are the

ROGER H. KENNETT • Department of Human Genetics, University of Pennsylvania School of Medicine, Philadelphia, Pennsylvania 19104. KATHLEEN B. BECHTOL • The Wistar Institute of Anatomy and Biology, Philadelphia, Pennsylvania 19104. THOMAS J. MCKEARN • Cytogen Corporation, Princeton-Forrestal Center, Princeton, New Jersey 08540.

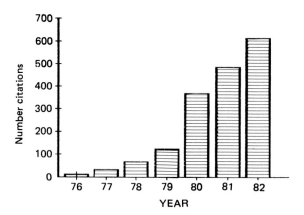

FIGURE 1. The number of publications citing Kohler and Milstein's (1975) original paper on mono-clonal antibodies in the years 1976–1982 as listed in the *Science Citation Index*. This does not, of course, include every publication using monoclonal antibodies, but does provide an indication of the rapid rate with which this technology has spread.

major components of the new rapid developments in biotechnology, will be combined to produce new progeny of which we may not even be aware.

In a recent listing of 141 biotechnology companies (Dorfman, 1982), 27 were listed as using hybridoma production, 43 recombinant DNA techniques, and 35 others were actually using both of these technologies. Ways in which the techniques are being used and will be used together in the future are discussed in Chapter 12 of this volume.

During the early stages of monoclonal antibody technology, it was, in general, immunologists who were aware of the implications and could take advantage of the production of hybridomas (Melchers *et al.*, 1978). Since those early years, it has spread to nearly every aspect of biomedical science. Section II provides a general overview of the various ways in which these reagents are being applied. As monoclonal antibody techniques evolved from an observation of basic science and developed as a technology, biologists, like physicists and chemists before them, found it necessary to resolve questions about the "interface" of business and academia. This aspect of monoclonal antibody technology and the resulting issues are discussed in Section III of this chapter.

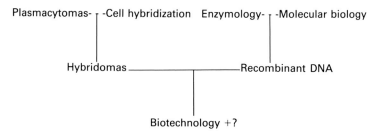

FIGURE 2. A genealogy of monoclonal antibodies. A general representation of the process by which advances in biotechnology have combined to produce new technologies.

During the past few years, the spread of monoclonal antibodies has been so rapid that it is nearly impossible to be aware of all the ways in which these reagents are being used. In our first volume on monoclonal antibodies, we could attempt to cover all the areas of application. By the time it was in print, there were already several aspects that were not included. At the time of preparing the present volume, the techniques have spread to the point that we cannot even consider being comprehensive, but must choose topics that illustrate in a general way the contributions that monoclonal antibodies have made to the biomedical sciences.

Some of the early enthusiasm for the potential of monoclonal antibodies was tempered by the awareness that monoclonal antibodies exhibited a new type of "cross-reactivity" (Lane and Koprowski, 1982). It was realized that even though they react with a single epitope, each antibody can react with more than a single molecule by detecting the same or a similar array of amino acids or carbohydrate moieties in different contexts.

As the technology has developed, it has become clear that the advantages of monoclonal antibody technology fall into general categories that we have tried to represent in the division of this volume.

1. Reactivity with a single epitope does allow the analysis of the fine antigenic structure of molecules and sometimes detection of previously undefined structural relationships.
2. The cloning step of hybridoma production allows one to prepare antibodies against specific molecules that exist in complex biological mixtures and then use the reagents to isolate the molecules and to analyze them in both the *in situ* and extracted form.
3. The availability of large amounts of the specific reagents in purified form that can be standardized and quality-controlled makes it possible to begin to apply these reagents in clinical settings. The specificity of the reagent allows one to make distinctions between "disease"-related epitopes and other "normal" epitopes that were not previously possible.
4. Finally, as in most areas of research, one of the most exciting aspects is that one cannot fully predict where the future will lead. Just as different areas of research combine to produce monoclonal antibody and recombinant DNA technology, so these two aspects of biotechnology are likely to combine with each other and with other aspects of biology to produce even more exciting and useful "surprises."

The topic of monoclonal antibodies and hybridomas has broadened so rapidly that it is impossible to cover the related area of T-cell hybridomas and T-cell lines comprehensively in this volume. We have included one chapter on this topic as a reminder that one can expect continuing developments in this area to combine with monoclonal antibody technology and DNA technology and produce results with considerable impact on biology and medicine. We can expect a continued progress in the isolation and characterization of lymphokines and other growth factors. Monoclonal antibodies and DNA technology will certainly continue to be used to isolate these molecules. By using the T-cell lines and hybrids as a source of mRNA for cloning, one can arrange to have bacteria or yeast make these factors, which can be used for analysis of immune mechanisms and growth control and then applied to therapy. We are planning a future volume in this series to cover these developments in more detail.

II. Monoclonal Antibodies—An Overview of Applications

Currently, the most extensive use of monoclonal antibodies is in research, though diagnostic applications are increasing, and applications in therapy are beginning to surface. A few examples will serve to illustrate the approaches used in the areas on which we have chosen to focus in this volume.

A. Characterization of the Fine Antigenic Structure of Macromolecules

Monoclonal antibodies have made it possible to analyze molecules on an epitope-by-epitope basis. One good example is the acetylcholine receptor (AchR) of the neuromuscular junction, which has been the subject of intensive study. Several animal toxins, such as α-bungarotoxin, specifically bind the receptor at its acetylcholine binding site. Such reagents have allowed affinity purification of the receptor from eel and ray electric organs. Highly purified AchR was thus available for immunizations and assays, and large numbers of specific monoclonal antibodies have been produced in several laboratories. The AchR molecular complex is made up of four polypeptide chains ($\alpha_2\beta\gamma\delta$). One outcome of the monoclonal antibody studies is a demonstration of relatively greater cross-reactivity between the α and β subunits and between the γ and δ subunits of the receptor. This has been interpreted to suggest a single ancestor polypeptide for each pair (Tzartos and Lindstrom, 1980).

The fine structure of the acetylocholine binding site of the receptor also has been further elucidated. Two molecules of α-bungarotoxin bind at or near the acetylcholine binding site on the receptor. It appears now that a monoclonal antibody can distinguish between the two α-bungarotoxin binding sites, that the two sites have different affinities for α-bungarotoxin, and that the antibody blocks binding at the high-affinity site only (Mihovilovic and Richman, 1982; Richman, Chapter 2 of this volume).

One of the early applications of monoclonal antibodies was defining antigenic sites on an antigenic variant of viruses, including flu, measles, and rabies. Monoclonal antibodies have provided reagents capable of distinguishing among strains of viruses isolated in different parts of the world. The reactivities of this world population of viruses with a panel of monoclonal antibodies can be used to ask how closely related the different isolates are to each other and to the strains used to produce vaccines. Laboratory variants of viruses have been obtained by negative selection with monoclonal antibodies (Koprowski and Wiktor, 1980; Gerhard *et al.*, 1980). The use of monoclonal antibodies makes it possible to relate single amino acid changes to changes in antigenic sites on the virus (Laver *et al.*, 1979). These studies, as well as similar studies on bacteria and parasites

(Phillips and Zodda, Chapter 10 of this volume), have implications for the utilization of monoclonal antibodies in medicine as well as providing information on the structure and biology of the microorganisms.

Monoclonal antibodies are being used to distinguish among related molecules in ways that polyclonal sera could not. For example, it is not yet known how many genes code for the different alkaline phosphatases found in various tissues. The molecules are so closely related that polyclonal sera in general fail to distinguish among them even after extensive absorption. In contrast, monoclonal antibodies have been found that distinguish among alkaline phosphatases of different tissue origin, among different alleles from the same tissue initially distinguished by different electrophoretic mobility, and among alleles of the same electrophoretic mobility that had not previously been detected (Slaughter et al., 1980; Harris, Chapter 3 of this volume).

Another example is the use of monoclonal antibodies to distinguish among different steroid hormones. Again, polyclonal sera can distinguish readily among steroid hormones and other molecules in, for example, a patient's serum. They are much less effective in distinguishing among different steroid hormones. However, with monoclonal antibodies that bind the distinguishing region of a particular steroid hormone, e.g., human chorionic gonadotropin, that hormone can be assayed separately from other structurally related steroid hormones. This greatly reduces the incidence of false positives sometimes found with immune sera.

Dr. Hakomori discusses in Chapter 4 the ways in which monoclonal antibodies against defined carbohydrate sequences have been useful and demonstrates the fine degree of specificity that these reagents allow.

In addition to detecting differences among related molecules, monoclonal antibodies have made it possible to detect epitopes shared by molecules that were not previously known to be structurally similar (Lin et al., Chapter 6 of this colume; Lampson, Chapter 7 of this volume).

B. Detection and Isolation of Antigens in Complex Biological Systems

One of the most useful applications of monoclonal antibody technology results from the ability to immunize animals with a complex mixture and obtain antibodies reacting with a single component of the mixture. This has enabled the detection and characterization of a large number of cellular components such as differentiation antigens and other membrane, cytoplasm, and nuclear components.

Monoclonal antibodies to the building blocks of the cytoskeleton provide reagents for immunofluorescent localization of each component under various morphological (e.g., flattened, spread versus round cells) and physiological (e.g., mitosis versus interphase) conditions. Microinjection of some of these monoclonal antibodies into living cells can specifically perturb the cytoskeletal molecule they bind and thus help to further elucidate the roles of the cytoskeletal components in the dynamic milieu of the functioning cell (Lin et al., Chapter 6 of this volume).

Monoclonal antibodies that perturb the cell-surface adhesion functions of cell–cell or cell–substrate interactions are helping to dissect the molecular composition of the adhesion process and to identify the several different mechanisms by which cells adhere (Horwitz *et al.*, Chapter 5 of this volume).

C. Toward Practical Applications in Medicine

Several monoclonal antibodies have been developed for screening tests for various neoplasia: In the case of prostate cancer, monoclonal antibody assays for serum levels of prostatic acid phosphatase (PAP) are currently available from both Hybritech and New England Nuclear. Such assays are more reliable than assays using immune sera, since the reagent is of constant quality from batch to batch (there is no variation in either the specificity or titer). A second reagent for early detection of prostate cancer is currently under development by Hybritech. It is a monoclonal antibody to prostate-specific antigen (PSA). Both the anti-PAP and anti-PSA are useful in monitoring the progress of treatment. However, as screening methods for early detection of the tumor, monoclonals to each antigen have been found to miss some stage 1 cases. Limited clinical tests indicate that the use of these two tests together can significantly improve the early detection of prostate cancer.

Monoclonal antibodies have proven useful in detecting human neuroblastoma cells. Monoclonal antibody PI153/3 reacts with neuroblastoma, retinoblastoma, and glioblastoma cell lines and with fetal brain. It does not react with a number of other tumors and normal tissues, including adult brain (Kennett and Gilbert, 1979). By immunoperoxidase staining of bone marrow samples, PI153/3 was found also to bind to tumor cells in bone marrow samples of patients with acute lympocytic leukemia (positive on non-B, non-T ALL and B-cell ALL but not T-cell ALL) and to a small population of putative immature lymphoid cells in some normal bone marrow samples (Jonak *et al.*, 1982).

It was possible to remove ambiguity in identifying the neuroblastoma cells by adding a second monoclonal antibody, P3B1-C3, to the test. P3B1-C3 does not react with neuroblastoma cells, but does react with all of the leukemia cells and immature lymphoid cells expressing the PI153/3 antigen. The pattern PI153/3 positive (PI153/3[+]), P3B1-C3 negative (P3B1-C3[−]) is expressed on neuroblastoma and retinoblastoma cells, in bone marrow samples, and in tumor biopsies from patients with these neoplasia. By double staining, it was shown that in PI153/3[+], P3B1-C3[+] bone marrow samples from all patients, both antigens are expressed on the surface of the same cell; no PI153/3[+], P3B1-C3[−] cells were found in these samples. Thus, the PI153/3[+], P3B1-C3[−] cell type is characteristic of neuroblastoma and related tumors (Jonak *et al.*, 1982). This illustrates the fact that even though monoclonal antibodies exhibit a limited specificity, the use of monoclonal antibodies for tumor detection is facilitated by the use of a panel of monoclonal antibodies.

In vivo inhibition of human melanoma growth in immunologically deficient nude (*nu/nu*) mice has been found to occur with five IgG2a monoclonal antibodies but not with 28 monoclonals of other antibody classes (IgG1, IgG2b,

IgG3, IgM, and IgA). The tumoricidal effect appears to be an IgG2a monoclonal antibody-dependent, macrophage-mediated cytotoxic activity (Herlyn and Koprowski, 1982). Chapters 8 and 9 in this volume discuss in more detail the use of monoclonal antibodies for detection and therapy of cancer.

In addition to their uses in these studies, monoclonal antibodies are also proving useful in studying the mechanism(s) involved in disease processes and in treatment. The binding specificity, affinity, and class of the antibodies have all been found to be important in determining the effect of the antibody. Some monoclonal antibodies that bind acetylcholine receptor have been found to mimic various aspects of myesthenia gravis. They induce short-term clinical effects identical to those caused by transfer of immune serum from animals with experimental autoimmune myesthenia gravis caused by immunization with purified acetylcholine receptor. Not all of the monoclonals that can cause this acute effect, which includes endplate necrosis and phagocytosis, bind to or near the acetylcholine binding site on the receptor (Richman *et al.*, 1980). Monoclonal antibodies of the IgG2a and IgG2b subclasses are, in general, more potent in producing the acute syndrome, while those of the IgG1 class are less effective (Richman, Chapter 2 of this volume). This may reflect a complement-mediated mechanism for the syndrome, since (1) IgG1 antibodies bind complement with low efficiency compared to IgG2a and IgG2b antibodies, and (2) the syndrome has been shown not to occur in complement-depleted animals (Lennon and Lambert, 1981).

The affinity of the monoclonal antibody is also an important factor in determining its ability to induce acute experimental myesthenia gravis. Monoclonal antibodies that are of low affinity for acetylcholine receptor *in situ* produce little or no clinical effect *in vivo*. The most efficient monoclonal antibodies for inducing the disease are those of intermediate affinity, while those of high affinity are markedly less potent. Previously, little correlation had been found between severity of symptoms and anti-acetylcholine receptor antibodies in the sera of patients with myesthenia gravis. With the new information gained with monoclonal antibodies, it is now time to reexamine this question (Richman, Chapter 2 of this volume).

D. *Developing Areas of Biotechnology*

The final section in the main body of this volume discusses aspects of biotechnology that are related to the initial rapid expansion of mouse monoclonal antibodies but include other aspects that add to or complement these techniques. A natural outgrowth of the original hybridoma technology is discussed by Buck *et al.* in Chapter 11. Chapter 12 discusses in more detail the uses of monoclonal antibodies in combination with molecular genetic techniques, as well as the production of continuous cell lines by transfection with tumor DNA rather than by somatic cell hybridization. Finally, the discussion of T-cell lines describes an area which has grown up along with monoclonal antibody production and which, in fact, complements it and will continue to do so as these two areas are combined to analyze lymphokines and T-cell function.

E. *Appendix to This Volume*

Finally, in the Appendix we include methods that are designed to be, in combination with those included in our first volume, helpful to those who are making monoclonal antibodies and will then need to characterize the antibodies and the antigens they detect, or who have the need to use *in vitro* immunization or to develop continuous B-cell or T-cell lines.

III. *Commercialization of Monoclonal Antibody Technology*

A. *Monoclonal Antibodies as Biotechnology*

Monoclonal antibody technology is an area of biological science with certain commercial potential. Indeed, to the members of the financial community, monoclonal antibody technology is generally viewed as similar to recombinant DNA technology since both of these areas initially involve the transfer of technical information from the biomedical academic institutions into industry, both technologies often deal in medically-related products, and both have resulted in the formation of a number of new companies begun for the express purpose of attempting their commercial exploitation. Despite these similarities, it is important to point out a number of ways in which monoclonal antibody technology is dissimilar to recombinant DNA technology. These include the much narrower focus of activities in the monoclonal antibody area, the fundamentally simpler selection and fusion techniques that monoclonal antibody technology employs, and the fact that no omnibus patent position exists in monoclonal antibody technology comparable to the position the Cohen–Boyer patent applications portend to hold in the recombinant DNA field.

The purpose of this section is to review some of the issues involved in the commercialization of monoclonal antibody technology. It should become apparent that there are many more questions than answers in this area, and it is hoped that this section will point out the substantial number of challenges and opportunities that await people who are willing to become active participants in this field.

B. *Philosophical Issues*

The dawning of the biotechnology era in the past 5–7 years has provided an initial opportunity for significant numbers of biological scientists to venture into the commercial arena. Because the major assets transferred by these scientists were intellectual properties as opposed to real properties, a number of philosophical issues have arisen. One of the more basic conflicts stems from the desire of private industry to have protection for its investments in technology. This protection has traditionally come from either securing patent protection or by maintaining trade secrets. In the former case, one openly discloses the technology that one possesses in exchange for a patent monopoly on this technology for the next 17 years. In the latter case, the companies seek to limit the availability of technical information and keep the technology (often a process) as a trade secret since they view that any disclosure of the information would be harmful and would render the technology unprotectable. Such attitudes of protectionism and secrecy stand in contrast to the philosophy of open discussion and disclosure that typifies the research in an academic setting. It is precisely this issue of ownership, patentability, or confidentiality of intellectual property that has proven to be perhaps the most awkward of barriers separating academia and industry.

A second issue of concern is the ownership of cell lines. Of particular concern are those cell lines that were generated by an academic investigator on an NIH grant and were then transferred or sold to some commercial organization for their exclusive marketing. The issue here is how one justifies the exclusive profit-taking of a private individual or company by way of a cell line generated on grants funded by taxpayer monies.

A third issue concerns those individuals who attempt to retain their full-time academic appointments in their attendant NIH funding bases while exercising significant managerial positions in privately held biotechnology companies. Surely, the prospects of serving two masters must complicate the day-to-day existence of such individuals.

The necessity of resolving the philosophical issues between industry and academia is heightened by the declining federal funding of basic research at the universities. In general, the research that is funded within industry tends to be more applications-oriented, with a goal of improving the efficiency of some manufacturing process or identifying some product applications for an already existing basic technology. This contrasts with the more basic or discovery research, which typically is conducted in an academic setting. This distinction is admittedly an oversimplification, but it permits the obvious suggestion that cooperative efforts between academia and industry should attempt to center the role of each party upon the tasks it does best and attempt to avoid redundant efforts.

C. Scientific Issues

If the application of monoclonal antibody technology to the commercial arena is to be successful in the long term, then the technology must be applied in a scientifically valid manner. One can argue that monoclonal antibody technology has but three basic advantages over conventional serology: (1) the monoclonal nature of the cell lines; (2) the high yield of immunoglobulin products from these hybridoma cells; and (3) the longevity of the cell lines. Functional implications derive from each of these primary properties. Hence, the monoclonal nature of the cell lines allows secretion of a single immunoglobulin product whose immunological specificity is very narrow. The high yield of secreted antibody by the hybridoma cell lines leads to a high specific antibody activity in the fluid surrounding the cells. The longevity of cell lines implies a stable source of the immunoglobulin, which further allows for careful characterization of the properties of this antibody.

Taken in its simplest form, then, one can ask whether a particular commercial application involving an antibody is better served if the antibody is monoclonal, present in high specific activity, or available as a standardized reagent. If the answer to all of these questions is negative, then one is hard pressed to see the need or the advisability of using a hybridoma antibody for the particular commercial application.

D. Business Issues

A biotechnology company, like any other organized human endeavor, requires a plan that includes the strategy and tactics for reaching a number of stated goals. The strategies employed by companies engaged in monoclonal antibody technology seem to fall into one of three categories: (1) development of monoclonal antibodies as replacement modalities for tests currently employing conventional antiserum; (2) development of monoclonal antibodies for new market applications wherein conventional antibodies have proven to be unsatisfactory; or (3) development of ancillary technology required for the efficient application of monoclonal antibodies in a particular market application.

The development of monoclonal antibodies as replacement modalities provides perhaps the fastest method for introducing a monoclonal antibody-based system into the current medical specialties marketplace. Examples of this include the introduction of a test for human IgE by Hybritech and an introduction of a test for the β subunit of chorionic gonadotropin (pregnancy test) by Monoclonal Antibodies, Inc. Such tests would be expected to face immediate competition from the conventional, preexisting antibody-based technologies and, unless the monoclonal antibody *per se* were to grant significant advantages to the user of the assay, it may be difficult to achieve a significant and sustained amount of product sales without substantial erosion of selling price.

Introduction of monoclonal antibodies as components of systems that represent new market applications will undoubtedly prove to be one of the major commercial uses for monoclonal antibody technology. Such applications have already emerged in the medical diagnostics setting (diagnosis of certain infectious diseases), in the therapeutic setting (immunotherapy of leukemias), in commercial processing (affinity chromatography of interferon), and as a research tools (identification of human lymphocyte subpopulations). In these cases, the monoclonal antibody-based systems do not face immediate competition from already existing antibody systems and, hence, the opportunity exists to quickly capture a large market share. Clearly, the same issues of relative worth of the system as compared to the conventional technology will determine the degree to which the particular market opportunities are realized. Also, in some cases, the new materials will be subjected to a more prolonged cycle of regulatory approval and there may be a longer period required for the education of the end-product users.

A number of organizations have already recognized and begun significant efforts in the area of developing ancillary technologies that are perceived to be necessary in order to implement monoclonal antibody technology. Included among these ancillary technologies are programs for the efficient covalent modification of immunoglobulins, programs for the efficient and economical scaleup of antibody production, programs to more rigidly ensure quality control of cell lines secreting monoclonal antibodies, and, finally, programs meant to produce monoclonal antibodies from nonrodent sources, such as humans. It is important to realize that the technical base for these ancillary programs may be in areas far removed from the conventional biological sciences. However, the successful conversion of programs from the research laboratory scale to the full commercial development scale will undoubtedly utilize several of these ancillary technologies.

E. Summary

The commercial development of monoclonal antibodies is in its infancy. Many new companies have sprung up and have attracted scientists with widely different industrial backgrounds. It is to be expected that some of the groups will fail in their plans to commercialize aspects of this technology. Those groups that do succeed commercially are likely to do so because they possess a balance of scientific and business skills and further possess the flexibility to adapt their strategies in the face of emerging competition. One might predict that the large number of startup companies in this area will consolidate with time into fewer groups, each with its own definable market niche. Time alone will tell how and when these transitions occur.

References

Dorfman, P. W. (ed.), 1982, GEN guide to biotechnology, *Genet. Eng. News* **2**:6–19.

Ephrussi, B., 1972, *Hybridization of Somatic Cells*, Princeton University Press, Princeton, New Jersey.

Gerhard, W., Yewdell, J., Frankel, M. E., Lopes, A. D., and Staudt, L., 1980, Monoclonal antibodies against influenza virus, in: *Monoclonal Antibodies. Hybridomas: A New Dimension in Biological Analyses* (R. H. Kennett, T. J. McKearn, and K. B. Bechtol, eds.), Plenum Press, New York, pp. 317–333.

Herlyn, D., and Koprowski, H., 1982, IgG2a monoclonal antibodies inhibit human tumor growth through interaction with effector cells, *Proc. Natl. Acad. Sci. USA* **79**:4761–4765.

Jonak, Z. L., Kennett, R. H. and Bechtol, K. B., 1982, Detection of neuroblastoma cells in bone marrow using a combination of monoclonal antibodies, *Hybridoma* **1**:349–368.

Kennett, R. H., 1979, Cell fusion, in: *Methods in Enzymology*, Volume LVIII (W. B. Jakoby and I. H. Pastan, eds.), Academic Press, New York, pp. 345–367.

Kennett, R. H., and Gilbert, F., 1979, Hybrid myelomas producing antibodies against a human neuroblastoma antigen present on fetal brain, *Science* **203:**1120–1123.

Kohler, G., and Milstein, C., 1975, Continuous culture of fused cells secreting antibody of predefined specificity, *Nature* **256:**495–497.

Koprowski, H., and Wiktor, T., 1980, Monoclonal antibodies against rabies virus, in: *Monoclonal Antibodies. Hybridomas: A New Dimension in Biological Analysis* (R. H. Kennett, T. J. McKearn, and K. B. Bechtol, eds.), Plenum Press, New York, pp. 335–351.

Lane, D., and Koprowski, H., 1982, Molecular recognition and the future of monoclonal antibodies, *Nature* **296:**200–202.

Laver, W. G., Air, G. M., Webster, R. G., Gerhard, W., Ward, C. W., and Dopheide, T. A., 1979, Antigenic drift in a type A influenza virus sequence differences in the hemagglutinin of Hong Kong (H3N2) variants selected with monoclonal antibodies, *Virology* **98:**226–237.

Lennon, V. A., and Lambert, E. H., 1981, Analysis of the antigenicity of acetylcholine receptor using monoclonal hybridoma antibodies, *Ann. N. Y. Acad. Sci.* **377:**143–157.

Melchers, F., Potter, M., and Warner, N. L., 1978, *Curr. Top. Microbiol. Immunol.* **81.**

Mihovilovic, M., and Richman, D. P., 1982, Monoclonal antibody to alpha-bungarotoxin binding site of *Torpedo* acetylcholine receptor modified cholinergic ligand binding to solubilized and membrane-bound acetylcholine receptor, *Soc. Neurosci. Abstr.* **8:**336.

Potter, M., 1972, Immunoglobulin-producing tumors and myeloma proteins of mice, *Physiol. Rev.* **52:**631–719.

Richman, D. P., Gonez, C. M., Berman, P. W., Burres, S. A., Fitch, F. W., and Arnason, B. G. W., 1980, Monoclonal anti-acetylcholine receptor antibodies can cause experimental myesthenia, *Nature* **386:**738–739.

Slaughter, C. A., Coseo, M. C., Abrams, C., Cancro, M. P., and Harris, H., 1980, The use of hybridomas in enzyme genetics, in: *Monoclonal Antibodies. Hybrodomas: A New Dimension in Biological Analyses* (R. H. Kennett, T. J. McKearn, and K. B. Bechtol, eds.), Plenum Press, New York, pp. 103–120.

Tzartos, S. J., and Lindstrom, J. M., 1980, Monoclonal antibodies used to prove acetylcholine receptor structure: Localization of the main immunogenic regions and detection of similarities between subunits, *Proc. Natl. Acad. Sci. USA* **77:**755–779.

PART II
CHARACTERIZATION OF THE DETAILED ANTIGENIC STRUCTURE OF MACROMOLECULES

2

Monoclonal Antibodies Directed against the Nicotinic Acetylcholine Receptor

David P. Richman

I. Introduction

A. The Neuromuscular Junction and Acetylcholine Receptor

The nicotinic acetylcholine receptor (AChR) is a transmembrane glycoprotein located at the neuromuscular junction (NMJ). This well-characterized receptor may be considered a model for the study of other neurotransmitter receptors and other cell membrane receptors, e.g., hormone receptors or antigen receptors. Similarly, the NMJ, because of its location remote from other synapses, represents a convenient model system for the study of synaptic transmission.

Knowledge of the biochemistry and functional behavior of AChR has been greatly enhanced by the existence of two exotic zoological phenomena, the electric organs of electric fishes and the paralytic venoms of elapid snakes. Electric organs of electric eels, e.g., *Electrophorus electricus,* and electric rays, e.g., *Torpedo californica,* have evolved from skeletal muscle by loss of the contractile elements. They represent an extremely rich source of the constituents of the nicotinic synapse and have been used to purify the enzyme acetylcholine esterase as well as AChR. Venoms of elapid snakes, especially the cobra *Naja naja* and the krait *Bungarus multicinctus,* act primarily by blocking neuromuscular transmission. This effect is mediated by polypeptide toxins present in the venoms that bind

David P. Richman • Department of Neurology, Division of the Biological Sciences, University of Chicago, and Pritzker School of Medicine, Chicago, Illinois 60637.

specifically, and with great affinity, to AChR. These 7000- to 8000-dalton toxins, e.g., naja toxin (NT) and α-bungarotoxin (αBT), have been employed as probes for AChR, and, in the case of NT, as an agent for affinity purification of AChR. The toxins bind AChR in a manner that blocks binding of the much smaller cholinergic ligands, so that these toxins in fact are markers for the cholinergic binding site of AChR. When AChR extracted from electric organ is purified on an affinity column made up of NT, large quantities (10–15 mg) of material of high purity (>90% of total protein) are obtained.

The ability to purify AChR has permitted extensive study of its biochemistry, molecular anatomy, and pharmacological and functional characteristics. Binding of cholinergic agonists induces the opening of a cation channel within the AChR molecule, with resultant depolarization of the postsynaptic membrane. The depolarization leads to a propagated action potential in the muscle membrane and eventually to muscle contraction. Information of this sort developed in the study of AChR is applicable to other ion channel-coupled neurotransmitter receptors at other synapses. In addition, data concerning receptor binding and activation are likely to be applicable to other cell surface receptors and, in a broader sense, represent a well-studied example of cell-to-cell communication.

AChR (for reviews see Barrantes, 1983; Briley and Changeux, 1977; Karlin, 1980; Raftery *et al.*, 1980) (from *Torpedo*) is an acidic glycoprotein (pI ≈ 5.0) with a molecular weight of about 250,000 daltons. Each molecule contains two acetylcholine binding sites and is made up of four glycopeptide chains, in the ratios $\alpha_2\beta\gamma\delta$. X-ray crystallographic and electron microscopic studies, as well as models derived from sequencing studies of the cloned genes of each subunit (Ballivet *et al.*, 1982; Devellers-Thiery *et al.*, 1983; Merlie *et al.*, 1983; Noda *et al.*, 1982, 1983; Stevens, 1982), suggest that AChR spans the entire postsynaptic membrane, with an overall length of 110 Å. The sugar-containing portions extend out 50 Å from the extracellular surface and the intracellular portions extends 15 Å from the inner surface of the membrane. Viewed on end, the molecule has a diameter of 80 Å and appears as a rosette of subunits around a negatively staining core—perhaps the ion channel. Two αBT molecules bind each AChR molecule. Binding of cholinergic agonists produces a two-stage conformational change in the molecule, which results in increased conductance through the ion channel.

AChR at the neuromuscular junction is the classic nicotinic cholinergic receptor. It binds nicotine but not muscarine. It is inhibited by the nondepolarizing competitive antagonist curare but not by atropine. It is also blocked by depolarizing antagonists, such as succinylcholine. In addition, αBT and NT bind the receptor almost irreversibly and block agonist and antagonist binding. There is suggestive evidence that some local anesthetics and animal toxins bind AChR at a different site. This is inferred because they apparently do not block cholinergic ligand binding, but rather induce increased ion channel conductance.

The NMJ consists of a motor axon terminal rich in mitochondria and acetylcholine-containing synaptic vesicles separated by a synaptic cleft from the specialized postsynaptic portion of the muscle referred to as the muscle endplate.

The endplate membrane is highly folded, with AChR located on the peaks of the membrane folds. The entire sarcolemmal membrane is coated by a basal lamina (basement membrane). In the valleys of the endplate membrane folds, the basal lamina contains acetylcholine esterase, the enzyme that hydrolyzes acetylcholine (ACh). The signal for muscle contraction begins with the release of ACh from the presynaptic membrane. ACh diffuses across the synaptic cleft and binds to AChR located in the endplate membrane (at the peaks of the folds), resulting in opening of the ion channel and depolarization of the endplate membrane. The ACh further diffuses into the "valleys" of the folded membrane and is hydrolyzed by acetylcholine esterase.

The amount of ACh contained in a single synaptic vesicle is referred to as a quantum and consists of about 10,000 molecules. In the resting state these quanta are spontaneously released from the terminal and produce small endplate membrane depolarizations referred to as miniature endplate potentials (MEPPs). Each individual action potential reaching the axon terminal releases about 100 quanta, with a resultant larger endplate depolarization referred to as an endplate potential (EPP). When a sufficient number of these EPPs are summed, threshold is reached for the generation of a muscle action potential, which is then propagated along the muscle membrane, triggering contraction. With sequential impulses arriving at the axon terminal, less ACh is released. After the first few impulses, further release of ACh is approximately one-third of the amount released initially. In the normal individual the amount of AChR activated is much above that needed for endplate depolarization (safety factor), so that the falloff in ACh release does not significantly reduce the muscle response.

B. Myasthenia Gravis and Experimental Myasthenia

Myasthenia gravis (MG) is a disease of motor weakness caused by abnormalities of the NMJ (for reviews see Drachman, 1978; Lindstrom, 1979, 1982; Lisak and Barchi, 1982). At the light microscopic level the NMJ in MG is normal; however, ultrastructurally, the normally highly folded endplate membrane is simplified and reduced in total area. There is also a reduction in the amount of AChR normally located primarily at the peaks of the folds. Physiologically, the spontaneously produced MEPPs are reduced in amplitude and repetitive stimulation of nerve results in a decrementing electrical response in muscle. In addition to the changes in the NMJ in MG, there are abnormalities of the thymus, either lymphoid follicular hyperplasia or frank neoplasia, and an increased occurrence of other autoantibodies and other presumably autoimmune syndromes.

The seminal observation of Patrick and Lindstrom (1973) of the animal model of MG, later referred to as experimental autoimmune myasthenia gravis (EAMG), induced by immunization with purified AChR led to an explosion in research activity and the development of new information concerning pathogenic mechanisms in MG. Patients with MG were found to have humoral and cellular immunity to purified AChR. However, anti-AChR titers correlate poorly with disease severity or activity. An extreme example of this is the fact that infants born of mothers with MG all have high anti-AChR titers, but only 12% develop neonatal MG. While factors intrinsic to the NMJ could play a role here, it is more likely that specific characteristics of the individual antibodies, or of other aspects of the immune response, are important.

The most highly studied variety of EAMG is that induced in rats by a single immunization with purified electric organ AChR along with complete Freund's adjuvant and pertussis vaccine (Lennon *et al.*, 1975, 1976). This illness is biphasic, with the first episode of weakness, associated with endplate necrosis and marked cellular infiltration of the endplate regions, occurring about 1 week after immunization. This acute phase clears, to be followed 2–3 weeks later by a chronic phase of weakness progressing to death, with a histological picture similar to MG, i.e., no cellular infiltration but marked simplification of endplate membrane. When serum from EAMG animals is injected into normal rats, only the acute phase occurs, beginning at 24–48 hr and clearing by the 5th day.

The widely held view is that neuromuscular transmission fails in MG, and in EAMG, because of a reduced amount of AChR at the NMJ (Lennon, 1978; Lindstrom, 1979). Both complement-mediated injury to the endplate membrane (Engel *et al.*, 1977) and increased AChR degradation by cross-linking antibodies (Kao and Drachman, 1977) have been proposed as the responsible mechanism for the reduction in AChR. A third possible means is pharmacological blockade of intact receptors.

C. Questions Addressed by Monoclonal Antibodies

The application of monoclonal antibody techniques to the study of AChR, a purified glycoprotein, is somewhat in contrast to the usual antigens studied by this technique. Rather than using the monoclonal antibody technology to study or isolate a relatively impure antigen present in small amounts, studies of AChR have applied the method to precise analysis of the structure and function of a relatively purified molecule and to analysis of the immunobiology of the autoimmune disease in which it is the antigen.

A number of probes of the AChR molecule are available, e.g., toxins, cholinergic ligands, agents that bind the ionic channel, and agents that bind to the sugar moieties. Monoclonal antibodies have been used to analyze other portions of the molecule with these as landmarks. A series of monoclonal antibodies, in conjunction with the other probes, can theoretically map the primary or tertiary structure of AChR. Fine analysis of the active regions of the molecule are also possible.

With respect to MG and EAMG, the autoimmune response may be analyzed in terms of the characteristics of antibody binding to AChR, the effector functions required of the binding antibodies, and the state of the immunoregulatory system, with special emphasis on the idiotype/antiidiotype network in these diseases.

II. Analysis of Acetylcholine Receptor by Monoclonal Antibodies

Monoclonal anti-AChR antibodies have been developed by a number of groups (Dwyer *et al.*, 1981; Froehner *et al.*, 1983; Gomez *et al.*, 1979a,b; James *et al.*, 1980; Lennon and Lambert, 1980; Mochly-Rosen *et al.*, 1979; Souroujou *et al.*, 1983; Tzartos and Lindstrom, 1980; Tzartos *et al.*, 1983; Vernet Der Garabedian and Morel, 1983; Watters and Maelicke, 1983). The majority of these have made use of a standard radioimmunoprecipitation assay to screen for anti-AChR monoclonal antibodies. This assay employs AChR labeled with [^{125}I]-αBT and therefore does not detect antibodies directed against the region of the molecule containing the cholinergic binding site. Other screening assays have included passive hemagglutination (Gomez *et al.*, 1979a,b) and immunoprecipitation with [^{125}I]-labeled AChR (Mochly-Rosen *et al.*, 1979; James *et al.*, 1980). By detecting antibodies against a random sample of AChR epitopes, the latter assays have produced a number of monoclonal antibodies directed at epitopes "near" the cholinergic binding site (Gomez *et al.*, 1979a,b, 1981; Gomez and Richman, 1981, 1982, 1983; James *et al.*, 1980; Mihovilovic and Richman, 1982, 1983, 1984; Mochly-Rosen and Fuchs, 1981; Watters and Maelicke, 1983; Yu *et al.*, 1979.

Anti-AChR monoclonal antibodies have been used for affinity purification of AChR from *Torpedo* electric organ using monoclonal antibodies bound to agarose (Lennon *et al.*, 1980). Elution of bound AChR from the affinity column was carried out at pH 10 with yields of AChR comparable to those obtained by affinity chromatography with NT columns. However, the specific activity of the AChR, in terms of αBT binding, was greatly reduced. This was apparently related to the high pH during elution, since reducing the time of exposure to high pH improved somewhat the specific activity of the product.

Analysis of AChR by monoclonal antibodies has involved a number of aspects of AChR structure. These have included studies of the "environment" of the molecule, e.g., *in situ* in membrane, in detergent-containing solution, at the NMJ, or elsewhere in the muscle fiber membrane (extrajunctional AChR); the pharmacology of the molecule, e.g., relation of binding to available pharmacological probes and to AChR function; the tertiary structure of AChR, i.e., the glycopeptide subunits; and cross-reactivity with AChR from different species. In general these studies have taken two, somewhat complementary, directions. The first group has been directed at analyzing the function of the AChR molecule, i.e., ligand binding and the subsequent events that lead to opening of the ion channel. The second group has been directed at mapping the primary structure of AChR.

In one study, 26 anti-AChR monoclonal antibodies raised against detergent-solubilized purified *Torpedo* AChR were studied for their ability to bind to endplate (junctional) AChR in muscle tissue sections from a wide range of species (Gomez *et al.*, 1981). Nineteen bound to endplates *in situ* in at least one species. In a study of 10 monoclonal antibodies raised against solubilized *Torpedo* AChR, six bound to membrane-bound *Torpedo* AChR with affinity equal to that of binding to AChR in solution (Gullick *et al.*, 1981). These data demonstrate that not all the AChR determinants are exposed either in tissue sections or in membrane fragments.

The earliest studies of the functional organization of AChR made use of the passive hemagglutination assay with sheep erythrocytes coated with detergent-purified *Torpedo* AChR (Gomez *et al.*, 1979a,b). Analysis of monoclonal antibodies in terms of their binding to the cholinergic binding site involved the ability of cholinergic ligands and toxins to inhibit hemagglutination. Twenty-five independent anti-AChR monoclonal antibodies were tested; their behavior segregated them into six groups (Gomez *et al.*, 1981; Gomez and Richman, 1984). Binding of five monoclonal antibodies was totally blocked by αBT but not by *d*-tubocurarine, benzoquinonium, carbamylcholine, or atropine. One monoclonal antibody was totally blocked by αBT and partially blocked by benzoquinonium. One monoclonal antibody was partially blocked by αBT and by carbamylcholine. Two monoclonal antibodies were partially blocked by αBT and by all the ligands. One had its titer *increased* in the presence of either αBT or benzoquinonium. The remaining 15 monoclonal antibodies had their binding unaffected by any of these agents.

In a separate study (James *et al.*, 1980) of five anti-AChR monoclonal antibodies using a radioimmunoprecipitation assay with [^{125}I]-labeled *Torpedo* AChR, two were totally blocked by *d*-tubocurarine and αBT and partially blocked by carbamylcholine. One was totally blocked by αBT, one was partially blocked by αBT, and the binding of one was unaffected by any of those agents. Another group (Mochly-Rosen and Fuchs, 1981), using a similar screening assay, found one of 32 anti-AChR monoclonal antibodies was blocked by αBT. This antibody was also totally blocked by *d*-tubocurarine, carbamylcholine, decamethonium, and acetylcholine.

More recently monoclonal antibodies have been used to provide a "fine analysis" of the cholinergic binding site of AChR. One monoclonal antibody whose binding is totally blocked by αBT and partially blocked by benzoquinonium was analyzed using an immunoprecipitation assay in which the amount of unprecipitated purified *Torpedo* AChR is measured by αBT binding (Mihovilovic and Richman, 1982, 1983, 1984). Data from this assay and from sucrose gradient sedimentation analysis of monoclonal antibody–AChR complexes showed that one antibody molecule binds one AChR molecule (two αBT binding sites). The antibody blocks only 50% of αBT binding to AChR by binding to only one of the two αBT binding sites on each AChR molecule. Its binding is not blocked by cholinergic agonists. It modifies *d*-tubocurarine binding to AChR, but not carbamylcholine binding. On the other hand, its effect on benzoquinonium binding to AChR resembles the effect on αBT. There are two binding sites for benzoquinonium on AChR, one of high affinity and one of low affinity. The high-affinity site is blocked by this antibody but not the low-affinity site (Mihovilovic and Richman, 1983). These results suggest that the αBT and benzoquinonium sites are related, that the two binding sites on each AChR do not behave identically, and that the monoclonal antibody can bind only one of them.

In addition, the binding of this monoclonal antibody affects AChR in a manner that prevents the rapid displacement of cholinergic ligands by αBT. Therefore it is likely that the conformational changes that AChR normally undergoes upon ligand binding are blocked or markedly slowed (Mihovilovic and Richman, 1982, 1984).

In a separate study (Watters and Maelicke, 1983) a group of six monoclonal antibodies were found to interact with the cholinergic ligand binding site. This analysis also demonstrated nonequivalence of the various ligand binding sites. One group of monoclonal antibodies blocked all cholinergic ligands, one group blocked all the bismethonium family of ligands, and one group blocked all but bismethonium compounds and *d*-tubocurarine.

A number of anti-AChR monoclonal antibodies block the function of the cholinergic ion channel (Donnelly *et al.*, 1983). The monoclonal antibody described above that blocks 50% of αBT binding also blocks agonist-induced ion fluxes. Three other monoclonal antibodies also interfere with fluxes, one by blocking agonist binding, one possibly by inhibiting agonist-induced conformational changes in AChR, and a third by possibly binding to the ion channel itself.

In order to analyze the primary structure of AChR, binding of monoclonal antibodies to isolated denatured glycopeptide subunits of *Torpedo* and *Electrophorus* AChR has also been studied (Tzartos and Lindstrom, 1980; Tzartos *et al.*, 1981). On the order of 30% of monoclonal antibodies raised against detergent-solubilized AChR bind denatured subunits. For the monoclonal antibodies cross-reacting with subunits, the binding affinity is usually much lower than for solubilized intact AChR. A few monoclonal antibodies were found to cross-react, at even lower affinity, with a second subunit. For monoclonal antibodies raised against isolated denatured subunits occasional cross-reaction between α and β subunits and between γ and δ subunits was found (Tzartos and Lindstrom, 1980). This observation has been interpreted as suggesting that each glycopeptide pair may have arisen from a single evolutionary ancestor, a conclusion supported by sequencing data from the cloned subunit genes (Ballivet *et al.*, 1982; Devellers-Thiery *et al.*, 1983; Merlie *et al.*, 1983; Noda *et al.*, 1982, 1983; Stevens, 1982).

Work is also ongoing to map the primary structure of the subunits (Gullick *et al.*, 1981; Gullick and Lindstrom, 1983). In this study, polypeptide fragments of isolated subunits are prepared by protease digestion and the ability of various monoclonal antibodies raised against intact solubilized AChR to bind the peptides determined.

In another study of 26 anti-*Torpedo* AChR antibodies their ability to cross-react with endplate AChR from muscle of a variety of vertebrate species has been determined (Gomez *et al.*, 1981). The number of monoclonal antibodies that bind to, or fail to bind to, both members of a given pair of species can be used as a measure of the evolutionary difference between the two species. More precisely, this is a measure of the evolutionary difference between the receptor molecules. If there is a descrepancy between the phylogenetic tree obtained for the species as a whole and the tree derived for the AChR, it indicates the previous presence of particular evolutionary pressures on AChR. The most significant discrepancy, as might be predicted, was found for elapid snakes (snakes producing neurotoxins), whose muscle AChRs are known not to bind to αBT. Monoclonal antibodies against other antigens may be used to carry out similar phylogenetic studies.

III. Monoclonal Antibodies and Myasthenia

We have developed 16 independent anti-AChR monoclonal antibodies, raised against solubilized *Torpedo* AChR, that induce myasthenia when injected into normal animals (Gomez *et al.*, 1979a; Yu *et al.*, 1979; Richman *et al.*, 1980; Gomez and Richman, 1984). These antibodies were obtained by fusion of spleen cells from immunized Lewis rats with either P3-X63-Ag8 or SP2/0-Ag14 cells. Most recent fusions have involved multiple-stage screening assays (Gomez and Richman, 1982, 1983, 1984). First anti-*Torpedo* AChR activity was determined using the passive hemagglutination assay described above. Supernatants from positive wells were then screened for cross-reactivity with *in situ* junctional AChR from mammalian muscle. The anti-*Torpedo* AChR-positive wells were also screened for activity against the cholinergic binding site by testing the ability of αBT to block hemagglutination.

These Lewis rat anti-AChR antibodies induce acute EAMG when injected into normal Lewis rats (Gomez *et al.*, 1979a; Yu *et al.*, 1979; Richman *et al.*, 1980). The disease is identical to the acute phase of EAMG induced in rats by active immunization with *Torpedo* AChR and identical to the acute disease induced by passive transfer of syngeneic EAMG serum (see Section I). Weakness appears from 18 to 24 hr after injection, peaks at 48 hr, and clears by 4–5 days. The severity ranges from cupped forepaws and weakened grip, to abnormal gait, to inability to stand or walk, to respiratory failure and death. Electrophysiological studies reveal decremental evoked electromyographic responses to repetitive nerve stimulation and diminished MEPP amplitudes (Burres *et al.*, 1981; Gomez *et al.*, 1981). Weakness and the electrophysiological abnormalities are repaired by the cholinesterase inhibitor prostigmine.

The only histological abnormalities in these animals are those in muscle (Richman *et al.*, 1980; Gomez *et al.*, 1982, 1984). Focal mononuclear cell infiltrations are present in the regions of endplates. The cells stain for acid phosphatase activity and are probably macrophages. Cholinesterase staining regions (endplates) are frequently separated from the underlying muscle fiber with occasional interposition of macrophages. Some macrophages are seen within muscle fibers. Ultrastructural studies reveal many structurally normal endplates invaded by or separated from the underlying muscle fibers by macrophages (Gomez *et al.*, 1982, 1984). Occasionally macrophages are within the synaptic cleft between nerve terminal and endplate membrane. In some animals degenerating postsynaptic membrane is seen *in situ* or within macrophages.

Similar clinical and electrophysiological findings have been reported by another group (Lennon and Lambert, 1980). Total body AChR was measured in their animals and was found to be reduced by about 60%. In other studies, clinical weakness in mice after injection of mouse anti-AChr monoclonal antibodies (Dwyer *et al.*, 1981) and mildly diminished AChR content in rats after injection of rat monoclonal antibodies (Tzartos and Lindstrom, 1980) have been reported.

These observations represent the first demonstration of the ability of monoclonal antibodies to induce an autoimmune state, one severe enough to lead to death. It implies that loss of regulation of a single immunocyte clone can lead to autoimmune disease. The recently described peripheral neuropathy in patients with monoclonal gammopathy, in which the monoclonal Ig binds to a myelin component, probably represents a naturally occurring example of this situation (Latov *et al.*, 1980). Only two of the monoclonal antibodies that have induced EAMG bind at or near the cholinergic binding site (Richman *et al.*, 1980). It therefore appears that this acute state, characterized by endplate necrosis and phagocytosis, does not require binding to the pharmacologically active portion of the AChR molecule. Moreover, this syndrome does not occur in animals depleted of complement (Lennon and Lambert, 1981).

Studies of monoclonal antibodies developed using the immunoprecipitation assay with AChR complexed to $[^{125}I]$-αBT have demonstrated, through inhibition studies, that 60% apparently bind to a portion of the α subunit denoted the "main immunogenic region" (MIR) (Conti-Tronconi *et al.*, 1981; Tzartos and Lindstrom, 1980; Tzartos *et al.*, 1981, 1982). Since these monoclonal antibodies bind to sites distinct from the cholinergic ligand binding site portion of the α chain, the relationship between MIR and functionally important regions of AChR is presently unknown.

Dose–response studies of antibody-induced EAMG were carried out using 14 SP2/0-derived antibodies (Gomez and Richman, 1984). Doses ranged from 0.25 to 50 mg/kg. The results revealed a wide range (more than 50-fold) in potencies. Monoclonal antibodies of subclasses IgG2a and IgG2b were included in the groups of high and intermediate potency. Two antibodies of subclass IgG1 were of low potency, an observation raising the question of whether the low complement-fixing ability of this subclass is important in EAMG. Two-monoclonal antibodies bound to *in situ* endplate AChR with extremely low avidity. These were the least potent in inducing EAMG, with doses of greater than 50 mg/kg (resulting in extremely high serum titers) leading to no clinical or electrophysiological abnormalities. Animals receiving these antibodies did have rare cellular infiltrates in muscle. On the other hand, antibodies with the highest avidity had only intermediate potency; those with intermediate avidity were the most potent. The data suggest two conclusions: first, low avidity results in low potency. (Data on a P3-derived anti-AChR antibody, BK60D, support that view. The monoclonal antibody does not induce EAMG; it does bind to *solubilized* mammalian AChR, but at 1/150 the affinity for solubilized *Torpedo* AChR; and it does not stain mammalian endplates in the relatively insensitive immunofluorescence assay. Low avidity could explain its inability to cause EAMG or to stain endplates.) A second conclusion is that high potency is related to intermediate rather than high avidity. It seems that in MG special attention to the antibodies with intermediate avidity may enable better correlations between antibody titer and disease state.

The fact that many of our anti-*Torpedo* AChR monoclonal antibodies bind to chicken endplate AChR allowed us to study the *in vivo* effects of a broader range of antibodies in this species than was possible in rats. Specifically, we were able to study the effect of antibodies that are totally blocked by αBT. In fact, we could study their effect in a situation in which antibodies directed against sites elsewhere on the AChR molecule produced no disease (Gomez and Richman, 1982, 1983). In chickens these rat antibodies produce no inflammatory changes in muscle, in contrast with their effect in rats. The αBT-blockable antibodies (those directed against sites related to the cholinergic binding site) produced paralysis in chickens beginning within 1 hr of intravenous injection and resulting in death within 16 hr. Decrementing electromyographic responses were marked, and both clinical and electromyographic abnormalities were repaired by prostigmine injection. *No* histological abnormalities were observed. None of the nonblockable antibodies had this effect. The conclusion that this severe paralysis was the result of pharmacological blockade of intact AChRs was supported by observations that blockable monoclonal antibodies applied *in vitro* to normal muscle produced diminished MEPP amplitudes within 30 min. Current theories of MG propose that the neuromuscular blockade results from reduced amounts of AChR at the NMJ. The present obervations suggest that the pharmacological blocking effects of antibody on intact AChR play a role as well.

Acute EAMG mimics the clinical findings in MG (but not the time course); however, the chronic phase of EAMG (induced by immunization with AChR in adjuvant) demonstrates histological changes more typical of the human disease. We have succeeded in inducing chronic EAMG in rats by repeated injection of a high-potency monoclonal antibody over a period of 2–9 months (Gomez *et al.*, 1982, 1984). The serum anti-AChR titer was maintained at the peak level obtained following a single injection. The animals were not clinically weak, there was no EMG decremental response, and light microscopic examination of muscle was normal. However, ultrastructural findings were similar to those of MG. Most of the neuromuscular junctions demonstrated simplified postsynaptic folds with abnormal synaptic clefts, sometimes containing electron-dense material. No cellular infiltrates were found. Very recent experiments have revealed similar ultrastructural abnormalities, but to a lesser extent, 21 days after a single injection of either of two monoclonal antibodies. The observations also demonstrate that the ultrastructural abnormality of MG need not be associated with clinical or EMG abnormalities, at least in rats.

These studies also highlight the fact that the acute phase of EAMG is transient and does not recur. In these multiple injected animals, the acute phase occurs after the first injection, lasts for only a few days, and does not recur with subsequent injections. We have studied this phenomenon in more detail (Corey *et al.*, 1984) and determined that subsequent injection of a second monoclonal antibody of different Ig subclass and idiotype, also does not result in a second episode of acute EAMG. To date, we have been unable to transfer this "resistance" with spleen cells.

The rat anti-AChR monoclonal antibodies have also been used to analyze the epitopes against which the anti-AChR antibodies are directed in MG (James *et al.*, 1982; Tzartos *et al.*, 1982). The ability of serum from individual patients to block binding of particular anti-AChR monoclonal antibodies was used as an indication of the presence in that serum of antibodies directed against the epitope defined by the monoclonal antibody. The analysis revealed epitope profiles in MG patients that were essentially identical to those of animals with EAMG.

The EAMG-inducing antibodies may be used to assess immune regulation as well, since they provide an exceptional opportunity to analyze the idiotype/antiidiotype network in EAMG. They are excellent reagents for raising antiidiotypic sera or monoclonal antibodies. In a study of five anti-AChR monoclonal antibodies, four cross-reacted with isogeneic antisera raised against any of them (Lennon and Lambert, 1980). In another study, using heterologous antiidiotypic sera raised against each of another group of five anti-AChR monoclonal antibodies, one antiserum cross-reacted with all the monoclonal antibodies and the other antisera cross-reacted with none (DeBaets *et al.*, 1982).

We have produced a series of isogeneic anti-Id monoclonal antibodies, some directed against the antigen binding site and others not. In the one anti-Id monoclonal antibody studied to date, cross-reaction with other EAMG-inducing monoclonal antibodies was found only against a monoclonal antibody having similar binding characteristics to the original monoclonal antibody but of a different Ig class (Table I).

The presence of public, and possibly dominant, idiotypes in MG patients is suggested by the observation (Dwyer *et al.*, 1983) that 40% of MG sera contain antiidiotypic activity directed against an idiotype defined by a mouse anti-AChR monoclonal antibody. In addition, there appeared to be a negative correlation

TABLE I

Effect of Various Anti-AChR Monoclonal Antibodies on Binding of Biotin-Labeled Anti-AChR Monoclonal Antibody 371A to Anti-Id Monoclonal Antibody GG-A

Inhibitor	Binding of biotinylated 371A[a]
—	0.141
371A	0.012
421H	0.010
132A	0.121
265A	0.148
63E	0.136
460D	0.137
D547[b]	0.148
SP2/0 supernatant	0.141
CM[b]	0.121

[a]Mean OD_{410} (of four replicates) of reaction product of alkaline phosphatase-labeled avidin.
[b]Antibody against an unrelated antigen.

between total anti-AChR titer and the antiidiotype titer. These observations hold out the promise of effective treatment of this autoimmune state by manipulation of the idiotype/antiidiotype network.

The studies described here represent the application of monoclonal antibody technology to a special situation: an autoimmune disease in which the antigen is obtainable in large quantities and has been well characterized. These new probes, however, have added substantially to our knowledge of the antigen and of the pathogenesis of the autoimmune state.

IV. Summary

AChR is a well-characterized transmembrane glycoprotein receptor and is the target of the autoimmune response in MG. In addition, an animal model, EAMG, has been developed by immunization with purified AChR. Monoclonal antibodies against AChR have been used to study AChR structure and function. Some antibodies bind to determinants present *in situ* and cross-react with *in situ* AChR from a number of species. Some bind in relation to the pharmacologically active portion of AChR. These new reagents have produced additional information on the fine structure of the active region of the molecule and on AChR function. A number of anti-AChR monoclonal antibodies also cross-react with denatured glycopeptide subunits of AChR and peptide fragments, and thereby represent new probes of AChR primary structure.

A number of the anti-AChR monoclonal antibodies that bind *in situ* to rat junctional AChR induce acute EAMG in normal rats. Studies of the epitopes bound, binding avidity, and immunoglobulin subclass have provided information on the immunobiological characteristics of this syndrome. Monoclonal antibodies directed against the cholinergic binding site of AChR induce a hyperacute paralysis. Chronic injection of monoclonal antibody results in the typical histological abnormality of chronic EAMG and MG, but without clinical or electrophysiological abnormalities. Studies of cross-reactive idiotypes among anti-AChR antibodies and anti-AChR sera demonstrate the presence of public idiotypes.

References

Ballivet, M., Patrick, J., Lee, J., and Heinemann, S., 1982, Molecular cloning of cDNA coding for the γ subunit of *Torpedo* acetylcholine receptor, *Proc. Natl. Acad. Sci. USA* **79:**4466–4470.

Barrants, F. J., 1983, Recent developments in the structure and function of the acetylcholine receptor, *Int. Rev. Neurobiol.* **24:**259–341.

Briley, M. S., and Changeux, J. P., 1977, Isolation and purification of nicotinic acetylcholine receptor and its functional reconstruction into a membrane environment, *Int. Rev. Neurobiol.* **20:**31.

Burres, S. A., Crayton, J. W., Gomez, C. M., and Richman, D. P., 1981, Myasthenia induced by monoclonal anti-acetylcholine receptor antibodies: Clinical and electrophysiological aspects, *Ann. Neurol.* **9:**563–568.

Conti-Tronconi, B., Tzartos, S., and Lindstrom, J., 1981, Monoclonal antibodies as probes of acetylcholine receptor structure. 2. Binding to native receptor, *Biochemistry* **20:**2181–2191.

Corey, A. L., Richman, D. P., Shuman, C. A., Gomez, C. M., and Arnason, B. G. W., 1984, Refractoriness to a second episode of experimental myasthenia: Relationship to exacerbating/remitting nature of myasthenia gravis, *Neurology*, in press.

DeBaets, M. H., Theofilopoulos, A. N., Blonda, A., Lindstrom, J. M., and Weigle, W. O., 1982, Idiotypic analysis of monoclonal anti-acetylcholine receptor antibodies, *Fed. Proc.* **41:**547.

Devellers-Thiery, A., Giraudat, J., Bentaboulet, M., and Changeux, J.-P., 1983, Complete mRNA coding sequence of the acetylcholine binding α-subunit of *Torpedo marmorata* acetylcholine receptor: A model for the transmembrane organization of the polypeptide chain, *Proc. Natl. Acad. Sci. USA* **80:**2067–2071.

Donnelly, D., Farach, M. C., Ferragut, J. A., Mihovilovic, M., Gonzalez-Ros, J. M., and Martinez-Carrion, M., 1983, Effect of acetylcholine receptor–monoclonal antibody complexes on receptor function, *Biochemistry* **22:**34A–35A.

Drachman, D., 1978, Myasthenia gravis, *N. Engl. J. Med.* **298:**136–141.

Dwyer, D. S., Kearney, J. F., Bradley, F. J., Kemp, G. E., and Oh, S. J., 1981, Interaction of human antibody and murine monoclonal antibody with muscle acetylcholine receptor, *Ann. N. Y. Acad. Sci.* **377:**143–157.

Dwyer, D. S., Bradley, R. J., Urquhart, C. K., and Kearney, J. F., 1983, Naturally occurring anti-idiotypic antibodies in myasthenia gravis patients, *Nature* **301:**611–614.

Engel, A. G., Lambert, E. H., and Howard, F. M., 1977, Immune complexes (IgG and C₃) at the motor endplate in myasthenia gravis: Ultrastructural and light microscopic localization and electrophysiological correlations, *Mayo Clin. Proc.* **59:**267–280.

Froehner, S. C., Douville, K., Klink, S., and Culp, W. J., 1983, Monoclonal antibodies to cytoplasmic domains of the acetylcholine receptor, *J. Biol. Chem.* **258:**7112–7120.

Gomez, C. M., and Richman, D. P., 1981, Inability of some anti-AChR monoclonal antibodies to induce myasthenia, *J. Neuropathol. Exp. Neurol.* **41:**300.

Gomez, C. M., and Richman, D. P., 1982, Acetylcholine receptor monoclonal antibodies specific for the alpha-bungarotoxin site induce paralysis, *Neurology* **32:**A221.

Gomez, C. M., and Richman, D. P., 1983, Anti-acetylcholine receptor antibodies directed against the binding site induce a unique form of experimental myasthenia. *Proc. Natl. Acad. Sci. USA* **80:**4089–4093.

Gomez, C. M., and Richman, D. P., 1984, Experimental autoimmune myasthenia gravis produced by monoclonal anti-acetylcholine receptor antibody: Identification of antibodies with widely differing capacities for induction of autoimmune disease, submitted.

Gomez, C. M., Richman, D. P., Berman, P. W., Burres, S. A., Arnason, B. G. W., and Fitch, F. W., 1979a, Monoclonal anti-acetylcholine receptor antibodies: Evidence for multiple pharmacologic specificities, *Fed. Proc.* **38:**143.

Gomez, C. M., Richman, D. P., Berman, P. W., Burres, S. A., Arnason, B. G. W., and Fitch, F. W., 1979b, Monoclonal antibodies against purified nicotinic acetylcholine receptor, *Biochem. Biophys. Res. Commun.* **88:**575–582.

Gomez, C. M., Richman, D. P., Wollmann, R. L., Berman, P. W., and Arnason, B. G. W., 1980, Passive transfer of experimental autoimmune myasthenia gravis using monoclonal anti-acetylcholine receptor antibodies, *Neurology* **30:**388.

Gomez, C. M., Richman, D. P., Berman, P. W., Crayton, J. W., Fitch, F. W., and Arnason, B. G. W., 1981, Monoclonal anti-acetylcholine receptor antibody: Studies of antibody specificity and effect of passive transfer, *Ann. N. Y. Acad. Sci.* **377:**97–109.

Gomez, C. M., Wollmann, R. L., and Richman, D. P., 1982, Monoclonal antibody to acetylcholine receptor produces simplified endplate architecture, *Neurology* **32:**A221.

Gomez, C. M., Wollmann, R. L., and Richman, D. P., 1984, Monoclonal antibody to acetylcholine receptor produces simplified endplate architecture, *Acta Neuropathol.*, in press.

Gullick, W. J., and Lindstrom, J. M., 1983, Mapping the binding of monoclonal antibodies to the acetylcholine receptor from *Torpedo californica*, *Biochemistry* **22:**3312–3320.

Gullick, W. J., Tzartos, S., and Lindstrom, J., 1981, Monoclonal antibodies as probes of acetylcholine receptor structure: 1. Peptide mapping, *Biochemistry* **20:**2173–2180.

James, R. W., Kato, A. C., Rey, M.-J., and Fulpius, B. W., 1980, Monoclonal antibodies against the neurotransmitter binding site of nicotinic acetylcholine receptor, *FEBS Lett.* **120:**145–148.

James, R. W., Lefvert, A.-K., Alliod, C., and Fulpius, B. W., 1982, Monoclonal anti-*Torpedo* receptor antibodies used to study antibody heterogeneity in myasthenic sera, *Neurochem. Int.* **4:**79–84.

Kao, I., and Drachman, D. B., 1977, Myasthenic immunoglobulin accelerates AChR degradation, *Science* **196:**526–529.

Karlin, A., 1980, Molecular properties of nicotinic acelylcholine receptors, in: *The Cell Surface and Neuronal Function* (C. W. Cotnian, G. Poste, and G. L. Nicolson, eds.), Elsevier/North Holland Bromesled Press, New York, pp. 191–260.

Latov, N., Sherman, W. H., Nemni, R., Galossi, G., Shyong, J. S., Penn, A. S., Chess, L., Olarte, M., Rowland, L. P., and Osserman, E. F., 1980, Plasma cell dyscrasia and peripheral neuropathy to peripheral nerve myelin, *N. Engl. J. Med.* **303:**618–621.

Lennon, V. A., 1978, The immunopathology of myasthenia gravis, *Hum. Pathol.* **9:**541–555.

Lennon, V. A., and Lambert, E. H., 1980, Myasthenia gravis induced by monoclonal antibodies to acetylcholine receptors, *Nature* **285:**238–240.

Lennon, V. A., and Lambert, E. H., 1981, Analysis of the antigenicity of acetylcholine receptor using monoclonal hybridoma antibodies, *Ann. N. Y. Acad. Sci.* **377:**143–157.

Lennon, V., Lindstrom, J., and Seybold, M., 1975, Experimental autoimmune myasthenia: A model of MG in rats and guinea pigs, *J. Exp. Med.* **141:**1364–1375.

Lennon, V., Lindstrom, J., and Seybold, M., 1976, Experimental autoimmune MG: Cellular and humoral immune responses, *Ann. N. Y. Acad. Sci.* **274:**283–299.

Lennon, V. A., Thompson, M., and Chen, J., 1980, Properties of nicotinic acetylcholine receptors isolated by affinity chromatography on monoclonal antibodies, *J. Biol. Chem.* **255:**4395–4398.

Lindstrom, J., 1979, Autoimmune response to acetylcholine receptors in myasthenia gravis and its animal model, *Adv. Immunol.* **27:**1–50.

Lindstrom, J., 1982, Structure of the acetylcholine receptor and specifities of antibodies to it in myasthenia gravis, *Ciba Found. Symp.* **90:**178–196.

Lisak, R. P., and Barchi, R. L., 1982, *Myasthenia Gravis*, Saunders, Philadelphia.

Merlie, J. P., Sebrane, R., Gardner, S., and Lindstrom, J., 1983, cDNA clone for the α subunit of the acetylcholine receptor from the mouse muscle cell line BC3H-1, *Proc. Natl. Acad. Sci. USA* **80:**3845–3849.

Mihovilovic, M., and Richman, D. P., 1982, Monoclonal antibody to α-bungarotoxin binding site of *Torpedo* acetylcholine receptor modifies cholinergic ligand binding to solubilized and membrane-bound acetylcholine receptor, *Soc. Neurosci. Abstr.* **8:**336.

Mihovilovic, M., and Richman, D. P., 1983, Monoclonal antibody (mcab) 247G: Example of a functional probe for the acetylcholine receptor (AcChR) molecule, *Soc. Neurosci. Abstr.* **9:**158.

Mihovilovic, M., and Richman, D. P., 1984, Modification of α-bungarotoxin and cholinergic ligand binding properties of *Torpedo* acetylcholine receptor by a monoclonal anti-acetylcholine receptor antibody, submitted.

Mochly-Rosen, D., and Fuchs, S., 1981, Monoclonal anti-acetylcholine-receptor antibodies directed against the cholinergic binding site, *Biochemistry* **20:**5920–5924.

Mochly-Rosen, D., Fuchs, S., and Esbhar, Z., 1979, Monoclonal antibodies against defined determinants of acetylcholine receptor, *FEBS Lett.* **106:**389–392.

Noda, M., Takahashi, H., Tanabe, T., Toyosato, M., Furutani, Y., Hirose, T., Asai, M., Inayama, S., Miyata, T., and Numa, S., 1982, Primary structure of α-subunit precursor of *Torpedo california* acetylcholine receptor deduced from cDNA sequence, *Nature* **299:**793–797.

Noda, M., Takahashi, H., Tanabe, T., Toyosato, M., Kikyotani, S., Hirose, T., Asai, M., Takashima, H., Inayama, S., Miyata, T., and Numa, S., 1983, Primary structure of β- and γ-subunit precursors of *Torpedo californica* acetylcholine receptor deduced from cDNA sequences, *Nature* **301:**251–254.

Patrick, J., an Lindstrom, J., 1973, Autoimmune response to acetylcholine receptor, *Science* **180:**871–872.

Raftery, M. A., Wizemann, V., and Blonchard, S. G., 1980, The use of photochemical probes for studies of structure and function of purified acetylcholine receptor preparations, *Ann. N. Y. Acad. Sci.* **346:**458.

Richman, D. P., Gomez, C. M., Berman, P. W., Burres, S. A., Fitch, F. W., and Arnason, B. G. W., 1980, Monoclonal anti-acetylcholine receptor antibodies can cause experimental myasthenia, *Nature* **386**:738–739.

Souroujon, M. C., Mochly-Rosen, D., Gordon, A. S., and Fuchs, S., 1983, Interaction of monoclonal antibodies to *Torpedo* acetylcholine receptor with the receptor of skeletal muscle, *Muscle Nerve* **6**:303–311.

Stevens, C. F., 1982, The acetylcholine receptor cloned east and west, *Nature* **299**:776.

Tzartos, S. J., and Lindstrom, J. M., 1980, Monoclonal antibodies used to probe acetylcholine receptor structure: Localization of the main immunogenic regions and detection of similarities between subunits, *Proc. Natl. Acad. Sci. USA* **77**:755–779.

Tzartos, S. J., Rand, D. E., Einarson, B. L., and Lindstrom, J. M., 1981, Mapping of surface structure of *Electrophorus* acetylcholine receptor using monoclonal antibodies, *J. Biol. Chem.* **256**:8635–8645.

Tzartos, S. J., Seybold, M. E., and Lindstrom, J. M., 1982, Specificities of antibodies to acetylcholine receptors in serum from myasthenia gravis patients measured by monoclonal antibodies, *Proc. Natl. Acad. Sci. USA* **79**:188–192.

Tzartos, S., Langeberg, L., Hochschwender, S., and Lindstrom, J., 1983, Demonstration of a main immunogenic region on acetylcholine receptors from human muscle using monoclonal antibodies to human receptor, *FEBS Lett.* **158**:116–118.

Vernet Der Garabedian, B., and Morel, E., 1983, Monoclonal antibodies against the human acetylcholine receptor, *Biochem. Biophys. Res. Commun.* **113**:1–9.

Watters, D., and Maelicke, A., 1983, Organization of ligand binding sites at the acetylcholine receptor: A study with monoclonal antibodies, *Biochemistry* **22**:1811–1819.

Yu, R., Richman, D. P., and Gomez, C. M., 1979, Immunohistochemical localization of acetylcholine receptors on rat myotube surface with monoclonal antibodies, *Soc. Neurosci.* **9**:490.

3

Monoclonal Antibodies to Enzymes

HARRY HARRIS

I. Introduction

The application of immunological methods to problems in enzymology has a long history and a very extensive literature. For the most part, this deals with studies using antisera raised against purified enzymes in animals of species other than those from which the enzymes were derived. The use of monoclonal antibodies is, of course, much more recent. Such antibodies have so far only been produced against a modest number of enzymes, though new reports are appearing at an increasing pace and there is little doubt that before long, such antibodies will become the reagents of choice for a wide variety of studies in enzyme immunochemistry. The analytic power of monoclonal antibodies in enzymology largely derives from the fact that each antibody is directed to an antigenic determinant that represents only a small region on the surface of the enzyme protein. Consequently, many antibodies with distinctive specificities can in principle be raised against a single enzyme. This contrasts with antisera, which contain a complex mixture of antibodies directed to different determinants on the enzyme surface and occurring in unknown proportions. The other important advantage is that monoclonal antibodies are single immunoglobulin species, which can, in principle, be produced in unlimited quantities by continued culture of the hybridoma cells that secrete them, whereas the antibody composition of antisera will vary in any particular animal during the course of immunization and will vary from animal to animal immunized with the same antigen.

    The aim of this chapter is to summarize the experience so far gained in the production of monoclonal antibodies to enzymes and the uses to which these

HARRY HARRIS • Department of Human Genetics, University of Pennsylvania School of Medicine, Philadelphia, Pennsylvania 19104.

reagents have been put in different types of investigations. The chapter is in two parts. The first part reviews the findings reported in the literature on a series of enzymes to which monoclonal antibodies have been raised for various purposes. The second part is an account of work from our own laboratory, which has been particularly directed to studying the potentialities of monoclonal antibodies as tools in enzyme genetics, using the human alkaline phosphatases as a model example.

II. Literature Review

Table I lists a series of enzymes against which monoclonal antibodies have been produced. Although numerically a very limited series, the list includes diverse examples of enzymes of different types from a wide range of species and tissue sources.

A. Hybridoma Production

The great majority of the antibodies were raised by the mouse hybridoma method (Kohler and Milstein 1975). In a few cases, rats were immunized, followed by fusion of their spleen cells with either rat (Choo et al., 1980) or mouse (Levey et al., 1981) plasmacytoma cells. There does not appear, however, to be any particular advantage in using rats except where the enzyme antigen comes from mouse, which was not the case in these particular examples.

Although in some cases highly purified enzyme preparations were used as immunogens (for references see Table I), in others successful production of enzyme-specific hybridomas was obtained by immunizing with only partially purified enzyme preparations, relatively crude membrane preparations, and indeed in some cases with whole cultured cells.

The immunization protocols varied in detail from one case to another. Immunization was generally started by injecting 15–125 μg of enzyme in incomplete Freund's adjuvant either intraperitoneally (i.p.) or subcutaneously (s.c.). This was usually followed by one or more injections of about the same amount of enzyme in complete Freund's adjuvant over the following 4–6 weeks. Finally, a similar dose of enzyme without adjuvant was given either intravenously (i.v.) or i.p. followed 2–5 (usually 3) days later by fusion of the spleen cells with plasmacytoma cells. Successful production of positive hybridomas was achieved in some cases without using either complete or incomplete Freund's adjuvant. Success was also obtained with various numbers of injections on various time scales. In many, though not all, cases the mouse serum was tested for antibodies to decide how long to pursue the immunization. In one case (α-glucosidase) successful production of positive hybridoma was only obtained when the hyperimmunization scheme proposed by Stahli et al. (1980) was used. In this scheme a series of weekly injections is followed by several daily i.v. injections prior to removal of the spleen and cell fusion.

Table I

Monoclonal Antibodies to Enzymes[a]

	Enzyme	Species	Tissue source	Antigen[a]	Screening procedure[b]	Applications[c]	References
1	Phenylalanine hydroxylase	Monkey	Liver	hpE	b	t, u, x	Choo et al. (1980, 1981), Cotton et al. (1980)
2	Phosphofructokinase	Human	Red cells	ppE	b	r, s, v	Vora et al. (1981, 1982), Vora and Francke (1981)
3	Tyrosine hydroxylase	Rat	Caudate nucleus and substantia nigra	ppE	a	w, x	Ross et al. (1981)
4	Glucose-6-phosphate dehydrogenase	Human	Red cells	hpE	a	x, z	Damiani et al. (1980)
5	Acetylcholinesterase	Rat	Liver	hpE	a	x, k	Dao et al. (1982)
		Human	Red cells	hpE	a	r, w, z	Fambrough et al. (1982)
6	Choline acetyltransferase	Bovine	Caudate nucleus	ppE	b	r	Levey et al. (1981), Levey and Wainer (1982)
		Drosophila melanogaster	—	ppE	b	r, x	Crawford et al. (1982)
7	Catalase T	Yeast (Saccharomyces cerevisiae)	—	hpE	b	—	Adolf et al. (1980)
8	Xanthine oxidase	Bovine	Milk	Fat-globule membrane	a	—	Mather et al. (1980)
9	5-aminolevulinate dehydrogenase	Spinach	—	ppE	c	u	Liedgens et al. (1980)
10	Guanylate cyclase	Rat	Lung	hpE	a	r, x, k	Lewicki et al. (1980), Brandwein et al. (1981)

(continued)

Table I (Continued)

	Enzyme	Species	Tissue source	Antigen[a]	Screening procedure[b]	Applications[c]	References
10	Guanylate cyclase (continued)	Rat	Brain	hpE	b	r, x, k	Nakene and Deguchi (1982)
11	β-D-Galactosidase	E. coli	—	hpE	c	x	Frackelton and Rotman (1980)
					a	x	Acolla et al. (1981)
12	Acid α-glucosidase	Human	Placenta	hpE	a	—	Hilkens et al. (1981)
13	RNA polymerase II	D. melanogaster	—	ppE	a	w	Kramer et al. (1980)
		Calf	Thymus	hpE	a	x, k	Christmann and Dahmus (1981)
14	S-Adenosylhomocysteine hydrolase	Human	Placenta	hpE	b	v	Hershfeld and Francke (1982)
15	γ-Cystathionase	Human	Liver	ppE	a	y	Glode et al. (1981)
16	Monoamine oxidase B	Human	Platelets	ppE	b	u, s	Denny et al. (1982)
17	5'-Nucleotidase	Rat	Liver	ppE	b	u, x	Siddle et al. (1981), Bailyes et al. (1982)
18	ATPase	Barley	Protoplast	Plasma membrane	a, b	x	Chin 1982
19	Cytochrome P-450 Phenobarbital induced	Rabbit	Liver	hpE	a	x, k	Park et al. (1980)
	3-Methyl cholanthrine induced	Rat	Liver	hpE	a	r, x, k	Park et al. (1982), Fujino et al. (1982)
20	3-Hydroxy-3-methyl glutaryl-CoA-reductase	Rat	Liver	hpE'	a	u, k	Clark et al. (1982)
21	Lysozyme c	Chicken	Egg white	hpE	a	r, x, z	Smith-Gill et al. (1982)

22	Urokinase	Human	Kidney	hpE	a	x	Herion et al. (1981)
		—	—	ppE	b	u, x, k	Kaltoft et al. (1982)
23	Alkaline phosphatase	Human	Placental	hpE	a	r, s, t, u, x	Slaughter et al. (1981, 1982), Gogolin et al. (1981, 1982), this chapter, Section III
		Human	Placental	hpE	a	t	Millan and Stigbrand (1981), Millan et al. (1982)
		Human	Cultured cells	Whole cells	b	—	Arklie et al. (1981)
		Human	Cultured cells	Whole cells	c	s	Wray and Harris (1982)
		Human	Liver	ppE	c	u	This chapter, Section III

[a]hpE, highly purified enzyme; ppE, partially purified enzyme.

[b]As indicated in the text; a, binding of antibody to antigen immobilized in microtiter wells; b, removal of enzyme activity from solution by antibody precipitated by staphylococcal bacteria with surface protein A, or anti-mouse immunoglobulin; c, binding of active enzyme by antibodies bound to microtiter wells.

[c]r, Interspecies comparisons; S, interlocus comparisons; t, interallelic comparisons; u, enzyme purification with monoclonal antibody affinity columns; v, gene mapping; w, immunocytochemical studies; x, effects on enzyme activity; y, immunoassay; z, antibody competition studies; k, comparisons of similar enzymes, e.g., soluble versus particulate (10), enzymes induced by different substances (19), enzyme changes by diet variation (4).

B. Hybridoma Screening

It is, of course, crucial in the production of monoclonal antibodies to a particular enzyme that there should be available a convenient procedure to screen the hybridoma culture fluids for the specific antibodies. Since generally only a small proportion of all the hybridomas generated will be secreting the desired specific antibody, it is desirable that the screening test should be carried out reasonably quickly to avoid the labor of maintaining the negative colonies for any length of time. The following three general approaches have been used in different cases (for references see Table I):

(a) Immobilization of antigen in wells of plastic microtiter plates followed by application of hybridoma culture fluids. Wells containing bound monoclonal antibody are then detected by the application of rabbit (or other species) anti-mouse immunoglobulin labeled either with ^{125}I or an enzyme such as peroxidase. Binding of the monoclonal antibody is then determined in a gamma counter or using suitable enzyme reagents in an ELISA. Some enzymes (e.g., alkaline phosphatase) do not readily bind to the plastic of the microtiter plate. In these cases, immobilization can be achieved by precoating the wells with antisera raised in rabbits to the purified enzymes (Slaughter et al., 1980, 1981).

Obviously, if impure enzyme has been used as the antigen for immunization of the mice, then positive hybridomas detected by this procedure may contain antibodies binding to impurity rather than the enzyme itself. Consequently, such hybridoma fluids need to be screened further by other methods (e.g., method b or c below) to detect those containing specific antibody to the enzyme.

(b) Incubation of hybridoma culture fluids with a standard amount of enzyme and then addition of staphylococcal bacteria with surface protein A or anti-mouse immunoglobulin to precipitate any enzyme–antibody complexes formed. Reduction of enzyme activity in the supernatant compared with the activity in a control lacking the particular culture fluid indicates the presence of a specific monoclonal antibody to the enzyme. In addition, or alternatively, determination of enzyme activity in the precipitate may be carried out, which is a modification of method c below. In some cases purified radioactively labeled enzyme has been used so that the enzyme can be identified in the precipitate by counting (Siddle et al., 1981) or by radioautography after SDS PAGE (Adolf et al., 1980; Denney et al., 1982).

In some studies, this type of screening was used but with omission of the second antibody or staphylococcal protein (Choo et al., 1980; Cotton et al., 1980; Chin, 1982). In cases where the monoclonal antibody–enzyme complex is soluble and does not precipitate, this procedure will detect only those monoclonal antibodies that significantly inhibit or enhance activity and others will be missed in the screen. However, some monoclonal antibodies against particular enzymes have been shown to be precipitating and in these cases the antibody will be detected in the screen irrespective of its direct effects on enzyme activity. In general it is better to use a precipitating second antibody or staphylococcal protein A in the screening procedure, and then examine the antibodies detected in separate experiments to determine their effects on enzyme activity or their ability to immunoprecipitate the enzyme.

(c) Application of hybridoma cell culture fluids to wells of microtiter plates (preferably precoated with rabbit anti-mouse immunoglobulin), followed by the application of enzyme so that the enzyme is bound in any wells containing immobilized specific monoclonal antibody. The enzyme activity of the immobilized enzyme–antibody complex is then detected using a standard enzyme assay procedure. The method is particularly convenient where the enzyme activity can be detected by a color change after incubation with an appropriate substrate. An alternative is to couple anti-mouse immunoglobulin to CNBr-activated paper disks and then put these in the wells of the microtiter plates, where the rest of the procedure can be performed (Frackelton and Rotman 1980).

It will be noted that method c, unlike methods a and b, depends on the retention of enzyme activity by the enzyme–monoclonal antibody complex. Where inhibition of enzyme activity by a monoclonal antibody occurs, method c is still probably applicable provided the inhibition is no greater than about 80% of the original activity. The occasional antibody that causes a complete or nearly complete inhibition of the enzyme activity would, however, be missed by this screening procedure.

Screening method c is particularly effective, and is quicker and more convenient to carry out than method b, for enzymes such as hydrolases (e.g., β-galactosidase, alkaline phosphatase) where artificial substrates producing distinctive colored or fluorescent products are available. For many other enzymes a variety of staining procedures suitable for the detection of the enzyme in complex mixtures after electrophoresis have been devised (Harris and Hopkinson, 1976) and these could no doubt be adapted for use in microtiter plates. Method c (like method b), is more convenient than method a in cases where only impure enzyme preparations are available for immunization, since hybridoma cell fluids containing antibodies against impurities will not generally be detected in the screen.

The brief descriptions of the three screening procedures (a, b, and c) provide only the basic principle of the methods. Detailed protocols for the washing procedures between each step in the assay and for the concentrations of the various reagents will be found in the original publications (references in Table I). In general such factors as the optimal concentrations of enzyme, dilution of antisera, and incubation times have to be worked out empirically for each new enzyme.

The screening methods (a, b, and c) have been adapted in various ways for comparing quantitatively the relative binding of particular monoclonal antibodies to different forms of the enzyme, such as allelic variants and homologous forms of the enzyme in different species, and examples of these procedures will be illustrated later in this chapter.

The monoclonal antibodies to the various enzymes listed in Table I were raised for a variety of purposes and have been used in different types of studies. These are indicated in Table I and some of them are briefly considered below.

C. Evolutionary Comparisons

Monoclonal antibodies are likely to prove of considerable interest in evolutionary studies of enzymes because antibodies directed to different determinants on the same enzyme protein can be tested for cross-reactivity with the homologous enzyme in other species. If the determinant detected by a particular antibody is represented in the homologous enzyme, albeit in a structurally modified form, cross-reactivity may be detected. The degree of binding of the antibody to the homologous enzyme compared with its binding to the enzyme against which it was raised should in principle provide an indication of the extent of structural change that has occurred in that particular region of the enzyme surface in the course of divergence of the enzyme structures in evolution. Each determinant is thought to involve only a small region of the enzyme surface, probably involving just a few amino acids (not necessarily sequential). Thus one should, in principle, be able to investigate evolutionary changes at a series of different sites on the surface of the enzyme molecule. This determinant-by-determinant approach using monoclonal antibodies contrasts with the more classical approach using polyclonal antisera, where the degree of relationship between homologous enzymes will in general represent the average of the effects of the series of different antibodies present in differing amounts in the polyclonal mixture.

So far, only a very modest amount of information about the potential of monoclonal antibodies for evolutionary studies of enzymes is available. However, the results do indicate that such a determinant-by-determinant comparison of homologous enzymes in different species will prove to be of great value. For example, when four monoclonal antibodies raised against human L (liver)-type phosphofructokinase were tested by an immunoprecipitation procedure (screening method b) against liver phosphofructokinase from monkey, dog, guinea pig, chinese hamster, cow, sheep, pig, mouse, rat, rabbit, chicken, turtle, and fish, one showed cross-reaction with liver phosphofructokinase from monkey and guinea pig but not from any of the other species; another cross-reacted with monkey, dog, and turtle phosphofructokinases but not with the enzyme from the other species; and two reacted only with human L-type phosphofructokinase (Vora et al., 1981). In the case of four monoclonal antibodies raised against monkey liver phenylalanine hydroxylase, two cross-reacted with human phenylalanine hydroxylase but not with the enzyme from rat or mouse, whereas two cross-reacted with the enzyme from all three species. It is noteworthy that one of the antibodies cross-reacting with the mouse phenylalanine hydroxylase had actually been raised by immunization of mouse (Choo et al., 1981). A monoclonal antibody raised against bovine choline acetyltransferase was found to cross-react weakly with the human and sheep enzyme but not with the enzyme from guinea pig, cat, rat, mouse, or chicken (Levey and Wainer 1982). Four monoclonal antibodies raised against rat guanylate cyclase, all cross-reacted with the enzyme from beef and pig but not rabbit, and at least one cross-reacted to a significant degree with the mouse enzyme (Lewicki et al., 1980). This antibody, like the others, had been raised by immunization in mouse.

Five monoclonal antibodies raised against human red cell acetylcholinesterase were shown by immunocytochemical studies to cross-react with human and monkey neuromuscular junctions, giving staining patterns corresponding to the distribution of junctional acetylcholinesterase (Fambrough *et al.*, 1982). When tested against neuromuscular junctions from rabbit, dog, guinea pig, and calf, two showed cross-reactivity with all four species; one reacted with rabbit, dog, and guinea pig but not calf; and one cross-reacted with rabbit but not the others. A monoclonal antibody raised against chicken lysozyme *c* was shown by competition studies to cross-react strongly with the lysozymes from seven different species of galliform (fowllike) birds, weakly with the enzyme from two other galliform species, but did not cross-react with duck lysozyme (Smith-Gill *et al.*, 1982). From a comparison of the known amino acid sequences of the lysozymes in these various species and from the known three-dimensional structure of the enzyme it was possible to identify one of the amino acids in the antigenic determinant to which this antibody is directed and to locate its site on the enzyme surface. Further examples of such interspecies comparisons are given in Section III with respect to the various alkaline phosphatases.

In general, cross-reactivity of a particular determinant over a wide range of species indicates that the determinant must have been relatively highly conserved in structure during the course of evolution, whereas a narrower range of species cross-reactivity implies a more rapid rate of evolutionary divergence.

Apart from its evolutionary interest, clear-cut differences in cross-reactivity profiles over a range of species with different monoclonal antibodies provides good evidence that the antibodies are directed to different determinants on the enzyme surface.

D. Effects on Enzyme Activity

Enzyme–antibody complexes formed by 18 different monoclonal antibodies raised against purified human placental alkaline phosphatase and originally detected by screening method a, which does not depend on the detection of enzyme activity, were all found to retain enzyme activity virtually intact (see Section III). A similar finding has been obtained with sets of monoclonal antibodies raised against human glucose-6-phosphate dehydrogenase (Damiani *et al.*, 1980), rat tyrosine hydroxylase (Ross *et al.*, 1981), rat guanylate cyclase (Lewicki *et al.*, 1980), and calf thymus RNA polymerase (Christmann and Dahmus, 1981). In other cases reaction of a monoclonal antibody with an enzyme results in inhibition or activation of enzyme activities. For example, of four antibodies raised against monkey phenylalanine hydroxylase, one was found to enhance activity by about 92%, two inhibited activity by about 62% and 11%, respectively, and one had no effect on activity (Choo *et al.*, 1981). Activation or partial inhibition of enzyme activity has been found with different monoclonal antibodies raised against a plant membrane ATPase (Chin, 1982). Partial inhibition of enzyme activity has also been reported for four monoclonal antibodies raised against chicken lysozyme *c* (Smith-Gill *et al.*, 1982). Occasionally an effectively complete inhibition of enzyme activity occurs. This was found to be the case with two antibodies raised against *Drosophila melanogaster* choline acetyltransferase (Crawford *et al.*, 1982). Inclusion of the substrate acetyl-CoA in the enzyme antibody reaction mixture at 10 times K_m substantially reduced the level of inhibition in both cases. Choline, however, asserted no protective effects. It was concluded in this case that the antibody was reacting at or near the acetyl-CoA binding region of the enzyme active site.

Among monoclonal antibodies raised against *Escherichia coli* β-galactosidase, several different types of effect on activity were noted (Frackelton and Rotman, 1980; Accolla *et al.*, 1981). About 4% showed some degree of inhibition and the rest little or no effect on the normal enzyme activity. However, a high proportion (about 50%) were found to enhance activity of different mutant forms of the enzyme with defective activity, an effect ascribed to conformational changes and previously recognized using polyclonal antisera. Single monoclonal antibodies may activate several different mutants and it appears that the determinant site for antibody binding is generally different from that of the mutational sites in cases showing this effect.

E. Gene Mapping

The chromosomal assignment of a gene coding for a particular enzyme expressed in cultured cells by the method of somatic cell hybridization requires a procedure that gives clear discrimination between the particular enzyme in the two species used to make the somatic cell hybrids. In many cases this discrimination is readily achieved by electrophoresis, and most chromosomal assignments of genes encoding enzymes have used this method. Where a clear electrophoretic separation cannot be achieved, immunological methods may be applied, but this requires that the antibodies used should have a high degree of specificity and in particular should react with the enzyme of the species with the enzyme to be assigned, but not with its counterpart in the other species. Monoclonal antibodies are reagents of choice because among those raised against the enzyme from one species at least some are likely to be unreactive with the enzyme of the other species used in the somatic cell hybridization. By this approach the loci coding for the L-type (Vora and Francke, 1981) and M-type (Vora *et al.*, 1982) subunits of phosphofructokinase and for *S*-adenosylhomocysteine hydrolase (Hershfeld and Francke, 1982) have been mapped to human chromosomes 21, 1, and 20, respectively.

F. Enzyme Purification Using Monoclonal Antibody Affinity Columns

Preparation of highly purified enzymes by standard biochemical procedures often presents considerable difficulties, particularly when the enzyme is relatively labile and where, as is generally the case, the enzyme protein represents only a very small fraction of the total protein in the starting material. The final stages of purification are usually the most difficult and often result in poor yields. Monoclonal antibodies coupled to activated sepharose provide a new tool with potentially a very wide application in enzyme purification. This is because, as pointed out earlier, it is not necessary to have a highly purified enzyme preparation in order to obtain an enzyme-specific monoclonal antibody.

The general method has so far been applied successfully to the purification of 5-aminolevulinate dehydratase from spinach (Liedgens *et al.*, 1980), phenylalanine hydroxylase from monkey liver (Choo *et al.*, 1981), monoamine oxidase B from human platelets (Denney *et al.*, 1982), γ-cystathionase from human liver (Glode *et al.*, 1981), 5'-nucleotidase from rat liver (Bailyes *et al.*, 1982), and human placental and liver alkaline phosphatases (this chapter, Section III). These studies, though each resulted in a successful outcome, have focused attention on a number of technical problems. These concern the choice of monoclonal antibody to use when several are available, the optimal relative amounts of antibody to activated sepharose to be used in constructing the affinity column, and the best method of elution of the bound antibody from the column. In one study where affinity columns were prepared with four different monoclonal antibodies to monkey phenylalanine hydroxylase (Choo *et al.*, 1981), it was found that efficient binding of the enzyme from crude liver extracts in 0.1 M Tris-HCl buffer, pH 8.6, was achieved in three cases and elution of the enzyme could be accomplished in two cases with reasonable yields (about 50%) by eluting with a high-pH buffer. In the other case, efficient binding was achieved only in the presence of L-phenylalanine, the enzyme substrate, and here elution was obtained simply by using an L-phenylalanine-free buffer. Elution from a monoclonal antibody affinity column of 5-aminolevulinate dehydratase (Liedgens *et al.*, 1980) and of urokinase (Kaltoft *et al.*, 1982) was obtained with low-pH buffers, of monoamine oxidase B from human platelets with 4.0 M KSCN (Denney *et al.*, 1982), of human liver alkaline phosphatase with 3.0 M NaCl (see Section III), and of γ-cystathionase (Glode *et al.*, 1980) and human placental alkaline phosphatase with high-pH buffer.

III. Enzyme Genetics

This section is concerned with work from our own laboratory aimed at exploring the uses of monoclonal antibodies in enzyme genetics. Three different though interrelated areas of the subject are considered: allelic variation, multilocus enzyme systems, and enzyme evolution.

A. Enzyme Variations

It is well known that an enzyme coded at a specific gene locus will very often occur in structurally different forms in different individuals. Such so-called allelic variants presumably arose by single-gene mutations in earlier generations, often a very long time ago. In most cases they probably represent the substitution of one amino acid for another in the sequence of the several hundred or so amino acids which make up the polypeptide chains of the particular enzymes. Thus the differences between the allelic forms generally reflect only slight changes in the overall structure of the enzyme protein. The extensive degree of allelic enzyme variation that we now know occurs in most natural populations was largely discovered by the technique of gel electrophoresis, though methods involving assays of enzyme activity, and kinetic and other types of investigation, have also been important. Immunological methods, however, have played only a very modest role in the development of this area. This is because, in the past, such studies could only be carried out using antisera raised against highly purified enzyme preparations. Such antisera are composed of a complex mixture of antibodies directed to a variety of different antigenic determinants on the enzyme surface (i.e., they are polyclonal). Each antigenic determinant represents only a small region of the enzyme. Thus, even though one or more of the antibodies present may discriminate between allelic forms of a given enzyme, differing by only one or very few amino acid substitutions, this discrimination will be effectively swamped by the many other antibodies in the antiserum that react with other determinants identical in the allelic forms of the enzyme. Attempts to absorb out cross-reacting antibodies have not generally proved fruitful in these circumstances and, in practice, antisera have not been of much help in discriminating between allelic variants. The main exception has been in the case of alleles causing enzyme deficiencies when the question was whether the allele produced a catalytically inactive enzyme protein (so-called cross-reacting material positive, CRM^+) or a true deficiency of the enzyme protein (CRM^-).

Monoclonal antibodies, in contrast, are each directed to a specific antigenic determinant. Thus in principle many monoclonal antibodies directed to different regions of the enzyme surface can be raised against any given enzyme. Consequently, it becomes practical to search for allelic differences on a determinant-by-determinant basis, using a panel of monoclonal antibodies raised against the particular enzyme.

A second major area of enzyme genetics concerns what have been called multilocus enzyme systems (Harris, 1979). It turns out that in the human and mammalian genome there are often two or more loci coding for structurally distinct enzymes that, however, resemble each other closely in their catalytic activities and in their overall structures. They are thought to have originated in evolution by gene duplication and to have subsequently diverged in their structures as a result of point mutations occurring in the course of evolution subsequent to the original duplication. Many examples of such multilocus enzyme systems are now known and classic immunological methods using polyclonal antisera have often been important in differentiating the various enzymes involved. However, one may anticipate that monoclonal antibodies will provide a further analytic tool.

A third area of the subject is concerned with enzyme evolution and involves comparisons of homologous enzymes in different species. Conventional antisera have been widely used in such studies, but again, one may expect monoclonal antibodies to provide a new dimension.

To investigate the various potentialities of monoclonal antibodies to studies in enzyme systems, we have chosen to use the human alkaline phosphatases as a model example. This is because these enzymes have been shown to encapsulate many of the central problems in the subject. They represent a typical multilocus enzyme system; one locus is highly polymorphic; and intriguing problems concerning their evolutionary relationships have come to light (Harris, 1982).

B. Alkaline Phosphatases (ALPs)

The alkaline phosphatases are membrane-bound glycoproteins that hydrolyze a wide range of phosphate esters and have high pH optima. Different forms occur in different tissues, and they are usually referred to as, e.g., liver, bone, kidney, intestinal, or placental ALPs (Fishman, 1974). The protein moieties of the various human ALPs are encoded by at least three gene loci: one for placental ALP, at least one for the intestinal ALPs (adult and fetal), and at least one for the liver, bone, and kidney ALPs (Mulivor et al., 1978a; Seargent and Stinson, 1979; McKenna et al., 1979).

C. Allelic Variation

Electrophoretic studies have shown that human placental ALP is highly polymorphic. Three common alleles (ALP_p^1, ALP_p^2, and ALP_p^3) at an autosomal locus, giving rise to six common phenotypes (1, 2-1, 2, 3-1, 3-2, 3), occur in most human populations and, in addition, an extensive array of so-called "rare" alleles, which are generally seen in heterozygous combination with one or another of the common alleles, have also been identified (Robson and Harris, 1965, 1967). In contrast, electrophoretic polymorphism has not been identified at the intestinal or liver/bone/kidney loci (Harris et al., 1974).

The first question we wished to ask was whether monoclonal antibodies will, in fact, discriminate allelic variants; if so, we wished to get some idea of how frequently such discriminating antibodies may be expected to occur among a set of monoclonal antibodies raised against a given enzyme. A panel of 18 monoclonal antibodies was obtained by the mouse hybridoma method using highly purified placental ALP preparations (from different placental ALP phenotypes) as immunogen (Slaughter et al., 1980, 1981, 1982). Screening for positive hybridomas was carried out by method a (see Section II). This involved immobilizing the enzyme in wells of PVC microtiter plates, applying the hybridoma culture fluids, and then detecting bound monoclonal antibody with either [125]I- or peroxidase-labeled rabbit anti-mouse immunoglobulin. It was found that ALP did not readily bind to the plastic, so immobilization was accomplished by precoating the plastic wells with anti-human placental ALP serum raised in rabbits against purified placental ALP. This was shown to give equal binding of the various ALP phenotypes to the plates.

In order to find out whether any of the monoclonal antibodies discriminate among the products of the different alleles detectable electrophoretically, ALP from a series of nearly 300 placentas was extracted and phenotyped by electrophoresis. This series contained representatives of each of the six common polymorphic types, though in differing numbers, reflecting the allele frequencies in the total sample. In addition, there were a number of different "rare variant" ALP phenotypes. In order to determine the relative reactivities of each of the monoclonal antibodies with each of the ALP phenotypes, a standard assay system based on the original hybridoma screening system was devised. In essentials, each microtiter plate received, in triplicate, 20 different ALPs each diluted to give the same activity and also 12 replicates of a single placental type 1 ALP, which was used as a standard on all plates. Also, 12 wells were used as blanks

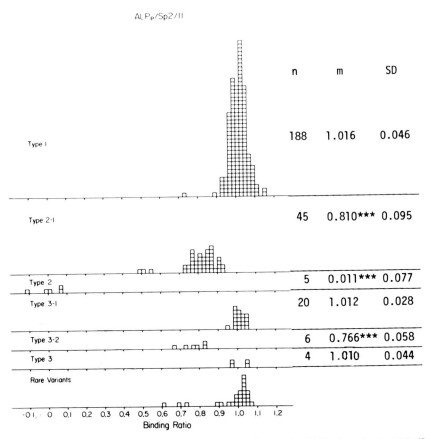

FIGURE 1. Histograms showing the distributions of binding ratios (BR) of antibody ALP$_p$/Sp2/11 with each of the six common ALP electrophoretic phenotypes and the rare variant phenotypes in a series of 295 placental ALPs from different individuals. Each square represents a single individual. The number of ALPs (n), mean BR (m), and standard deviation (SD) of BRs for each electrophoretic phenotype are shown. The significance of the difference for the mean of the type 1 samples and the mean for each of the other phenotypes was determined by t-tests. Significant differences $p <$ 0.0001(***) are indicated.

without added ALP but otherwise processed in the same way. Binding of the monoclonal antibodies to the varous ALPs in the individual wells was determined either by counting in a gamma counter where ^{125}I had been used to label the second antibody (Slaughter *et al.*, 1981) or by OD_{450} determination of peroxidase activity in a Multiscan apparatus (Flow Labs) where peroxidase-labeled second antibody was used (Slaughter *et al.*, 1982). The reactivity of a particular monoclonal antibody with a particular ALP sample was determined as a binding ratio (BR) defined as the mean of the values for the test sample divided by the mean of the values for the ALP type 1 standard, after subtraction of blanks. With this type of standardization, it was found that the BRs for different samples were essentially independent of variations in absolute counts or OD_{450} values from plate to plate or from day to day, of differing amounts of label in the second antibody, and of whether the second antibody was labeled with ^{125}I or peroxidase. A BR value close to 1.0 indicates no difference in binding relative to the standard, whereas a BR close to 0.0 indicates absence of binding.

Figure 1 illustrates the results obtained with one of the antibodies (ALP_p/Sp2/11) tested against 291 placental ALPs. It shows histograms of BR values for each of the common polymorphic types and for the rare variants. Each square represents the BR for a single individual. Means and standard deviations are shown for each of the common electrophoretic phenotypes, and the significance levels for the difference between the mean for the type 1 samples and the mean for each of the other phenotypes are also indicated. It will be seen that with this antibody there is virtually no binding with the ALP type 2 samples (homozygotes for allele ALP_p^2), and that the mean BRs for the heterozygous phenotypes 2-1 and 3-2 are significantly reduced compared with type 1 and also types 3-1 and 3. It will, however, be noted that the means for the 2-1 samples were not 50% of those for types 1 and 3 samples as might be expected, but were about 0.8. We will return to this unexpected finding later. It will also be seen from Figure 1 that some of the rare variant phenotypes showed reduced BRs. These had been found electrophoretically to be heterozygous for a rare allele and the ALP^2 allele. Thus it is apparent that antibody ALP_p/Sp2/11 discriminates between the product of the ALP_p^2 allele, with which it effectively fails to bind, and the products of alleles ALP_p^1 and ALP_p^3, to which it binds strongly.

Figure 2 illustrates the findings with another antibody, ALP_p/Sp2/3, which also discriminates between the product of the ALP_p^2 allele and the products of the other alleles. However, in this case, the discrimination is much less marked, since the mean BR for type 2 homozygotes is about 90% of the means for types 1 and 3. These differences, though small, are statistically highly significant. Evidently ALP_p/Sp2/3 does bind quite strongly to the product of allele ALP_p^2 but presumably with relatively reduced avidity compared with its binding to the products of ALP_p^1 and ALP_p^3.

Table II summarizes the main results obtained with 18 different monoclonal antibodies. Six of them discriminate among the products of the three common alleles, though to different degrees.

Another antibody (ALP_p/Sp2/4) apparently discriminates among different forms of ALP type 1 that have the same electrophoretic mobilities. This effect

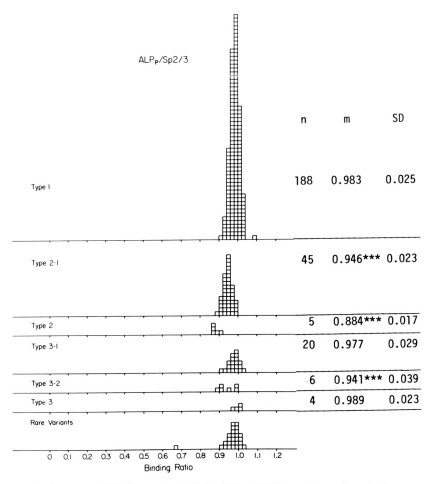

FIGURE 2. Histograms of binding ratios (BR) for ALPs of different electrophoretic phenotypes as in Fig. 1 except using antibody ALP$_p$/Sp2/3. Significant differences $p < 0.001$(***) indicated.

was noted when it was found that the variance of BRs for the ALP type 1 samples with this antibody was significantly much larger than the variances for the type 1 BRs with the other antibodies (Slaughter *et al.*, 1981). When we obtained this result, we thought it possible that it might be due to some kind of experimental variation for which we had not allowed. Alternatively, it could reflect real individual differences. That is, some type 1 ALPs might have high binding ratios and others low binding ratios. To test this, we repeated the whole experiment and found that there was highly significant correlation between the two sets of results, i.e., individuals with low values in the first experiment showed similarly low values in the second and the same was true for those showing intermediate or high values (Figure 3). This would not have been expected if the variation were due to random error in the BR determinations. The result indicates that there is

TABLE II
Discrimination of Common ALP Types by Monoclonal Antibodies[a]

Reactivity pattern	n	Ab.	BR	Data source
Reduced binding with type 2	4	Sp2/3	0.88[b]	Slaughter *et al.* (1981)
		Sp2 11	0.06[b]	Slaughter *et al.* (1981)
		Sp2/14	0.79[b]	Slaughter *et al.* (1982)
		Sp2/18	0.04[b]	Slaughter *et al.* (1982)
Reduced binding with type 3	2	P3/1	0.07[c]	Slaughter *et al.* (1981)
		Sp2/10	0.29[c]	Slaughter *et al.* (1982)
Heterogeneity of type 1	1	Sp2/4	—	Slaughter *et al.* (1981)
No discrimination of common ALP types	11	Sp2/2, Sp2/5, Sp2/6, Sp2/7, Sp2/8, Sp2/9, Sp2/12, Sp2/13, Sp2/15, Sp2/16, Sp2/17	—	Slaughter *et al.* (1981, 1982)

[a]The full designation (Slaughter *et al.*, 1982) of the various antibodies (Ab.) listed includes the prefix $ALP_p/$ since they were all raised using placental ALP as immunogen.
[b]BR with type 2.
[c]BR with type 3.

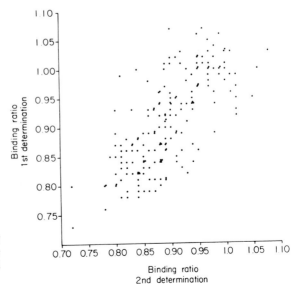

FIGURE 3. Correlation of binding ratios (BR) obtained in two separate determinations of type 1 placental ALPs with antibody $ALP_p/Sp2/4$.

a real heterogeneity among the type 1 ALPs. Possibly there are two different alleles both giving ALP products with the same electrophoretic mobility but differing slightly in their relative avidities for this particular antibody. If so, the distribution would represent three overlapping genotypes: low-binding homozygotes, heterozygotes, and high-binding homozygotes. The antibody is presumably directed at a determinant characteristic of the high-binding type since the combined type 1 mean was significantly greater than the means for the other common phenotypes (Slaughter *et al.,* 1981). Thus, in this case, there was presumptive evidence for allelic differences not reflected by electrophoretic differences.

The findings clearly demonstrate that allelic differences, presumably representing very small differences in overall structure, possibly only single amino acid substitutions, can be discriminated by different members of a panel of monoclonal antibodies raised against a particular enzyme. However, the results also demonstrate an unexpected phenomenon, which is likely to prove to be of very general significance. This concerns the different degrees of reactivity which particular allelic variants exhibit with different antibodies.

At the beginning of this work, it had been anticipated that most structural changes of single antigenic determinants on the surface of protein antigens would result in relatively large changes in the ability of the antibody to bind to the determinant, and this would give rise to "all-or-none" patterns of binding with enzyme proteins bearing nonidentical forms of any given determinant. This expectation was based upon the notion of an antigenic determinant as a very small feature of the protein's surface encompassing only about four amino acid residues (Sela, 1969). Almost any amino acid substitution within such a small site would result in a disturbance of the configuration of a large proportion of the atoms mediating antibody binding and hence be expected to give rise to a correspondingly marked loss of antigenicity. Three of the antibodies that discriminate among products of the common ALP_p alleles (antibodies $ALP_p/P3/1$, $ALP_p/Sp2/11$, and $ALP_p/Sp2/18$) show an "all-or-none" effect of this kind. In other cases, however, significant binding to an allelic product bearing a structurally altered determinant was found, although at a reduced level compared to standard control binding (Table II). In two of these cases (antibodies $ALP_p/Sp2/3$ and $ALP_p/Sp2/14$) the BR was reduced only to about 90% and 80% of the standard type 1 control, respectively, and in the third case (antibody $ALP_p/Sp2/10$) it was reduced to about 30%.

A number of possibilities could account for such findings. First, the number of amino acids on a protein antigen contributing to the total energy of binding with a monoclonal antibody may often be larger than anticipated. The net effect on a single amino acid substitution within a determinant may therefore be proportionally reduced. In this context, it may be relevant to note that the prototype studies of the sizes of antigenic determinants on proteins, especially the classic experiments of Sela and his colleagues (Sela, 1969), not only made use of antibodies that were heterogeneous, but also mainly considered antibodies against particular synthetic oligopeptide haptenic determinants, which may not be typical of proteins in general. Second, while some amino acid replacements, such as charged for uncharged or oppositely charged residues, will usually have a drastic affect on binding affinity, other, more "conservative" substitutions may have much smaller effects on BR. Third, reduction of affinity may arise from amino acid substitutions not only within the affected determinant itself, but also at a site or sites outside the determinant. Such substitutions may transmit conformational changes to the moieties within the determinant recognized by the antibody, thus giving a rise to a "poorer fit." Since, in principle, almost any degree of conformational change could arise in this way, an almost continuous spectrum of binding affinities may result. Another possibility, which cannot be formally excluded at this time, is that occasional monoclonal antibodies might recognize more than one determinant site on the same polypeptide chain of the antigen molecule. Such repeating determinants could, in principle, arise from internal homologies due to the existence of a series of homologous domains along the length of the polypeptide. If only one of such a series of domain sites were affected by an amino acid substitution, binding to the antigen would be reduced but not obliterated. Whatever the mechanisms most commonly involved, it appears probable from the present data that all degrees of reduction in BR are possible with different allelic variants of a protein antigen.

D. Heterozygotes

Placental ALP is dimeric, that is, it has two polypeptide chains per molecule. In a heterozygote, two sorts of polypeptide chains are being made, one by each allele, and when these combine to give dimers, one gets three types of molecules: two homodimers containing identical polypeptides determined by each of the alleles and a heterodimer containing the two different polypeptides. If a particular monoclonal antibody binds to the polypeptide product of one allele but not to that of the other, then one of the homodimers will show full binding and the other homodimer will show no binding. In the heterodimer, binding will occur to only one of the polypeptide subunits, so that the binding ratio should be around 0.5 if both polypeptides are present in similar amounts. In general, we found that heterozygotes give binding ratios intermediate between those for the two corresponding homozygotes, but there were some interesting and unexpected complexities. Table III shows the results with two antibodies, neither of which reacts with the type 2 homozygote; one gives about 80% binding in the heterozygote type 2-1 (and also 3-2), whereas the other gives about 50% binding. The 50% case is no surprise, but the 80% case is unexpected.

One possible explanation is that in this case the binding of the monoclonal antibodies to the individual subunits of the dimeric enzyme protein are not truly independent so that the probability of binding to the first subunit is greater than the probability of binding to the second subunit once the determinant on the first subunit has been occupied by an antibody. This would reduce the level of antibody binding to the homodimer with two polypeptide subunits containing a binding site relative to the binding with the heteromeric form containing only a single binding site. This may be occurring in the 80% case, but not in the 50%

TABLE III

Binding Ratios for Heterozygous ALP Types 2-1 and 3-2 with Antibodies $ALP_p/Sp2/11$ and $ALP_p/Sp2/18^a$

ALP type	$ALP_p/Sp2/11$			$ALP_p/Sp2/18$			Significance of difference between means^a p
	n	Mean BR	SD	n	Mean BR	SD	
2-1	45	0.810	0.095	20	0.489	0.106	<0.001
3-2	6	0.776	0.058	6	0.484	0.075	<0.001

^{a}Significances of differences between the mean BR for each phenotype with the two antibodies were estimated by t-tests (Slaughter *et al.*, 1981, 1982).

case, and the results are telling us something about the sites of the determinants on the subunits and the structures of the antibody–enzyme complexes. Probably different determinants are involved. They may be overlapping and include the same amino acid substitution, *or* they may be well separated on the subunit surface.

E. Electrophoresis

After reaction of placental ALP with each of the 18 anti-placental ALP monoclonal antibodies, there was virtually no change in enzyme activity. In addition, the antibodies were nonprecipitating. These properties allowed us to investigate the relative mobilities of the antibody–enzyme complexes compared with the uncomplexed enzymes in gel electrophoresis by staining for alkaline phosphatase activity (Gogolin *et al.*, 1981). The mobilities of the complexes in starch and polyacrylamide gels depend both on molecular size and on net charge. In enzyme electrophoresis in agarose gels, mobility differences are largely independent of molecular size, so that differences in mobility are essentially determined by differences in net charge at the pH being used. Monoclonal antibody–enzyme complexes must necessarily be larger than uncomplexed enzyme, and this tends to produce slower mobilities in starch and polyacrylamide gels. In agarose gel electrophoresis, increases or decreases in net charge reflected in corresponding changes in mobility are demonstrable when the same enzyme is treated with different antibodies.

Placental alkaline phosphatase in tissue extracts is mainly present in the dimeric form (A isozymes), but larger molecular size forms (B isozymes), which probably represent aggregates of the A forms possibly associated with other nonenzymic tissue components, also occur and are separated in starch and acrylamide gel electrophoresis (Robson and Harris, 1967; Doellgast *et al.*, 1977). In starch gel electrophoresis, the A isozymes were invariably retarded after complexing with antibody. The same was found in many cases for the B isozymes, but with certain antibodies somewhat increased mobility of the B isozymes was observed apparently because the retardation due to increased size was overriden in these cases by an increase in net negative charge (Gogolin et al., 1981). In acrylamide gel electrophoresis, both the A and B isozymes were invariably retarded.

The electrophoretic procedures were used to confirm the allelic discriminations demonstrated originally by the quantitative binding ratio technique. Typical examples of this with antibodies ALP_p/Sp2/11 and ALP_p/Sp2/18, both of which had been found in the binding ratio studies to be unreactive with the product of the ALP_p^2 allele, are illustrated in Figure 4.

Figure 4 also demonstrates the use of this technique to analyze one of the rare electrophoretic variants (P292). In the absence of antibody this variant showed a triple-banded electrophoretic phenotype, indicating that it represented a heterozygote for a rare allele and the common ALP_p^1 allele. The typical electrophoretic product of the ALP_p^2 allele was not present. However, the variant gave reduced BRs with antibody ALP_p/Sp2/11 and also with antibody ALP_p/Sp2/18. These findings suggested either that the product of the rare allele showed reduced or absent reactivity with these antibodies or that the product of the ALP_p^1 allele was, in this instance, atypical and had reduced reactivity with the antibodies. By electrophoretic comparisons of P292 and appropriate controls

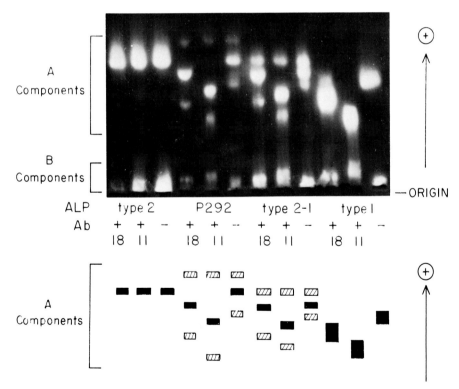

FIGURE 4. Photograph and diagram showing isozyme patterns after starch gel electrophoresis of placental ALPs (types 1, 2-1, and 2 and rare variant P292) before (−) and after (+) incubation with antibodies ALP_p/Sp2/18 and ALP_p/Sp2/11 (only the antibody numbers 18 and 11 are shown).

before and after incubation with the antibodies, it was found that the first of these two possibilities was correct. That is, the homodimeric product of the rare allele failed, like the product of ALP_p^2, to react with the antibody, whereas the homodimeric product of the presumed ALP_p^1 allele in the heterozygote reacted with the antibody in the same way as control type 1 ALP. Figure 4 shows the relevant electrophoretic comparisons. After incubation with the antibodies, the main, fast-moving isozyme (A isozyme) of the type 1 ALP control is retarded, but that of the type 2 ALP control is unaffected. In the 2-1 heterozygous control, a characteristic triple-banded pattern is seen. Here the most rapidly migrating band, which corresponds to the type 2 homodimer, is unaffected by the antibodies, but the slowest migrating band of the triplet, which corresponds to the type 1 homodimer, is retarded. The intermediate band, which represents a heterodimer, is also retarded relative to the corresponding band seen in the absence of antibody. The rare variant, P292, shows a typical heterozygous triple-banded pattern. The most rapidly migrating band represents the homodimer derived from the rare allele, and this is unaffected by incubation with the antibodies. The intermediate band of the triplet, presumably representing a heterodimer containing one subunit determined by the rare allele and one determined by the common ALP_p^1 allele, is retarded after incubation with the antibodies, and the slowest band of the triplet, which corresponds to the ALP type 1 homodimer, is also retarded. Thus the fast-moving component in P292, which appears to represent the homodimeric product of a rare allele, resembles the homodimeric product of the ALP_p^2 allele by showing no significant reactivity with either antibody $ALP_p/Sp2/18$ or antibody $ALP_p/Sp2/11$. However, it differs electrophoretically from the homodimeric product of allele ALP_p^2.

F. Intestinal ALPs

As noted earlier, there are at least three gene loci that code for the protein moieties of various human ALP glycoproteins: one for placental ALP, at least one for intestinal ALP, and at least one for liver/bone/kidney ALP. Two distinct forms of intestinal ALP, adult and fetal, have been identified (Mulivor *et al.*, 1978b). They are indistinguishable in terms of a number of properties that distinguish them sharply from placental ALP and the liver, bone, and kidney ALPs—for example, thermostability, specific inhibition with various inhibitors, such as phenylalanine, homoarginine, or phenylalanylglycylglycine, and cross-reaction with antiserum to placental ALP. But they differ in their electrophoretic characteristics. The fetal form is faster at alkaline pH. If it is treated with the enzyme neuraminidase, which removes negatively charged sialic acid residues, its mobility is retarded. The adult form is unaffected by neuraminidase because it contains no sialic acid residues. However, even after removal of sialic acid residues, the anodal mobility of the fetal form is still slightly greater than that of the adult form (Mulivor *et al.*, 1978b). It is not clear at present whether this difference arises because the two enzymes are coded at different loci which are expressed differently during development, or whether they are due to differences in their carbohydrate moieties other than sialic acid; that is, whether they arise by so-called posttranslational changes.

If one makes antiserum in rabbits against purified placental ALP, it does not cross-react against liver/bone/kidney ALPs, but it does cross-react with the intestinal ALPs (Lehmann 1975). However, using the Ouchterlony double-diffusion technique, one can show that this is a reaction of only partial identity. Furthermore, one can absorb out the cross-reacting antibodies with intestinal ALP, leaving an antiserum that reacts only with placental ALP. This implies that among the collection of antibodies that make up the heterogeneous polyclonal antiserum made to placental ALP, some also react with intestinal ALP, while others do not. The question therefore arises whether, among the monoclonal antibodies raised against purified placental ALP, any will be found that cross-react with intestinal ALP.

To examine this question, ascites fluids containing the different monoclonal antibodies raised against placental ALP were incubated with adult and fetal intestinal ALPs and then examined electrophoretically. One of the antibodies showed marked cross-reaction with adult intestinal ALP (Figure 5) and also with fetal intestinal ALP. We then wished to compare the relative reactivities of the adult and fetal forms with one another and also with the placental enzyme. To do this, we developed a method, which we have called electrophoretic titration (Gogolin *et al.*, 1982). In essentials, this involves incubating a standard amount of

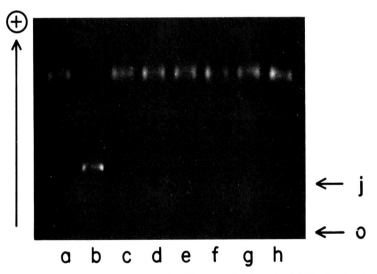

FIGURE 5. Polyacrylamide gel electrophoresis of human adult intestinal ALP after incubation with six different monoclonal antibodies raised against purified human placental ALP. Channels a and h contain adult intestinal ALP without antibody; channels b–g contain adult intestinal ALP after incubation with mouse ascites fluids containing antibodies $ALP_p/Sp2/5$, $ALP_p/Sp2/2$, $ALP_p/Sp2/11$, $ALP_p/Sp2/3$, $ALP_p/Sp2/4$, and $ALP_p/P3/1$, respectively. Only $ALP_p/Sp2/5$ shows binding (retardation) to intestinal ALP. The letters o and j indicate the origin and the junction between the 9.5% and 5% polyacrylamide layers.

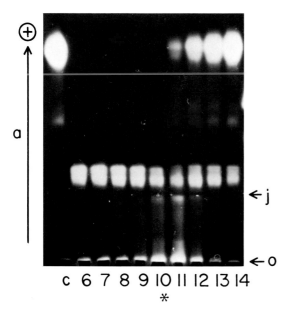

FIGURE 6. Electrophoretic titration of human placental ALP (type 1) in polyacrylamide gel. Channel c contains uncomplexed placental ALP (control). The other channels are the same ALP after incubation with serial (one in two) dilutions of antibody $ALP_p/Sp2/5$. Numbers 6–14 indicate the dilution of the antibody in the series 2^x, where x = 6–14. The asterisk indicates the endpoint of the titration. Letters o and j as in Figure 5.

enzyme with serial (one in two) dilutions of antibody and examining each mixture by electrophoresis so that one can visibly distinguish free enzyme from the enzyme–antibody complexes. The endpoint of the titration is defined as the highest dilution of antibody at which no free enzyme is seen under the standardized conditions used. A typical example of such a titration is shown in Figure 6. In the case of the particular antibody that cross-reacted with adult and fetal intestinal ALPs, the titration endpoints for placental, adult, and fetal intestinal ALPs were, respectively, 1/1024, 1/128, and 1/1 (Gogolin *et al.*, 1982). This implied that the relative amounts of antibody required to fully complex the same quantity of enzyme (in terms of activity per milliliter) was in the ratio placental ALP, adult intestinal ALP, fetal intestinal ALP of 1 : 8 : 1028. The finding that placental ALP was more reactive with this antibody than either of the intestinal ALPs was not surprising because the antibody had been raised using placental ALP as immunogen. However, the marked difference in reactivity of adult and fetal intestinal ALP was unexpected and implied that the antibody was detecting a structural difference between the two forms.

One possible difficulty about the interpretation of this result arises from the fact that we use the same amount of enzyme activity for each enzyme. If the enzymes had different specific activities (i.e., activity per unit weight of protein), the results would not necessarily indicate differences in avidity, because smaller amounts of enzyme protein would have been used to give the same activity for the forms with the highest specific activity. This, in turn, would require smaller amounts of antibody to reach the endpoint of the titration. Earlier data on specific activities suggested that both the adult and fetal forms of intestinal ALP have higher specific activities than placental ALP. However, more recent data indicate that, at most, only small differences in specific activity exist (less than twofold, which would correspond to less than one dilution in the electrophoretic titration).

The various ALPs are glycoproteins, so that the determinants to which a particular monoclonal antibody is directed can, in principle, be either in the protein or the carbohydrate moieties of the molecules or may indeed involve both the protein and carbohydrate structures. The particular antibody that, unlike the others, cross-reacts strongly with the intestinal ALPs showed no discrimination among the various allelic types of placental ALP. The absence of any discrimination by this antibody among the various allelic types of placental ALP suggests that if it is indeed directed against a region in the protein moiety of the molecule, then this region is highly conserved among individuals in the species. This would fit with the finding that it also cross-reacts with intestinal ALP, suggesting that the determinant is relatively highly conserved in evolution. However, the results are also consistent with the possibility that the antibody is directed to a determinant in the carbohydrate part of the molecule. If this is so, it would imply that the differences in reactivity between the adult and fetal forms are due to differences in the structures of the carbohydrates. One such difference, namely the presence of sialic acid residues in the fetal but not in the adult form of the enzyme, has been shown *not* to be the main cause of the large difference in reactivity of the two forms with the antibody. More detailed studies on the rest of the carbohydrate moieties and their effects on reactivity are clearly required.

G. Evolutionary Studies

Our earlier studies on the evolution of alkaline phosphatases had been carried out biochemically using criteria such as thermostability, or sensitivity to inhibition with a series of amino acid or peptide inhibitors that sharply distinguish the three main forms of human ALPs (placental, intestinal, and liver/bone/kidney), and with polyclonal antiserum raised against purified human placental ALP (Goldstein and Harris, 1979; Goldstein *et al.,* 1982; Harris, 1982). We found that the ALP expressed in placentas from a series of nonhuman primates and lower mammals was quite different from human placental ALP. Instead, it closely resembled the liver/bone/kidney ALP found in these species and also in humans. The only exceptions were placentas from the Great Apes (chimpanzee and orangutan), where typical human-type placental ALP was found. Thus, expression of the human placental ALP locus in placenta appeared to be a relatively recent event in mammalian evolution, possibly arising from a recent duplication and/or a mutation profoundly altering the regulatory systems that presumably control the expression of these enzymes in different tissues. In surveying an extensive range of tissues from these various species, we did not find an ALP with the characteristic biochemical features of the human placental ALP. However, to our surprise, an unusual ALP closely resembling it was found in substantial amounts in lungs from several Old World monkeys, though not in any other tissue from these or other species. This ALP was very thermostable, like human placental ALP, but it was quite strikingly different in its sensitivity to certain inhibitors, a finding which indicated that the structures of the binding sites for these inhibitors were different. However, quite remarkably, the heat-stable Old World monkey lung ALP cross-reacted with polyclonal antiserum raised in rabbits against purified human placental ALP, giving precipitin lines of apparent identity with human placental ALP in Ouchterlony double-diffusion plates. Thus, despite the biochemical differences, these ALPs are clearly very closely related immunologically to human placental ALP.

It was of obvious interest to see how our panel of 18 monoclonal antibodies reacted with these heat-stable Old World monkey ALPs—whether they all reacted uniformly or whether a distinctive profile of reactivities could be detected. Preliminary studies, using the electrophoretic system described earlier, showed that while most of the antibodies cross-reacted, some failed to show any cross-reaction at all by this method. We then set out to determine quantitatively the degree of cross-reactivity of each monoclonal antibody with each Old World monkey lung ALP relative to its reactivity with human placental ALP.

This was done by a new method in which the monoclonal antibodies were immobilized in wells of microtiter plate, thermostable lung ALPs and also human placental ALPs applied in standard amounts, and finally the amount of ALP bound determined in terms of the enzyme activity of the enzyme–antibody complex. The result in each case was expressed as the activity given by the particular lung ALP divided by the activity with human placental ALP under the same conditions, so-called relative reactivity (RR).

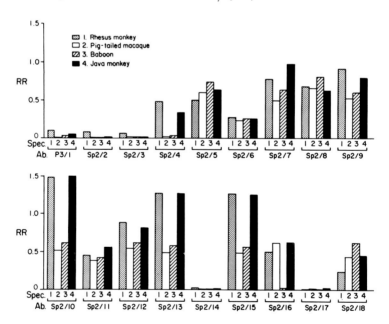

FIGURE 7. Relative reactivity (RR) determinations (see text) of heat-stable (65°C, 1 hr) lung ALPs from four Old World monkeys with 18 different monoclonal antibodies raised against purified human placental ALP.

Figure 7 shows the RR values for each of four Old World monkey lung ALPs with each of the 18 monoclonal antibodies (Rogers and Harris, 1982). A wide range of values is seen. At one extreme there is apparently little or no binding (RR close to zero); at the other extreme the binding appears to be as strong as, and in some cases even stronger than, with human placental ALP. The majority of values are in the intermediate ranges, which suggests that antigenic sites homologous to those to which the various antibodies are directed on human placental ALP also occur on these Old World monkey lung ALPs, but have, in most cases, a somewhat reduced avidity for the antibodies. This is presumably the consequence of amino acid substitutions that have occurred during their divergent evolutions. In general, there is a good correlation of the reactivity values for the various antibodies among the ALPs from the different Old World monkey species. However, in some cases, a particular antibody discriminates quite sharply between the species. This is illustrated in Figure 8, which shows the RR values obtained for the thermostable lung ALPs from baboon and pig-tailed macaque tested against the 18 monoclonal antibodies raised against human placental ALP. The values obtained for the antibodies are highly correlated, but in one case, marked cross-reactivity was found in the pig-tailed macaque ALP but none in the baboon ALP. Other examples of this phenomenon are seen in Figure 7.

The results show that the antigenic determinants to which the 18 monoclonal antibodies raised using human placental ALP as immunogen are, in 13 of the cases, also represented in the Old World monkey thermostable lung ALPs, but the degree to which they are modified, as judged by their relative reactivities with the different antibodies, varies, and in some cases a determinant may be recognized by one of the antibodies in one of the closely related species and not in another. Presumably the differences in reactivity of the different determinants between the human placental ALP and the Old World monkey ALPs are due to amino acid substitutions that have differentiated the different ALPs during the course of evolution, though they may also reflect polymorphism (allelic variation) within certain of the species.

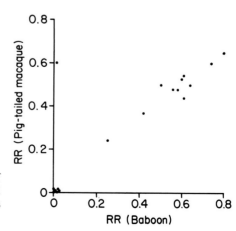

FIGURE 8. Correlation of RR values (see text) of heat-stable lung ALPs from baboon and pig-tailed macaque with 18 different monoclonal antibodies raised against purified human placental ALP.

Much remains to be done, but it is clear that panels of monoclonal anti-bodies of this sort are likely to provide a very powerful tool in evolutionary studies of enzymes. Presumably the antigenic sites that have been most highly conserved will show higher relative reactivities than those that have been less well conserved, so that, in principle, it should become possible, using the various antibodies, to trace the evolution of different antigenic sites on the surface of enzyme molecules.

H. Immunoaffinity Enzyme Purification

In our original studies, the monoclonal antibodies had been raised using a highly purified placental ALP as immunogen. This had been prepared by con-ventional biochemical procedures that involved, after extraction of the enzyme from the tissue, an extensive series of separations involving concanavalin A–Sepharose affinity chromatography, DEAE ion-exchange chromatography, and gel-filtration chromatography (Slaughter *et al.*, 1982). Once monoclonal antibodies had been obtained, we prepared an immunoaffinity column by react-ing mouse ascites fluid containing one of the antibodies with CNBr-activated sepharose 4B, and found that this enabled us to purify the enzyme in a single step starting from crude placental extract. Elution from the column was with 1.0 N NH_4OH, the fractions being neutralized immediately after elution. About 9 mg of purified enzyme was obtained starting from approximately 200 g of placenta. Its specific activity was essentially the same as the original purified preparation and it gave a single protein band on SDS PAGE electrophoresis.

In subsequent work on liver and intestinal ALPs we found that purification by conventional methods was much more difficult than with placental ALP, because the enzymes are much less stable, present in lesser amounts in the tissues, and tend to be contaminated with other tissue proteins that are not easily separated by standard biochemical techniques. Therefore we used only partially purified enzyme preparations as immunogens to produce monoclonal anti-bodies using method c (see Section II) to screen the hybridomas for specific anti-ALP antibodies. These monoclonal antibodies were then used to prepare immu-noaffinity columns from which highly purified preparations of these ALPs were obtained. Figure 9 illustrates a purification of liver ALP on such a column. In this case it was found necessary to partially separate the ALP in the crude liver extract by chromatography on DEAE and concanavalin A–Sepharose prior to applying the enriched but impure preparation to the immunoaffinity column. Elution from the immunoaffinity column was with 3 M NaCl at pH 8.0.

Our own experiences and those reported in the literature by others (see Section II) concerning the use of monoclonal antibody immunoaffinity columns in enzyme purification make it clear that the method is of great value. However, various problems arise in practice and it is worth drawing attention to the chief difficulties. There are three main areas of uncertainty, which require systematic investigation in each case. The first concerns the question as to which of a set of

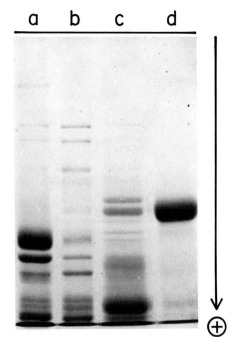

Figure 9. SDS polyacrylamide electrophoresis of proteins showing purification of human liver ALP using a monoclonal antibody immunoaffinity column (Meyer *et al.*, 1982). The proteins were stained with coomassie blue. (a) Crude liver extracts, (b) after elution from DEAE column, (c) after elution from concanavalin-A–Sepharose column, (d) after elution from monoclonal antibody sepharose 4B affinity column.

monoclonal antibodies raised against a given enzyme will give efficient binding to the immunoaffinity column and also efficient release without denaturation when an appropriate eluting reagent is applied. In most cases, efficient binding has been obtained, but satisfactory elution has been unobtainable with some antibodies and erratic with others unless narrowly defined conditions, both in the preparation of the column and in the elution procedures, are adhered to. Our own impression is that the antibody should not have too high an avidity for the enzyme, but the precise factors required are unclear. The second problem is the proportion of antibody to CNBr-activated sepharose to be used in constructing the columns. Our own impression is that too large an amount of antibody results in excessively tight binding of the ALP and consequently failure in elution, whereas too little antibody restricts capacity. The third problem concerns the method of elution. High-pH or low-pH eluants have been successful in different cases, as have high concentrations (e.g., 3–4 M) of salts such as NaCl or KCNS at neutral or near neutral pH. The choice obviously depends on the known properties and characteristics of the particular enzyme, but the appropriate eluant has largely to be determined empirically.

Immunoaffinity columns prepared with monoclonal antibodies represent an important new tool in enzyme purification, particularly for enzymes in which the final stages of purification are difficult by conventional procedures. In effect they provide a new strategy for enzyme purification because highly specific antibodies can be prepared with only partially purified preparations and then used to make affinity columns to obtain the highly purified enzymes.

IV. Concluding Remarks

It will be apparent that monoclonal antibodies represent a powerful new tool in enzyme immunochemistry. They have a great variety of different applications, and in conclusion it is perhaps worth summarizing these briefly. Examples of many of these applications with the relevent literature references have been indicated in Table I.

1. Immunological discrimination of allelic variants of a given enzyme.
2. Immunological characterization and discrimination of the products of different loci in multilocus enzyme systems.
3. Assignment of genes encoding particular enzymes to specific chromosomes or regions of chromosomes in somatic cell hybrid studies.
4. Immunological studies of enzyme evolution on a determinant-by-determinant basis.
5. Purification of enzymes by monoclonal antibody immunoaffinity chromatography.
6. Studies on the tissue or cellular locations of different enzymes by immunocytochemistry.
7. Specific quantitative immunoassay of enzymes in complex mixtures (e.g., crude tissue extracts or serum).
8. Immunological comparisons of similar enzymes present in different forms (e.g., soluble versus particulate), or induced under different conditions.
9. Elucidation of the surface topology of the antigenic determinant sites of a given enzyme and its correlation with its functional characteristics and with its three-dimensional structure.
10. Studies on the carbohydrate moieties of enzyme glycoproteins.

Acknowledgments

The work from the author's laboratory was supported by NIH Grants GM 27018 and GM 20138.

References

Accolla, R. S., Cina, R., Montesoro, E., and Celada, F., 1981, Antibody-mediated activation of genetically defective *Escherichia coli* β-galactosidases by monoclonal antibodies produced by somatic cell hybrids, *Proc. Natl. Acad. Sci. USA* **78:**2478–2482.

Adolf, G. R., Hartter, E., Ruis, H., and Swetly, P., 1980, Monoclonal antibodies to yeast catalase T, *Biochem. Biophys. Res. Commun.* **95:**350–356.

Arklie, J., Trowsdale, J., and Bodmer, W. F., 1981, A monoclonal antibody to intestinal alkaline phosphatase made against D98/Ah-2 (HeLa) cells, *Tissue Antigens* **17:**303–312.

Bailyes, E. M., Newby, A. C., Siddle, K., and Luzio, J. P., 1982, Solubilization and purification of rat liver 5'-nucleotidase by use of a zwitterionic detergent and monoclonal antibody immunoadsorbent, *Biochem. J.* **203:**245–251.

Brandwein, H., Lewicki, J., and Murad, F., 1981, Production and characterization of monoclonal antibodies to soluble rat lung guanylate cyclase, *Proc. Natl. Acad. Sci.* **78:**4241–4245.

Chin, J. J. C., 1982, Monoclonal antibodies that immunoreact with a cation-stimulated plant membrane ATPase, *Biochem. J.* **203:**51–54.

Choo, K. H., Myer, J., Cotton, R. G. H., Camakaris, J., and Danks, D. M., 1980, Isolation of a phenylalanine hydroxylase-stimulating monoclonal antibody by rat-myeloma–rat-spleen-cell fusion, *Biochem. J.* **191:**665–668.

Choo, K. H., Jennings, I. G., and Cotton, R. G. H., 1981, Comparative studies of four monoclonal antibodies to phenylalanine hydroxylase exhibiting different properties with respect to substrate dependence, species-specificity and a range of effects on enzyme activity, *Biochem. J.* **188:**527–535.

Christmann, J. L., and Dahmus, M. E., 1981, Monoclonal antibody specific for calf thymus RNA polymerases II_o and II_a, *J. Biol. Chem.* **256:**11798–11803.

Clark, R. E., Martin, G. G., Barton, M. C., and Shapiro, D. J., 1982, Production and characterization of monoclonal antibodies to rat liver microsomal 3-hydroxy-3-methylglutaryl-coenzyme A reductase, *Proc. Natl. Acad. Sci. USA* **79:**3734–3738.

Cotton, R. G. H., Jennings, I. G., Choo, K. H., and Fowler, K., 1980, Isolation and characterization of a myeloma–spleen-cell hybrid producing antibody to phenylalanine hydroxylase, *Biochem. J.* **191:**777–783.

Crawford, G., Slemmon, J. R., and Salvaterra, P. M., 1982, Monoclonal antibodies selective for *Drosophila melanogaster* choline acetyltransferase, *J. Biol. Chem.* **257:**3853–3856.

Damiani, G., Frascio, M., Benatti, U., Morelli, A., Zocchi, E., Fabbi, M., Bargellesi, A., Pontremoli, S., and DeFlora, A., 1980, Monoclonal antibodies to human erythrocyte glucose 6-phosphate dehydrogenase, *FEBS Lett.* **119:**169–173.

Dao, M. L., Johnson, B. C., and Hartman, P. E., 1982, Preparation of a monoclonal antibody to rat liver glucose-6-phosphate dehydrogenase and the study of its immunoreactivity with native and inactivated enzymes, *Proc. Natl. Acad. Sci. USA* **78:**2840–2844.

Denney, R. M., Fritz, R. R., Patel, N. T., and Abell, C. W., 1982, Human liver MOA-A and MAO-B separated by immunoaffinity chromatography with MAO-B specific monoclonal antibody, *Science* **215:**1400–1403.

Doellgast, G. J., Speigel, J., Guenther, R. A., and Fishman, W. H., 1977, Studies on human placental alkaline phosphatase. Purification by immunoabsorption and comparison of the 'A' and 'B' forms of the enzyme, *Biochim. Biophys. Acta* **484:**59–78.

Fambrough, D. M., Engel, A. G., and Rosenberry, T. L., 1982, Acetylcholinesterase of human erythrocytes and neuromuscular junctions: Homologies revealed by monoclonal antibodies, *Proc. Natl. Acad. Sci. USA* **79:**1078–1082.

Fishman, W. H., 1974, Perspectives on alkaline phosphatase isozymes, *Am. J. Med.* **56:**617–650.

Frackelton, A. R., Jr., and Rotman, B., 1980, Functional diversity of antibodies elicited by bacterial β-D-galactosidase, *J. Biol. Chem.* **255:**5286–5290.

Fujino, T., Park, S. S., West, D., and Gelboin, H. V., 1982, Phenotyping of cytochromes P-450 in human tissues with monoclonal antibodies, *Proc. Natl. Acad. Sci. USA* **79:**3682–3686.

Glode, L. M., Epstein, A., and Smith, S. G., 1981, Reduced γ-cystathionase protein in human malignant leukemia cell lines as measured by immunoassy with monoclonal antibody, *Cancer Res.* **41:**2249–2254.

Gogolin, K. J., Slaughter, C. A., and Harris, H., 1981, Electrophoresis of enzyme monoclonal antibody complexes: Studies of human placental alkaline phosphatase polymorphism, *Proc. Natl. Acad. Sci.* **78:**5061–5065.

Gogolin, K. J., Wray, L. K., Slaughter, C. A., and Harris, H., 1982, A monoclonal antibody that reacts with non-allelic enzyme glycoproteins, *Science* **216:**59–61.

Goldstein, D. J., and Harris, H., 1979, Human placental alkaline phosphatase differs from that of other species, *Nature* **280:**602–605.

Goldstein, D. J., Rogers, C., and Harris, H., 1982, Evolution of alkaline phosphatase in primates, *Proc. Natl. Acad. Sci. USA* **79:**879–883.

Harris, H., 1979, Multilocus enzymes in man, in: *Human Genetics: Possibilities and Realities*, Ciba Foundation Symposium 66, pp. 187–204.

Harris, H., 1982, Multilocus enzyme systems and the evolution of gene expression: The alkaline phosphatases as a model example, in: *The Harvey Lectures,* Volume 76, Academic Press, New York, pp. 95–124.

Harris, H., and Hopkinson, D. A., 1976, *Handbook of Enzyme Electrophoresis in Human Genetics,* North-Holland, Amsterdam.

Harris, H., Hopkinson, D. A., and Robson, E. B., 1974, The incidence of rare alleles determining electrophoretic variants: Data on 43 enzyme loci in man, *Ann. Hum. Genet., Lond.* **37:**237–253.

Herion, P., Glineur, C., Dranssen, J. D., Urbain, J., and Bollen, A., 1981, Monoclonal antibodies against urokinase, *Biosci. Rep.* **1:**885–892.

Hershfield, M. S., and Francke, U., 1982, The human genes for *S*-adenosylhomocysteine hydrolase and adenosine deaminase are syntenic on chromosome **20:** *Science* **216:**739–742.

Hilkens, J., Tager, J. M., Buijs, F., Brower-Kelder, B., van Thienen, G. M., Tegelairs, F. P. W., and Hilgers, J., 1981, Monoclonal antibodies against human acid α-glucosidase, *Biochim. Biophys. Acta* **678:**7–11.

Kaltoft, K., Nielsen, L. S., Zeuthen, J., and Dano, K., 1982, Monoclonal antibody that specifically inhibits a human M_r 52,000 plasminogen-activating enzyme, *Proc. Natl. Acad. Sci. USA* **79:** 3720–3723.

Kohler, G., and Milstein, C., 1975, Continuous cultures of fused cells secreting antibodies of pre-defined specificity, *Nature* **256:**495–497.

Kramer, D., Haars, R., Kabisch, R., Will, H., Bautz, F. A., and Bautz, E. K. F., 1980, Monoclonal antibody directed against RNA polymerase II of drosophila melanogaster, *Molec. Gen. Genet.* **180:**193–199.

Lehmann, F.-G., 1975, Immunological relationship between human placental and intestinal alkaline phosphatase, *Clin. Chim. Acta* **65:**257–269.

Levey, A. I., and Wainer, B. H., 1982, Cross-species and intraspecies reactivities of monoclonal antibodies against choline acetyltransferase, *Brain Res.* **243:**469–473.

Levey, A. I., Aoki, M., Fitch, F. W., and Wainer, B. H., 1981, The production of monoclonal antibodies reactive with bovine choline acetyltransferase, *Brain Res.* **218:**383–387.

Lewicki, J. A., Brandwein, H. J., Waldman, S. A., and Murad, F., 1980, Purified guanylate cyclase: Characterization iodination and preparation of monoclonal antibodies, *J. Cyclic Nucleotide Res.* **6:**283–296.

Liedgens, W., Grutzmann, R., and Schneider, H. A. W., 1980, Highly efficient purification of the labile plant enzyme 5-aminolevulinate dehydratase (EC 4.2.1.24) by means of monoclonal antibodies, *Z. Naturforsch.* **35:**958–962.

Mather, I. H., Nace, C. S., Johnson, V. G., and Goldsby, R. A., 1980, Preparation of monoclonal antibodies to xanthine oxidase and other proteins of bovine milk-fat-globule membrane, *Biochem. J.* **188:**925–928.

McKenna, M. J., Hamilton, T. A., and Sussman, H. H., 1979, Comparison of human alkaline phosphatase isoenzymes. Structural evidence for three protein classes, *Biochem. J.* **181:**67–73.

Millan, J. L., and Stigbrand, T., 1981, "Sandwich" enzyme immunoassay for placental alkaline phosphatase, *Clin. Chem.* **27/12:**2014–2018.

Meyer, L. J., Lafferty, M. A., Raducha, M. G., Foster, C. J., Gogolin, K. J., and Harris, H., 1982, Production of a monoclonal antibody to human liver alkaline phosphatase, *Clin. Chem. Acta* **126:**109–117.

Millan, J. L., Beckman, G., Jeppsson, A., and Stigbrand, T., 1982, Genetic variants of placental alkaline phosphatase as detected by a monoclonal antibody, *Hum. Genet.* **60:**145–149.

Mulivor, R. A., Plotkin, L. I., and Harry Harris, 1978a, Differential inhibition of the products of the human alkaline phosphatase loci, *Ann. Hum. Genet. Lond.* **42:**1–13.

Mulivor, R. A., Hannig, V. L., and Harris, H., 1978b, Developmental change in human intestinal alkaline phosphatase, *Proc. Natl. Acad. Sci. USA* **75:**3909–3912.

Nakane, M., and Deguchi, T., 1982, Monoclonal antibody to soluble guanylate cyclase of rat brain, *FEBS Lett.* **140:**89–92.

Park, S. S., Persson, A. V., Coon, M. J., and Gelboin, H. V., 1980, Monoclonal antibodies to rabbit liver cytochrome P450 LM2, *FEBS Lett.* **116:**231–235.

Park, S. S., Fujino, T., West, D., Guengerich, F. P., and Gelboin, H. V., 1982, Monoclonal antibodies that inhibit enzyme activity of 3-methylcholanthrene-induced cytochrome P-450, *Cancer Res.* **42:**1798–1808.

Robson, E. B., and Harris, H., 1967, Further studies on the genetics of placental alkaline phosphatase, *Ann. Hum. Genet. London* **30:**219–232.

Robson, E. B., and Harris, H., 1965, Genetics of the alkaline phosphatase polymorphism of the human placenta, *Nature* **207:**1257–1259.

Rogers, C. E., and Harris, H., 1982, Differentiation of immunochemically related enzymes in different primate species by monoclonal antibodies, *FEBS Lett.* **146:**93–96.

Ross, M. E., Reis, D. J., and Tong, H. J., 1981, Monoclonal antibodies to tryosine hydroxylase: Production and characterization, *Brain Res.* **208:**493–498.

Seargeant, L. E., and Stinson, R. A., 1979, Evidence that three structural genes code for human alkaline phosphatases, *Nature* **281:**152–154.

Sela, M., 1969, Antigenicity: Some molecular aspects, *Science* **166:**1365–1374.

Siddle, K., Bailyes, E. M., and Luzio, J. P., 1981, A monoclonal antibody inhibiting rat liver 5′-nucleotidase, FEBS Lett. **128:**103–107.

Slaughter, C. A., Coseo, M. C., Abrams, C., Cancro, M. P., and Harris, H., 1980, The use of hybridomas in enzyme genetics, in: *Monoclonal antibodies. Hybridomas: A New Dimension in Biological Analyses* (R. H. Kennett, T. J. McKearne, and K. B. Bechtol, eds.), Plenum Press, New York, pp. 103–120.

Slaughter, C. A., Coseo, M. C., Cancro, M. P., and Harris, H., 1981, Detection of enzyme polymorphism by using monoclonal antibodies, *Proc. Natl. Acad. Sci.* **78:**1124–1128.

Slaughter, C. A., Gogolin, K. J., Coseo, M. C., Meyer, L. J., Lesko, J., and Harris, H., 1983, Discrimination of human placental alkaline phosphatase allelic variants by monoclonal antibodies, *Am. J. Hum. Genet.* **35:**1–20.

Smith-Gill, S. J., Wilson, A. C., Potter, M., Prager, E. M., Feldman, R. J., and Mainhart, C. R., 1982, Mapping the antigenic epitope for a monoclonal antibody against lysozyme, *J. Immunol.* **128:**314–322.

Stahli, C., Staehelin, T., Miggiano, V., Schmidt, J., and Haring, P., 1980, High frequencies of antigen-specific hybridomas: Dependence on immunization parameters and prediction by spleen cell analysis, *J. Immunol. Methods* **32:**297–304.

Vora, S., and Francke, U., 1981, Assignment of the human gene for liver-type 6-phosphofructokinase isozyme (PFKL) to chromosome 21 by using somatic cell hybrids and monoclonal anti-L antibody, *Proc. Natl. Acad. Sci. USA* **78:**3738–3742.

Vora, S., Wims, L. A., Durham, S., and Morrison, S. L., 1981, Production and characterization of monoclonal antibodies to the subunits of human phosphofructokinase: New tools for the immunochemical and genetic analysis of isozymes, *Blood* **58:**823–829.

Vora, S., Durham, S., DeMartinville, B., George, D. L., and Francke, U., 1982, Assignment of the human gene for muscle-type phosphofructokinase (PFKM) to chromosome 1 (region cen Q32) using somatic cell hybrids and monoclonal anti-M antibody, *Somatic Cell Genet.* **8:**95–104.

Wray, L., and Harris, H., 1982, Demonstration using monoclonal antibody of inter-locus heteromeric isozymes of human alkaline phosphatase, *J. Immunol. Methods* **55:**13–18.

4

Monoclonal Antibodies Directed to Cell-Surface Carbohydrates

SEN-ITIROH HAKOMORI

I. Introduction

Cell surface carbohydrates in glycolipids and glycoproteins represent a large variety of antigens (for reviews, see Marcus and Schwarting, 1976; Watkins, 1980; Hakomori, 1981a; Marcus et al., 1981). Typical glycosphingolipid antigens are listed in Table I. Some carbohydrate sequences in glycolipids are also found in the peripheral region of side-chain carbohydrates in glycoproteins (Tonegawa and Hakomori, 1977; Fukuda et al., 1979; Järnefelt et al., 1978), while others are highly characteristic for glycolipids. However, carbohydrate antigens exclusively present in glycoproteins are not known. Furthermore, carbohydrate antigens in glycoproteins are poorly immunogenic. Therefore, only glycolipid antigens and their monoclonal antibodies will be discussed in this chapter. Cell surface glyco-lipids have also been implicated as regulators of cell proliferation, as mediators of cell–cell interactions (for a review, see Hakomori, 1981b), and as receptors for certain bioactive factors (Fishman and Brady, 1976). Therefore, antibodies to glycolipids are also useful in studying the function of glycolipids in membranes.

Antibodies directed to a pure glycolipid (Koscielak et al., 1968; Naiki et al., 1974; Hakomori, 1972; Nagai and Ohsawa, 1974; Laine et al., 1974) or an oligosaccharide–carrier protein complex (Zopf and Ginsburg, 1975; Zopf et al., 1975) have been prepared for studies of carbohydrate distribution in tissues and cells (Marcus and Janis, 1970; Suzuki and Yamakawa, 1981) as well as for studies of changes of carbohydrates associated with the cell cycle (Wolf and Robbins, 1974; Lingwood and Hakomori, 1977), cell contact (Hakomori and Kijimoto,

SEN-ITIROH HAKOMORI • Division of Biochemical Oncology, Fred Hutchinson Cancer Research Center, and University of Washington, Seattle, Washington 98104.

TABLE I
Glycosphingolipid Antigens and Specific Cell Surface Markers[a]

Blood group antigens
ABH; Le[a]; Le[b]; Ii; PP$_1$P[k]
Heterophile antigens
Forssman; Hanganutziu–Deicher (HD)
Lymphoid subpopulation and NK cell markers
Differentiation antigen
Forssman; Ii; F9; TerC; SSEA-1; SSEA-3; SSEA-4
Glycolipids reacting with "autoantibodies" or antiglycolipid
antibodies causing autoimmune diseases
Glycolipid tumor-associated antigens

[a]For the references for each item, see Table IV of the review
by Hakomori (1981b); Marcus and Schwarting (1976).

1972), oncogenic transformation (Hakomori *et al.*, 1968), and their functional modification (Lingwood *et al.*, 1978). Following the introduction of the hybridoma technique for the preparation of monoclonal antibodies by Köhler and Milstein (1975, 1976), various antibodies directed to glycolipids or to the carbohydrates of glycoproteins have been prepared. A relatively small number of monoclonal antibodies have been prepared by immunizing BALB/c mice with a purified glycolipid or a mixture of glycolipids plus carrier macromolecules or particles (Young *et al.*, 1979, 1981; Hakomori *et al.*, 1983a,b; Abe *et al.*, 1984; Fukushi *et al.*, 1984). Immunization with an oligosaccharide–protein complex has been used in recent studies (Mandal and Karush, 1981; Terashima *et al.*, 1982). In addition, a great number of monoclonal antibodies directed to whole cells, including various tumor cells, have been prepared, and many of them have been identified as being directed to glycolipids or to glycoprotein carbohydrates at the cell surface (Solter and Knowles, 1978; Stern *et al.*, 1978; Eisenbarth *et al.*, 1979; Nudelman *et al.*, 1980; Voak *et al.*, 1980; Magnani *et al.*, 1981; Brockhaus *et al.*, 1981 Hakomori *et al.*, 1981; Pukel *et al.*, 1982; Nudelman *et al.*, 1982, 1983; Kannagi *et al.*, 1982b, 1983a).

The occurrence of human plasmacytomas secreting IgM or IgA is well known clinically and is described as Waldenström macroglobulinemia (Bergsagel, 1977). These were the first monoclonal anticarbohydrate antibodies produced by plasmacytomas before the hybridoma technique was introduced. Some of these myeloma proteins react with specific carbohydrate sequences in glycolipids or glycoproteins at the cell surface.

This chapter will review four areas of study on anticarbohydrate monoclonal antibodies: (1) work on naturally occurring myeloma proteins recognizing specific carbohydrate sequences; (2) research on monoclonal antibodies prepared by the hybridoma technique after immunization with glycolipid preparations and oligosaccharide–protein complexes; (3) work on various anticarbohydrate monoclonal antibodies prepared by the hybridoma technique using whole cells as immunogens; and (4) the possible application of these antibodies, and prospects for work in these areas.

II. Naturally Occurring Monoclonal Myeloma Immunoglobulins Directed to Specific Carbohydrate Sequences

A number of patients with Waldenström macroglobulinemia have been characterized as secreting IgM or IgA myeloma proteins that are directed to a specific carbohydrate sequence. Interestingly, these antibodies are directed to glycolipids or glycoproteins of a patient's own erythrocytes and tissues and therefore can be regarded as autoantibodies. Characteristically, the antibody reactivity is obvious at 4°C, but is greatly diminished at room temperature, and is essentially absent at 37°C. They are, therefore, cold-reactive antibodies. The pathogenesis for the occurrence of such anticarbohydrate antibodies is not known. Immunoglobulins can be classified into three types with regard to their specificity: (1) Ii specificities, (2) specificities directed to sialosyl residues, and (3) specificities toward other carbohydrate residues.

A. Monoclonal IgM with Ii Specificities

A large portion of the IgM produced by Waldenström macroglobulinemia patients has been characterized as having a specificity for the I antigen, i.e., (1) they strongly agglutinate adult erythrocytes at low temperature, and (2) they do not agglutinate fetal or umbilical cord erythrocytes or the adult erythrocytes of very rare individuals with blood group i phenotype (the incidence was initially reported to be five out of 22,000). In contrast, some IgM antibodies in patients with Waldenström macroglobulinemia show anti-i specificity, i.e., (1) they strongly agglutinate the rare human erythrocytes of individuals with blood group i phenotype, as well as fetal and umbilical cord erythrocytes of the majority of the human population, which are not agglutinated by anti-I antibodies, and (2) they do not agglutinate erythrocytes of most of the adult population, which are agglutinated by anti-I antibodies (for review, see Race and Sanger, 1975; Prokop and Uhlenbruck, 1965).

The chemical basis of Ii specificity has been studied by Marcus et al. (1963) and Feizi et al. (1971a,b). These studies suggested that the Ii-specific structures are composed of galactose and N-acetylglucosamine, and the I-active structure can be regarded as the precursor of blood group ABH antigens. The extensive studies by Feizi et al. (1971a,b) indicated that some sugar sequences, resulting from the Smith degradation of blood group ABH substances, inhibit various anti-I activities. Best-characterized of these carbohydrate sequences is

Galβ1→4GlcNAcβ1→6Galβ1→R, which reacts specifically with anti-I "Ma" anti-body. The structure represents the branching point of the carrier carbohydrate chain for blood group ABH determinants (Feizi *et al.*, 1971a). However, the structural basis for the specificities of the individual anti-I and anti-i antibodies was not characterized until recently, when Ii-active glycolipid haptens from bovine and human erythrocyte membranes were extensively purified and char-acterized (Watanabe *et al.*, 1975, 1979; Niemann *et al.*, 1978; Feizi *et al.*, 1979). Thus, a large variety of anti-I antibodies have been characterized as being di-rected to various domains within the branched carbohydrate structure called lacto-*N*-*iso*octaosyl, as shown in Table II and Figure 1. Interestingly, some of the monoclonal antibodies recognize the β1→6 linked side chain, others recognize the β1→3 linked side chain, and a few are directed to both the β1→6 linked and β1→3 linked side chains of this structure (Watanabe *et al.*, 1979; Feizi *et al.*, 1979). The specificity of the antibodies and the structures recognized by the antibodies have been reviewed (Hakomori, 1981a; Feizi, 1981).

The specificity of anti-i antibodies has now been characterized as being the unbranched, linear structure composed of repeating *N*-acetyllactosamine units. In contrast to anti-I antibodies, whose specificities can be classified into three categories of branched structures (Table II), many anti-i specificities are indis-tinguishable. Most anti-i activity is (1) within two repeating units of *N*-acetyllac-tosamine, (2) abolished by elimination of the terminal β-Gal residue, (3) lost by hydrazinolysis of the *N*-acetyl group of the GlcNAc residue, and (4) inhibited by fucosyl 1→2 substitution of the terminal Gal, but less inhibited by sialosyl 2→3 substitution (Niemann *et al.*, 1978) (Table III).

TABLE II

Three Classes of I-Active Structures Recognized by Three Classes of Anti-I Monoclonal
Antibodies

1. Anti-I Phi, Da, Sch, Low:
   Galβ1→4GlcNAcβ1
                       ↘
                        $^{6}_{3}$Galβ1→4GlcNAcβ1→3Galβ1→4Glcβ→Cer
                       ↗
   Galβ1→4GlcNAcβ1

2. Anti-I Ma, Woj:
   Galβ1→4GlcNAcβ1
                       ↘
                        $^{6}_{3}$Galβ1→4GlcNAcβ1→3Galβ1→4Glcβ→Cer
                       ↗
   GlcNAcβ1

3. Anti-I Gra, Ver, Ful, Step:
      GlcNAcβ1
                       ↘
                        $^{6}_{3}$Galβ1→4GlcNAcβ1→3Galβ1→4Glcβ→Cer
                       ↗
   Galβ1→4GlcNAcβ1

FIGURE 1. Minimum essential structure for the expression of I and i specificities. Anti-i monoclonal antibodies, such as Den, McD, Tho, and Hog, recognize two repeating *N*-acetyllactosamine structures without branching. Elimination of the terminal Gal and the *N*-acetyl group of GlcNAc results in a complete loss of the activity. In contrast, various anti-I antibodies recognize the branched lacto-*iso*octaosyl structure having 1→3 and 1→6 *N*-acetyllactosamines. Antibodies Phi, Da, Sch, and Low require two terminal residues, whereas antibodies Step and Gra mainly recognize the β1→3 linked *N*-acetyllactosamine residue. In contrast, the antibodies Ma and Woj recognize the β1→6 *N*-acetyllactosamine branch. These results are a summary of Niemann *et al.* (1978), Watanabe *et al.* (1979), and Feizi *et al.* (1979).

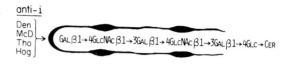

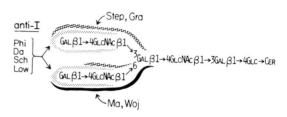

TABLE III

Essential Structure Recognized by Monoclonal Anti-i Antibodies

Essential active structure
  Galβ1→4GlcNAcβ1→3Galβ1→4GlcNAcβ1→3Galβ1→4Glcβ→Cer

Inactive analogues
  GlcNAcβ1→3Galβ1→4GlcNAcβ1→3Galβ1→4Glcβ→Cer
  Galβ1→4GlcNAcβ1→3Galβ1→4Glcβ→Cer
  Galβ1→4GlcNAcβ1→6Galβ1→4GlcNAcβ1→3Galβ1→4Glcβ→Cer

B. *Immunoglobulin Directed to Sialosyl Residues of Glycoproteins or Glycolipids*

In contrast to anti-Ii antibodies, some of the immunoglobulins present in sera of patients with Waldenström macroglobulinemia agglutinate fetal cord and adult erythrocytes equally well, and the agglutination is inactivated by treatment with sialidase as well as various proteases. The specificity of the antibodies is therefore considered to be directed to the sialosyl residues of glycoproteins. The reactive site is called Pr, and the antibody is called anti-Pr, according to the designation of Roelcke (1974) and Roelcke *et al.* (1974). One of the anti-Pr antibodies was identified as IgA(κ) (Roelcke, 1973).

The activity of the human erythrocyte antigen Sa, which reacts with a human monoclonal IgM, was abolished by sialidase treatment, but its reactivity was only partially reduced by protease treatment (Roelcke *et al.*, 1980). A cold

TABLE IV
*Reactivities of Various Monoclonal Antibodies Directed to
Sialosyl Residues of Glycolipids and Glycoproteins[a]*

	Expression on RBC		Effect of enzymes on RBC	
Antigen	Adult	Newborn (fetus)	Proteases	Sialidase
Pr 1,2,3	+	+	↓	↓
Pr a	+	+	↓	−
Sa	+	+	↓	↓
Gd	+	+	−	↓
F1	+	−	−	↓

[a]According to Roelcke (1974). (↓) Decreased or abolished by enzyme treatment; (−) unchanged by enzyme treatment.

agglutinin that recognizes protease-insensitive sialosyl residues was called anti-Gd (Roelcke *et al.*, 1977). The anti-Gd antibodies seem to react with gangliosides having a long carbohydrate chain with a NeuAcα2→3Gal terminus, such as sialosyl-lacto-N-*nor*hexaosylceramide (NeuAcα2→3Galβ1→4GlcNAcβ1→3Galβ1→4GlcNAcβ1→3Galβ1→4Glc→Cer). The antibody did not react with a ganglioside with a NeuAcα2→6Gal residue (Kundu *et al.*, 1982). The anti-Pr and anti-Sa antibodies may recognize any type of sialosyl residue (Table IV), including NeuAcα2→6Gal, NeuAcα2→3Gal, and NeuAcα2→3GalNAc, and NeuAcα2→6GalNAc residue, irrespective of the location and linkage of the residue to protein or glycolipid.

Tsai *et al.* (1977) described an IgM(κ) antibody from a patient with Waldenström macroglobulinemia that can be classified as having anti-Pr$_2$ specificity according to Roelcke's classification (Roelcke, 1974). The antibody showed the ability to bind specifically to N-acetylneuraminosyl residues in glycoproteins and glycolipids. The antibody did not react with glycolipids having N-glycolylneuraminic acid (see Table V). Since IgM itself is a glycoprotein containing sialosyl

TABLE V
Sialosyl Glycolipids That Are Recognized by Monoclonal Antibody MKV[a]

	Minimum concentration in hemagglutination inhibition[b]
NeuAcα2→3Galβ1→4Glc→Cer	0.2
NeuAcα2→3Galβ1→4GlcNAcβ1→Galβ1→4Glc→Cer	0.2
NeuNGcα2→3Galβ1→4Glc→Cer	No reaction (>100)
NeuNGcα2→3Galβ1→4GlcNAcβ1→3Galβ1→4Glc→Cer	No reaction (>100)

[a]According to Tsai *et al.* (1977).
[b]In μg/ml inhibiting hemagglutination caused by MKV monoclonal antibody 1.0 μg/ml.

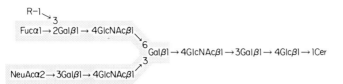

FIGURE 2. The structural domain recognized by the antibody F1. The immunoblastoma antibody F1 recognizes a branched structure that is similar to the structure recognized by anti-I antibodies (see Figure 1 legend). However, the F1 antibody, in contrast to the anti-I antibody, requires two different termini: one, a fucosyl $\alpha 1 \rightarrow 2$ residue, and the other, a sialosyl $\alpha 2 \rightarrow 3$ residue. [Based on Kannagi et al. (1983c).]

residues, the IgM may react not only with the sialosyl residues in glycolipids and glycoproteins at the cell surface, but may also react with its own sialosyl residues. The antibody was characterized as showing a cryoprecipitable property. Apparently, the physical basis for its precipitation in the cold is the intermolecular immune binding of the N-acetylneuraminosyl residue (Tsai et al., 1977).

More recently, Roelcke (1981) described a cold agglutinin, F1, that reacts with adult erythrocyte antigens and is inactivated by sialidase treatment. It resembles anti-I antibodies in reacting more strongly with adult erythrocytes than with umbilical cord erythrocytes; however, unlike I, the F1 antigen is destroyed by sialidase treatment. The antigen is also distinctive from Pr, Gd, and Sa. Differential properties and specificities of antibodies directed to various types of sialosyl residues are summarized in Table IV. A recent study on the specificity of the F1 antibody indicates that it recognizes binary determinants located at the termini of a branched lacto-*iso*octaosyl structure, i.e., the fucosyl residue at the $Gal\beta 1 \rightarrow 4GlcNAc\beta 1 \rightarrow 6$ side chain and the sialosyl residue at the $Gal\beta 1 \rightarrow 4GlcNAc\beta 1 \rightarrow 3$ side chain (Kannagi et al., 1983c) (see Figure 2).

C. Monoclonal IgM Antibody Directed to Globoside and Forssman Antigen

An IgM(κ) antibody directed to globoside and Forssman hapten was reported in one case of macroglobulinemia (McG). The antibody agglutinates sheep erythrocytes and reacts to liposomes containing Forssman glycosphingolipid (Joseph et al., 1974; Alving et al., 1974). It was later found that the antibody also agglutinates human erythrocytes, and the agglutination is strongly inhibited by globoside (Naiki and Marcus, 1977). Thus, the specificity of the IgM is obviously directed to globoside, as well as to Forssman. Interestingly, the antibody does not react to a new glycolipid having the sequence $GalNAc\beta 1 \rightarrow 3Gal\beta 1 \rightarrow 4GlcNAc\beta 1 \rightarrow 3Gal\beta 1 \rightarrow 4Glc \rightarrow Cer$ (Kannagi and Hakomori, unpublished observation). Therefore, the antibody may recognize not only the terminal GalNAc, but also the internal $Gal\alpha 1 \rightarrow 4Gal$ structure in globoside and in Forssman antigen, as shown in Table VI.

TABLE VI

The Structure Recognized by IgM Monoclonal Antibody McG[a]

	Reactivity
GalNAcβ1→3Galα1→4Galβ1→4Glc→Cer $\Big\}$ GalNAcα1→3GalNAcβ1→3Galα1→4Galβ1→4Glc→Cer	+++
GalNAcβ1→4Galβ1→4Glc→Cer $\Big\}$ GalNAcβ1→3Galβ1→4GlcNAcβ1→3Galβ1→4Glc→Cer	−

[a]Joseph *et al.* (1974); Naiki and Marcus (1977).

D. A Monoclonal IgM(λ) Antibody Directed to Type 1 Chain (Lacto-N-Tetraose)

A bronchogenic lung carcinoma case with a gammopathy complication producing an antibody directed to the type 1 chain sugar sequence (Galβ1→3GlcNAcβ1→3Galβ1→R) was reported (Kabat *et al.*, 1982). This antibody, IgM^{Woo}, is an IgM(λ) and does not agglutinate O erythrocytes, unlike cold-reactive anti-Ii antibodies, which are IgM(κ). It is suggested that the antibody, reactive at 37°C, inhibits lung cancer growth, since the type 1 chain sugar sequence may be greatly increased in cancer tissue due to its inability to complete ABH blood group antigen.

III. Monoclonal Anticarbohydrate Antibodies Prepared by Hybridoma Technique

A. Hybridomas Prepared by Immunization with Glycolipids or Carbohydrate–Protein Complexes

Only a few hybridoma cell lines have been established from mice immunized with a purified glycolipid or oligosaccharide–protein complex (Young *et al.*, 1979, 1981; Mandal and Karush, 1981; Terashima *et al.*, 1982; Hakomori *et al.*, 1983a,b; Fukushi *et al.*, 1984; Abe *et al.*, 1984). The antibodies produced by these hybridoma cell lines are directed to ganglio-*N*-triaosylceramide (asialo-GM$_2$), glycolipids having sialosyl 2→6Gal, *N*-acetyllactosaminyl, fucosyl-*N*-acetyllactosaminyl (type 2 chain H or X hapten), di- or trifucosyl type 2 chain (X hapten with internal Fucα1→3GlcNAc), Le^a, type 1 chain A, protein complex with lactosyl, and lacto-*N*-biosyl I (Galβ1→3GlcNAc).

The structures recognized by two monoclonal antibodies directed to ganglio-*N*-triaosylceramide were best characterized by their reactivity with various derivatives of this antigen glycolipid. The IgM antibody produced by hybridoma 2D4 may recognize the primary hydroxyl group (C6) side of the pyranose ring of the terminal GalNAc residue, while the IgG antibody produced by hybridoma D11G10 may recognize the acetamido group (C2) side of the pyranose ring of the GalNAc residue. This assumption is based on the data shown in Table VII (Young *et al.*, 1979). Surprisingly, the IgM antibody (2D4) reacts with the "x_2 glycolipid," which has the GalNAcβ1→3Galβ1→4GlcNAcβ1→3Gal sequence, but it does not react with globoside (see Table VIII). The IgM antibody, therefore, may recognize (1) the C6 side of the GalNAc pyranose ring, (2) the penultimate β-Gal (not α-Gal), and (3) perhaps the internal Glc or GlcNAc configuration as well. The functional group that might be recognized by the IgM as compared to the IgG3 antibody is illustrated in Figure 3.

Many monoclonal antibodies are directed predominantly toward terminal sugar residues, such as the 2D4 antibody mentioned above, and the IB9 antibody directed to NeuAcα2→6Gal (or GalNAc) residue (Hakomori *et al.*, 1983a,b). The IB9 antibody reacts with any type of ganglioside or sialosylglycoprotein having the above structure, but does not react with those having NeuAcα2→3 or 4Gal structure.

Recognition of not only the terminal sugar residue, but also the internal sugar linkage by a monoclonal antibody has been demonstrated by the reactivity of anti-type 2 chain H (produced by clone BE2), anti-*N*-acetyllactosamine (produced by clone 1B2) (Young *et al.*, 1980), and anti-type 1 chain A (produced by clone AH21) (Abe *et al.*, 1984). For example, the BE2 antibody does not react with the sugar sequence Fucα1→2Galβ1→3GalNAc, and reacts weakly with Fucα1→2Galβ1→3GlcNAc, but reacts strongly with Fucα1→2Galβ1→4GlcNAc (for details see Tables VII and IX). Internal recognition of globoside and Forssman antigens by a monoclonal IGM (McG) has been clearly described (see Section IIC). The antibody directed to the embryonic antigen SSEA-3 shows the most typical internal recognition (see Section IIIB1).

Since "hybridomas" are prepared by cell fusion of immune mouse spleen lymphocytes with "HAT-sensitive" NS-1 myeloma cells, the incidence of successful isolation of hybridomas may largely depend on the immune response of mice. Some carbohydrate chains in glycolipids are strongly immunogenic in mice, whereas many others are only weakly immunogenic, or not immunogenic at all. We have tried to obtain monoclonal antibodies by hybridomas directed to GM_1, GM_2, or GM_3 gangliosides, asialo-GM_1 (ganglio-*N*-tetraosylceramide), and globosides, but these efforts have all failed, although a large variety of immunization methods with these glycolipid antigens have been tried. On the other hand, monoclonal antibodies directed to asialo-GM_2 (ganglio-*N*-triaosylceramide), lactoneotetraosylceramide and other lacto-series glycolipids, including blood group ABH, Le^a, Le^b, and X and Y determinants, have been successful, as shown in Table VII. While globoside is hardly immunogenic in mice, a new type of extended globo-series glycolipid (Table X) is highly immunogenic and constitutes SSEA-3 and SSEA-4 (see Section IIIB1). Therefore, the success or

TABLE VII

Specificities and Properties of Monoclonal Antibodies Produced by Hybridoma Prepared following Immunization with Glycolipids or Carbohydrate–Protein Complex

Antibodies	Specificities and properties

1. Anti-GgOs$_3$Cer (ganglio-*N*-triaosyl-ceramide)
(Young *et al.*, 1979)
GalNAcβ1→4Galβ1→4Glc→Cer
   Clone 2D4   IgM(μ + κ)
   Antigen: purified GgOs$_3$Cer adsorbed
   on *Salmonella minnesota*
	Reactivity not influenced by de-*N*-acetylation and re-*N*-acylation of GalNAc residue; reactivity abolished by oxidation of primary OH of GalNAc by galactose oxidase
	→ Recognition of the acetamide group of GalNAc residue

Clone D11G10 IgG3(γ3 + κ) Antigen: the same as above	Reactivity not influenced by oxidation of primary OH of GalNAc by galactose oxidase; reactivity abolished by modification of *N*-acetyl group of GalNAc → Recognition of the acetamide group of GalNAc residue

2. Anti-*N*-acetyllactosaminyl structure
(Young *et al.*, 1981)
Galβ1→4GlcNAcβ1→3Gal→R
   Clone 1B2   IgM
   Prepared by immunization with lacto-*N*-norhexaosylceramide (i-active glycolipid)
	Reacts with *N*-acetyllactosaminyl structure (type 2 chain), i.e., lacto-*N*-neotetraosylceramide (paragloboside) and lacto-*N*-norhexaosylceramide; no reaction with type 1 chain lacto-*N*-tetraosylceramide

3. Anti-type 2 H structure
(Young *et al.*, 1981)
Fucα1→2Galβ1→4GlcNAcβ1→3Gal→R
   Clone BE2   IgM
   Prepared by immunization with total neutral glycolipid of human erythrocytes
	Reacts with glycolipids having type 2 chain H structure (H1, H2, H3); Fucα1→2Galβ1→4GlcNAcβ1→3Gal→R; a weak reaction with type 1 chain H structure (H5); Fucα1→2Galβ1→3GlcNAcβ1→3Gal→R; no reaction with ganglio-series H, Fucα1→2Galβ1→3GalNAcβ1→4Gal→R

4. Anti-Le^a structure
(Young *et al.*, 1983)
Galβ1→3GlcNAcβ1→3Gal→R
       4
       ↑
     Fucα1	

Table VII (*Continued*)

Antibodies	Specificities and properties
4. Anti-Le^a structure (*continued*)	
Clones Ca3-F4 (IgG1), CA4-C4 (IgG2a)	Directed to a complete Le^a structure
Clone BC9-E5 (IgG3), DG4-1 (IgG1) Prepared by immunization with meconium glycolipids	Directed toward Fucα1$\rightarrow$4GlcNAcβ1 residue, i.e., do not require the terminal Galβ1$\rightarrow$3 substitution

5. Anti-type 1 chain A
(Abe *et al.*, 1984)
    Clone AH21 IgM
    Prepared by immunization with a ceramide hexasaccharide having type 1 chain isolated from MKN45 tumor cells
	Does not cross-react with type 2 chain A; does not agglutinate blood group A erythrocytes

6. Anti-type 2 chain A (unpublished observation) Prepared by immunization with a ceramide hexasaccharide having type 2 chain	Does not cross-react with type 1 chain A

7. Antibody to NeuAcα2$\rightarrow$6Gal residue
(Hakomori *et al.*, 1983a,b)
    Clone 1B9
    Prepared by immunization with NeuAcα2$\rightarrow$6Galβ1$\rightarrow$4GlcNAcβ1$\rightarrow$3Galβ1$\rightarrow$4Glc$\rightarrow$Cer
	Cross-reacts with NeuAcα2$\rightarrow$6GalNAc structure, but does not cross-react with NeuAcα2$\rightarrow$3Gal or sialic acid

8. Antibody to V^{3}III^{3}Fuc$_2$nLc$_6$ (difucosylated type 2 chain)
(Fukushi *et al.*, 1984)
    Clones FH4, 5
    Prepared by immunization with V^{3}III^{3}Fuc$_2$nLc$_6$ and selected by this glycolipid
	Does not cross-react with V^{3}FucnLc$_6$ or III^{3}FucnLc$_4$

9. Antilactose (Mandal and Karush, 1981) Galβ1$\rightarrow$4Glc Various clones IgM, IgG	Specificity was not determined, but confirmed the higher affinity in IgG than in IgM
10. Anti-lacto-N-biose I antibodies (Terashima *et al.*, 1982) Galβ1$\rightarrow$3GlcNAc Antigen: *p*-aminophenyl-lacto-N-biose Z coupled to bovine serum albumin	Not reactive with Galβ1$\rightarrow$4GlcNAc

TABLE VIII

The Common Structure Recognized by IgM 2D4 Monoclonal Antibody[a]

	Reactivity
GalNAcβ→4Galβ1→4Glcβ1→1Cer	+++
GalNAcβ1→3Galβ1→4GlcNAcβ1→3Galβ1→4Glcβ1→1Cer	+++
GalNAcβ1→3Galα1→4Galβ1→4Glcβ1→1Cer	−

[a]Young *et al.* (1979); Kannagi and Hakomori (unpublished).

failure of establishing hybridomas to produce monoclonal antibodies reflects the ability of mice to respond to antigenic stimulation. This principle is important for understanding the antigenic analysis of cell surface glycolipids as well.

Certain hybridoma antibodies directed to a defined structure can be selected by the glycolipid with that defined structure. A typical example is the preparation of the FH4 antibody that specifically reacts to a difucosylated type 2 chain ($III^3V^3Fuc_2nLc_6$), but does not react to monofucosylated type 2 chain ($V^3FucnLc_6$, $III^3FucnLc_4$) (Fukushi *et al.*, 1984). Mice were immunized with $III^3V^3Fuc_2nLc_6$, spleen cells were harvested and fused with NS-1 myeloma, and the hybridoma was selected by positive reactivity with $III^3V^3Fuc_2nLc_6$ and negative reactivity with $V^3FucnLc_6$ and $III^3FucnLc_4$. The epitope structures of these antibodies as compared with that of anti-X-hapten antibodies are shown in Figure 4.

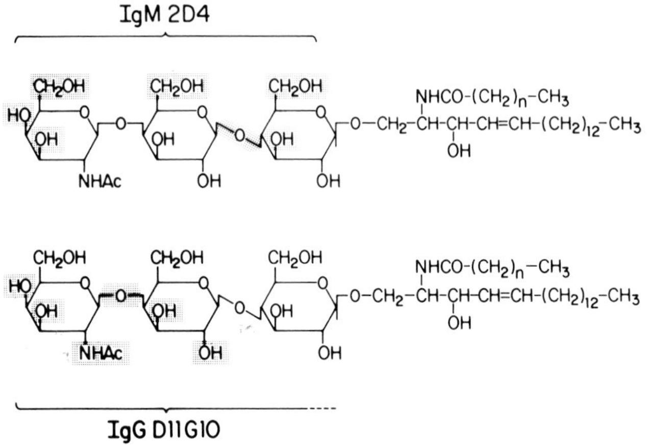

FIGURE 3. Structures recognized by two monoclonal antibodies directed to ganglio-*N*-triaosylceramide (asialo-GM$_2$). Since the IgM 2D4 antibody reacts with de-*N*-acetylated compounds as well as x$_2$ glycolipids (see text), and its reactivity is abolished by oxidation of the primary hydroxyl group, the IgM antibody may recognize the shaded function in the upper structure. In contrast, the reactivity of the IgG3 antibody is abolished by de-*N*-acetylation, but not by oxidation of the primary hydroxyl group. Therefore, the IgG3 antibody may recognize the shaded function in the lower structure.

TABLE IX

Structure Recognized by 1B2 and BE2 Monoclonal Antibodies[a]

	Reactivity
1B2	
Galβ1→4GlcNAcβ1→3Galβ1→4GlcNAcβ1→3Galβ1→4Glcβ1→1Cer	+++
Galβ1→4GlcNAcβ1→3Galβ1→4Glcβ1→1Cer	+++
Galβ1→3GlcNAcβ1→3Galβ1→4Glcβ1→1Cer	−
Galβ1→3GalNAcβ1→4Galβ1→4Glcβ1→1Cer	−
NeuAc2→3Galβ1→4GlcNAcβ1→3Galβ1→4Glcβ1→1Cer	−
Fucα1→2Galβ1→4GlcNAcβ1→3Galβ1→4Glcβ1→1Cer	−
BE2	
Fucα1→2Galβ1→4GlcNAcβ1→3Galβ1→4Glcβ1→1Cer	+++
Fucα1→2Galβ1→4GlcNAcβ1→3Galβ1→4GlcNAcβ1→3Galβ1→4Glcβ1→1Cer	+++
Fucα1→2Galβ1→4GlcNAcβ1 ↘ $^3_6$ Galβ1→4GlcNAcβ1→3Galβ1→4Glcβ1→1Cer Fucα1→2Galβ1→4GlcNAcβ1 ↗	+++
Fucα1→2Galβ1→3GlcNAcβ1→3Galβ1→4Glcβ1→1Cer	−
Fucα1→2Galβ1→3GalNAcβ1→4Galβ1→4Glcβ1→1Cer	−

[a]Young *et al.* (1981).

TABLE X

Specificities and Properties of Monoclonal Anticarbohydrate Antibodies Directed to Specific Types of Cells and Cell Lines

Class of antigen structure series	Cells used as immunogen (host animals)	Specificity defined	Reference	
			Hybridoma established	Structures defined
I. Globo series	Human Burkitt lymphoma (rat)	Globotriaosylceramide (Gb₃) (Table XVII)	Wiels et al. (1981)	Nudelman et al. (1983)
	Mouse spleen (rat)	Forssman Gb₅	Stern et al. (1978)	Stern et al. (1978)
	Influenza virus (human lymphocytes stimulated by influenza virus with NS-1)	Forssman Gb₅ (Table X)	Nowinski et al. (1980)	Nowinski et al. (1980)
	Mouse early embryo (4–8-cell stage) (mouse)	SSEA-3, extended globo series (Table XII)	Shevinsky et al. (1982)	Kannagi et al. (1983a)
	Human teratocarcinoma 2102 (mouse)	SSEA-4, sialosylgalactosyl globoside (Table XII)	Kannagi et al. (1983d)	Kannagi et al. (1983d)
II. Ganglio series	Mouse lymphoma L5178 (mouse)	E(IgM) ganglio-N-triaosyl-ceramide	Urdal et al. (1982)	Urdal et al. (1982)
	Human melanoma (mouse)	GD₃ Ganglioside (Table XIII)	Dippold et al. (1980), Yeh et al. (1982)	Pukel et al. (1982), Nudelman et al. (1982)
	Human peripheral blood B-lymphocytes of melanoma patients transformed by EB virus	GM₂ Ganglioside (oncofetal antigen I-1), GD₂ Ganglioside (oncofetal antigen I-2)	Irie et al. (1982) Irie et al. (1982)	Cahan et al. (1982) Tai et al. (1983)
	Chicken embryo retina cells (mouse)	GQ Ganglioside	Eisenbarth (1979)	Eisenbarth (1979)
III. Lacto series	Mouse teratocarcinoma F9 (mouse syngeneic)	SSEA-1 (as X hapten; Table XI)	Solter and Knowles (1978)	Gooi et al. (1981), Hakomori et al. (1981), Kannagi et al. (1982b)
	Human gastric cancer (mouse), human colonic cancer (mouse)	WGHS 29; ZWG 13, 14, 111 (as X hapten; Table XIX, Fig. 4)	Koprowski et al. (1979)	Brockhaus et al. (1982)

	Human lung cancer cell lines	J525A3, J34F8, J38F12 (as X hapten; Table XIX, Fig. 4)	Cuttitta et al. (1981)	Huang et al. (1983a)
	Human promyelocytic leukemia HL60	My-1 (as X hapten; Table XIX, Fig. 4)	Civin et al. (1981)	Huang et al. (1983b)
	As above	VEP8, VEP9 (as X hapten; Table XIX, Fig. 4)	—	Gooi et al. (1983a)
	As above	IG10 (as X hapten; Table XIX, Fig. 4)	—	Urdal et al. (1983)
	Human colon adenoma (mouse)	Y Hapten (Table XIX)	Brown et al. (1983)	—
	Human lung cancer (mouse)	Y Hapten (Table XIX)	Anger et al. (1982)	Lloyd et al. (1983)
	Human gastric cancer (mouse)	Y Hapten (Table XIX)	—	Abe et al. (1983)
	Human teratoma (primitive endoderm)	Type 1 chain (Galβ1→3GlcNAc)	Williams et al. (1982)	Gooi et al. (1983b)
	Human epidermoid carcinoma A431 cells; the antibody (101) specifically precipitated soluble EGF receptor	Type 1 chain H (Fucα1→2Galβ1→GlcNAc)	Richert et al. (1983)	Fredman et al. (1983)
	Human erythrocytes, human cancer cells	A Determinant	Voak et al. (1980)	Voak et al. (1980)
	Human erythrocytes	B Determinant	Sacks and Lennox (1981)	Sacks and Lennox (1981)
	Human colorectocarcinoma	Le^b Determinant (Table XV)	Koprowski et al. (1979)	Brockhaus et al. (1981)
	Human nonlymphoblastic	Lactosylceramide (Galβ1→4Glc→Cer)	Andrews et al. (1983)	Symington et al. (1984)
	Human colorectocarcinoma	N-19-9 sialosyl Le^a (Table XIV)	Koprowski et al. (1979)	Magnani et al. (1982)
IV. Other carbohydrate antigens	Human desialylated erythrocytes	T Antigen (Galβ1→3GalNAcα1→Cer or Thr)	Rahman and Longenecker (1982)	Rahman and Longenecker (1982)
	Various human malignant cells	Ca-1 Antigen, probably sialosyloligosaccharide	Ashall et al. (1982)	Bramwell et al. (1983)

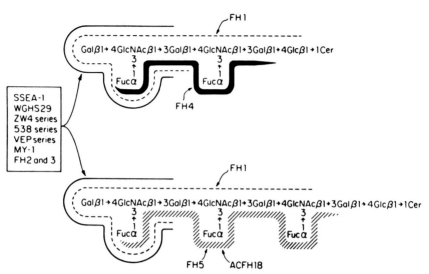

FIGURE 4. Domains recognized by various monoclonal antibodies in fucosylated type 2 chain. The epitope structure of antibodies FH1–5 and ACFH-18 as compared to various other monoclonal antibodies directed to the X determinant is shown. Various monoclonal antibodies, including FH2 and FH3, are directed to the X determinant, in contrast to FH1, which recognizes internal repeating type 2 chain as well. FH4 recognizes two fucosyl residues (shown as a solid zone), and FH5 and ACFH18 recognize three fucosyl residues linked to type 2 chain (shown as a shaded zone).

B. Monoclonal Antibodies Prepared by Immunization with Specific Types of Cells

Immunogenicity of membrane glycolipids and glycoproteins of animal cells has been more clearly demonstrated in recent years through the monoclonal antibody technique than through similar studies in the past. The classic studies of Witebsky (1929) and Hirszfeld et al. (1929) reported the presence of tumor-distinctive lipid antigens that elicited a complement-fixing antibody when rabbits were immunized with tumor tissue homogenates. Rapport and Graf (1961, 1969) identified various glycolipid immunogens demonstrating tissue specificity. Antibody response to the glycolipid fraction of cells or tissues used as immunogens was demonstrated by the complement fixation reaction. The presence of tumor-associated glycolipid antigens has been repeatedly demonstrated on a chemical as well as immunochemical basis (see for review Hakomori and Young, 1978; Hakomori and Kannagi, 1983; Sundsmo and Hakomori 1976; Rosenfelder et al., 1977; Young and Hakomori, 1981). Since the introduction of the monoclonal antibody technique the same approach has been found to be extremely useful for detecting the presence of cell-type-specific glycolipids and glycoproteins, and the approach has been applied to studies in three major areas: (1) analysis of the antigenic composition of the early embryo and teratocarcinoma, (2) analysis of tumor antigens, and (3) analysis of blood group and cell-type-specific antigens.

1. Glycolipid Antigens in Early Mouse Embryo and Teratocarcinoma

Since this area has been well described in the literature, only a few monoclonal antibodies directed to glycolipids will be mentioned. The first monoclonal anticarbohydrate antibody was prepared from hybridomas with rat spleen cells immunized with mouse spleen cells (Stern *et al.*, 1978). The antibody was found to be directed to a Forssman antigen. This monoclonal antibody characteristically reacts with teratocarcinoma stem cells and with early mouse embryo at the morula stage, and is maximally expressed at the early blastocyste stage (Willison and Stern, 1978). The finding was further confirmed by chemical analysis of teratocarcinoma stem cells, which contained ceramide pentasaccharide Forssman antigen and a shorter chain Forssman antigen. In addition, globoside (globotetraosylceramide) and globotriaosylceramide, the precursors of Forssman glycolipids, have also been found in teratocarcinoma and are expressed maximally at the premorula stage (Willison *et al.*, 1982).

A monoclonal antibody directed to the undifferentiated mouse teratocarcinoma F9 was established and called stage-specific embryonic antigen 1 (SSEA-1) (Solter and Knowles, 1978). SSEA-1 is maximally expressed at the morula to early blastocyste stages, particularly at the inner cell mass, but declines at the later stages of the blastocysts. The antigen was identified as a glycolipid having N-acetyllactosaminyl structure and was susceptible to endo-β-galactosidase of *Escherichia freundii* (Nudelman *et al.*, 1980). The antibody also reacted with meconium glycoprotein with Ii activity, but the activity was inhibited by a fucosylated oligosaccharide with the X-hapten sequence, i.e., Galβ1→4[Fucα1→3]Galβ1→R (Gooi *et al.*, 1981). The antigen was subsequently identified as a group of glycolipids with the common X-hapten structure, shown in Table XI (Hakomori *et al.*, 1981; Kannagi *et al.*, 1982b). These glycolipids are widely distributed in various human tissues. Some of them increase greatly in human cancer and have been characterized as having the unusual polyfucosylated structure with the X determinant (see also Table XI; Hakomori *et al.*, 1981). The X structure seems to be strongly immunogenic to mice, and many "tumor-specific" monoclonal antibodies have now been found to be directed to this structure (see next subsection).

Another type of monoclonal antibody prepared by immunization of murine early embryo has been established, called stage-specific embryonic antigen 3 (SSEA-3). It reacts with unfertilized egg and zygote and the two- to four-cell stage embryo, is maximally expressed at the eight-cell stage, and disappears at the morula and blastocyste stages. The antigen reactive to this antibody is also expressed on undifferentiated human teratocarcinoma 2102. The antibody reacts weakly with globoside (GalNAcβ1→3Galα1→4Galβ1→4Glc→Cer) and strongly with a new globo-series glycolipid having Galβ1→3 or NeuAcβ2→3Galβ1→3 substitutions. Therefore, the SSEA-3 antibody recognizes the internal structure of extended globo-series glycolipids. The epitope structure is shown underlined in Table XII. Another established monoclonal antibody prepared by immunizing mice with human teratocarcinoma 2102 was found to be directed to the NeuAcα2→3Galβ1→3-substituted globoside structure and is called SSEA-4 (Table XII).

TABLE XI

Glycolipids Carrying the X Determinant and Internal Fucosyl Residues and Their Reactivity to SSEA-1, FH4, and FH5 Monoclonal Antibodies[a]

Structure	SSEA-1	FH4	FH5	Accumulation in tumor
Galβ1→4GlcNAcβ1→3Galβ1→4Glc→Cer 　　　　3 　　　　↑ 　　　Fucα1	−[b] +[c]	−	−	+++
Galβ1→4GlcNAcβ1→3Galβ1→4Glc→Cer 　　　　3 　　　　↑ 　　　Fucα1	+++	−	±	−
Galβ1→4GlcNAcβ1→3Galβ1→4Glc→Cer 　　　　3　　　　　　　　　　3 　　　　↑　　　　　　　　　　↑ 　　　Fucα1　　　　　　　　Fucα1	+++	+++	+++	+++
Galβ1→4GlcNAcβ1→3Galβ1→4GlcNAcβ1→3 Galβ1→4Glc→Cer 　　　　3 　　　　↑ 　　　Fucα1	+++	+	+	−
Galβ1→4GlcNAcβ1→3Galβ1→4GlcNAcβ1→3Galβ1→4Glc→Cer 　　　　　　　　　　　　3 　　　　　　　　　　　　↑ 　　　　　　　　　　Fucα1	+++	ND	ND	+
Galβ1→4GlcNAcβ1→3Galβ1→4GlcNAcβ1→3Galβ1→4Glc→Cer 　　　　3　　　　　　　　　　　　　3 　　　　↑　　　　　　　　　　　　↑ 　　　Fucα1　　　　　　　　　　Fucα1	+++	+++	+++	+++

[a]From Kannagi et al. (1982b); Hakomori et al. (1982); Fukushi et al. (1984). ND, Not determined.
[b]Low density.
[c]High density.

TABLE XII

Glycolipid Structure Defined by the Monoclonal SSEA-3 and SSEA-4 Antibodies[a]

Structure	SSEA-3	SSEA-4
GalNAcβ1→4Galβ1→4Glc→Cer	−	−
GalNAcβ1→3Galα1→4Galβ1→4Glc→Cer	+	−
Galα1→3GalNAcβ1→3Galα1→4Galβ1→4Glc→Cer	+++	−
NeuAcα2→3Galβ1→3GalNAcβ1→3Galα1→4Galβ1→4Glc→Cer	+++	+++
Fucα1→2Galβ1→3GalNAcβ1→3Galα1→4Galβ1→4Glc→Cer	+	−

[a]Kannagi *et al.* (1983a, 1983d).

2. Monoclonal Antibodies Recognizing Tumor-Associated Glycolipid Antigens

(a) Melanoma Antigen. Two monoclonal antibodies (IgG3 R24; IgM 4.2) specifically directed to human melanoma cells have been independently identified in two different laboratories as being directed to a glycolipid (Dippold *et al.*, 1980; Yeh *et al.*, 1982). The antigen defined by R24 was identified as a ganglioside with the same TLC mobility and carbohydrate composition as GD3 ganglioside (Pukel *et al.*, 1982). The antigen specifically reacting with the 4.2 antibody was characterized by methylation and enzymatic degradation as NeuAcα2→8NeuAcα2→3Galβ1→4Glc→Cer (Table XIII). In contrast to brain GD3, melanoma GD3 contains a much higher proportion of longer chain fatty acids. The 4.2 antibody did not react with various other gangliosides, including GT1a

TABLE XIII

Ganglioside Structure Defined by the Human Melanoma-Specific Monoclonal Antibody 4,2[a]

Structure	Reactivity
NeuAcα2→3Galβ1→4Glc→Cer	−
NeuAcα2→8NeuAcα2→3Galβ1→4Glc→Cer[b]	+++
NeuAcα2→8NeuAcα2→3Galβ1→3GalNAcβ1→4Galβ1→4Glc→Cer 3 ↑ (GT1a) NeuAcα2	−
NeuAcα2→8NeuAcα2→3Galβ1→3GalNAcβ1→4Galβ1→4Glc→Cer 3 ↑ (GQ1b) NeuAcα2 8 ↑ NeuAcαα	−

[a]Yeh *et al.* (1982); Nudelman *et al.* (1982).
[b]Ceramide contains long-chain fatty acids.

and GQ1b, which had the same sugar sequence as GD_3 (NeuAcα2→8NeuAcα2→3Gal) (Nudelman *et al.*, 1982). The GD_3 ganglioside is present in small quantities in brain and in various other tissues and organs (Brunngraber, 1979). A relative abundance of this glycolipid in retina tissue has been described (Holm *et al.*, 1972). Nevertheless, the antibody has been characterized as being highly specific to human melanoma cells and tissues. The reason for the melanoma specificity of GD_3 gangliosides is not known. It could be their high concentration and density at the melanoma cell surface and the specific organization of GD_3 at the melanoma cell surface due to its different ceramide composition, which may enhance the reactivity of GD_3 on the melanoma cell surface. The effect of ceramide structure on the immunogenicity and antigenicity of glycolipids recently has been disclosed (Kannagi *et al.*, 1982a, 1983b).

(b) Glycolipid Antigens of Colorectal Adenocarcinoma. A number of monoclonal antibodies directed to human colorectal adenocarcinoma have been prepared (Koprowski *et al.*, 1979, 1981). One of the antibodies was found to be highly specific for a number of colorectocarcinoma tissues. The binding of the antibody to carcinoma tissue extract was inhibited by serum from patients with adenocarcinoma of the colon, but not by serum from patients with other bowel diseases or from healthy volunteers (Koprowski *et al.*, 1981). The specific antigen defined by this monoclonal antibody was identified as monosialoganglioside (Magnani *et al.*, 1981). The structure was recently identified as a sialosyl-Le[a], the isomer of sialosyl-X (Magnani *et al.*, 1982) (see Table XIV). The glycolipid with sialosyl-X structure was previously isolated and characterized from normal human kidney by Rauvala (1976), but sialosyl-Le[a] must be highly specific for neoplastic tissue.

Four monoclonal antibodies produced by hybridomas obtained from a mouse immunized with human adenocarcinoma cell line SW1116 (Koprowski *et al.*, 1979) have been characterized as being directed to Le[b] antigen (Brockhaus *et al.*, 1981) (see Table XV). The apparent specificity of antibodies for colorectocarcinoma cell lines, as described by Koprowski *et al.* (1979), may be explained by the high levels of Le[a]- and Le[b]-active glycolipids that occur in some adenocarcinomas, regardless of the Lewis blood group status of the donor (Hakomori and Andrews, 1970).

TABLE XIV

Fucoganglioside Structure Defined by the Human Colorectal Adenocarcinoma-Specific Monoclonal Antibody 1116NS-52a[a]

Structure	Reactivity
NeuAc2→3Galβ1→4GlcNAcβ1→3Galβ1→4Glc→Cer 3 ↑ Fucα1	−
NeuAc2→3Galβ1→3GlcNAcβ1→3Galβ1→4Glc→Cer 4 ↑ Fucα1	+++

[a]Magnani *et al.* (1981, 1982).

TABLE XV

Structure of Le^b Glycolipid Defined by Monoclonal Antibody Directed to Human Colorectocarcinoma Cell Lines

Structure	Reactivity
Fucα1→2Galβ1→3GlcNAcβ1→3Galβ1→4Glc→Cer 4 ↑ Fucα1	+++
Fucα1→2Galβ1→3GlcNAcβ1→3Galβ1→4Glc→Cer 3 4 ↑ ↑ GalNAcα1 Fucα1	−

A large increase in gangliosides with the NeuAcα2→6Gal residue in colonic and liver cancer has been observed, and the monoclonal antibody IB9, directed to this structure, has been established (Hakomori *et al.*, 1983b). Two types of gangliosides accumulating in various human cancers detected by this antibody have been isolated and their structures characterized as shown in Table XVI.

(c) Monoclonal Antibodies with Tumor Selectivity Directed to the X-Hapten Structure (Galβ1→4[Fucα1→3]GlcNac). Although the X-hapten structure (or X determinant) is widely distributed in human glandular tissue, and fucosyl α1→3GlcNAc transferase is known to be present in normal serum (Watkins, 1980), many hybridomas producing "tumor-selective" antibodies directed to this structure have been isolated. Three monoclonal antibodies prepared by immunization with small cell lung cancer (NCI-H69) react with three major types of human lung cancer cells (small cell, adenocarcinoma, and squamous carcinoma), but not with a large variety of other human malignant cells, nonmalignant human cell lines, and normal human tissues (Cuttitta *et al.*, 1981). Many of these antibodies have been found to be directed to the X determinant (Huang *et al.*, 1983a). Four hybridomas obtained from mice immunized with human colon or stomach adenocarcinomas produce antibodies directed to the X determinant

TABLE XVI

Two Gangliosides Accumulating in Human Cancer and Defined by the Monoclonal Antibody IB9[a]

Galβ1→4GlcNAcβ1→3Galβ1→4Glc→Cer
6
↑
NeuAcα2

Galβ1→4GlcNAcβ1→3Galβ1→4GlcNAcβ1→3Galβ1→4Glc→Cer
6   3
↑   ↑
NeuAcα2   Fucα1

[a]Hakomori *et al.* (1983b).

TABLE XVII
Glycolipid Structures Defined by Monoclonal Antibody to Daudi
Burkitt Lymphoma[a]

Structure	Reactivity
Galβ1→4Glc→Cer	−
Galα1→4Galβ1→4Glc→Cer	+++
Galα1→3Galβ1→4Glc→Cer	−
GalNAcβ1→3Galα1→4Galβ1→4Glc→Cer	−
GlcNAcβ1→3Galβ1→4Glc→Cer	−
GalNAcβ1→4Galβ1→4Glc→Cer	−

[a]Nudelman *et al.* (1983).

(Brockhaus *et al.*, 1982). The accumulation of a ceramide pentasaccharide with X structure (Yang and Hakomori, 1971) and the presence of a polyfucosylated type 2 chain structure (Hakomori *et al.*, 1981, 1983a) have been observed in various types of human adenocarcinoma (Table XI). These chemical changes of glycolipid pattern may well be correlated with the reactivity of these monoclonal antibodies, and are regarded as the basis for important characteristic membrane changes. Recently, monoclonal antibodies (FH4, FH5, and ACFH18) that preferentially recognize di- and trifucosyl type 2 chain structures have been established (Fukushi *et al.*, 1984). A preferential reactivity of such antibodies with specific types of cells, including cancer cells, is expected.

(d) The Burkitt Lymphoma Glycolipid Antigen. The monoclonal antibody (38.13) defining the antigen specifically expressed on Burkitt tumor cells irrespective of their possessing Epstein–Barr virus (EBV) genome has been established (Wiels *et al.*, 1981). This antigen is not detectable on EBV-positive lymphoblastoid cell lines, normal antigen-activated lymphocytes, or fresh malignant cells from patients affected with a variety of lymphoproliferative disorders (Wiels *et al.*, 1981). Further extensive studies on the distribution of this antigen in a large number of Burkitt lymphoma lines, lymphoblastoid cell lines, and their hybrids indicate that the antigen is expressed in a large variety of B-cell neoplasms (Klein *et al.*, 1983). The antigen has been identified as a simple glycolipid, a ceramide trihexoside, with the structure shown in Table XVII (Nudelman *et al.*, 1983). This glycolipid is a normal tissue component and is widely distributed in a large variety of normal cells and tissues. The reason this type of common structure was recognized as a Burkitt lymphoma-specific antigen is not clear at this time. The phenomenon may well be due to the fact that Burkitt lymphoma cells (Daudi) used as immunogen contained a large quantity of the glycolipid as compared to other, normal tissue. It is known that this glycolipid is cryptic at the erythrocyte surface, although the glycolipid can be detected chemically in significant quantity in normal human erythrocytes (Marcus *et al.*, 1976, 1981). In individuals with a rare genetic trait, blood group P[k], the chemical quantity of this glycolipid is many times higher than in normal erythrocytes. Therefore, P[k] erythrocytes react very well with anti-P[k] antibodies. Norman human erythrocytes, from P$_1$ or P$_2$ populations, do not react with anti-P[k] antibodies, although normal erythrocytes

contain a much lower, but still significant, quantity of ceramide trihexoside (Marcus *et al.*, 1976, 1981). Similarly, a small quantity of ceramide trihexoside in various normal cells may not be recognized by Burkitt lymphoma-specific antibodies.

3. Other Monoclonal Antibodies Reacting with Cell-Type-Specific Glycolipid Antigens

A large number of hybridomas that produce monoclonal antibodies directed to various cell surface components have been isolated. Some of them are directed to specific glycolipid antigens characteristic of the type of cells used for immunization. However, only a relatively small number of these antibodies have been characterized.

(a) Human Monoclonal Antibodies Directed to Forssman Antigen. Nowinski *et al.* (1980) have established a hybridoma cell line, H1-C4, by hybridization of human lymphocytes and mouse myeloma NS-1. The human lymphocytes were obtained from the spleen of a patient at surgery, and the splenic cells were minced, gently suspended in Hank's saline solution, and then, after washing by centrifugation, resuspended in culture medium and stimulated by influenza virus. The *in vitro*-stimulated lymphocytes were then fused with NS-1 cells in 40% polyethylene glycol for 12 min at $250 \times g$. Clones were isolated through antibody-binding assays in microtiter plates. One clone produced a human IgM antibody reacting specifically with influenza virus membrane, as well as with one glycolipid Forssman antigen. No other glycolipids reacted with this antibody (see Table XVIII).

(b) Monoclonal Antibody Directed to Chicken Embryo Retinal Cells. A hybridoma producing an antibody (A2 B5) was established from a fusion of spleen cells of mice immunized with chicken embryo retinal cells with NS-1. The antigen reacting to this antibody was associated with plasma membranes of a neuron cell body and was found to specifically react with the GQ ganglioside fraction of bovine brain. The reactivity with GQ was determined by inhibition of antibody cytotoxicity, rather than direct-binding assay (Eisenbarth *et al.*, 1979). Further verification of the specificity of the antibody may be necessary.

TABLE XVIII

Glycolipid Structure Defined by Human Monoclonal IgM Antibody[a]

Structure	Reactivity
(asialo-GM$_1$) Galβ1→3GalNAcβ1→4Galβ1→4Glc→Cer	−
(globoside) GalNAcβ1→3Galα1→4Galβ1→4Glc→Cer	−
GalNAcα1→3GalNAcβ1→3Galα1→4Galβ1→4Glc→Cer	+++
GlcNAcβ1→3Galβ1→4Glc→Cer	−
GalNAcα1→3Galβ1→4GlcNAcβ1→3Galβ1→4GlcNAcβ1→3Galβ1→4 Glc→Cer	−

$$GalNAc\alpha1→3Gal\beta1→4GlcNAc\beta1→3Gal\beta1→4GlcNAc\beta1→3Gal\beta1→4\ Glc→Cer$$
$$2$$
$$\uparrow$$
$$Fuc\alpha1$$

[a]Nowinski *et al.* (1980).

TABLE XIX

Various Monoclonal Antibodies Directed to Type 1 and Type 2 Chains and Their Fucosylated Derivatives

		Monoclonal antibody	References
Type 1 chain terminus (Le^c)	Galβ1→3GlcNAcβ1→R	FC10,2	Gooi et al. (1983b)
Type 2 chain terminus	Galβ1→4GlcNAcβ1→R	1B2	Young et al. (1981)
Type 1 chain H (Le^d)	Galβ1→3GlcNAcβ1→R 　　　　2 　　　　↑ 　　　Fucα1	101	Fredman et al. (1983)
Type 2 chain H	Galβ1→4GlcNAcβ1→R 　　　　2 　　　　↑ 　　　Fucα1	BE2	Young et al. (1981)
Le^a	Galβ1→3GlcNAcβ1→R 　　　　　　4 　　　　　　↑ 　　　　　Fucα1	CF4-C4; CF4-F4	Young et al. (1983)

	Structure	Antibodies	References
Le^b	Galβ1→4GlcNAcβ1→R 2↑ 3↑ Fucα1 Fucα1	1116NS-10	Brockhaus et al. (1981)
X	Galβ1→4GlcNAcβ1→R 3↑ Fucα1	SSEA-1	Gooi et al. (1981), Hakomori et al. (1981), Kannagi et al. (1982b)
		WGHS29; ZWG13,14,111 J525 series My-1 VEP8,9 1G10	Brockhaus et al. (1982) Huang et al. (1983a) Huang et al. (1983b) Gooi et al. (1983a) Urdal et al. (1983)
Poly X (see Figure 3)	Galβ1→4GlcNAcβ1→3Galβ1→4GlcNAcβ1→3Gal 3↑ 3↑ Fucα1 Fucα1	FH4; FH5	Fukushi et al. (1984)
Y	Galβ→4GlcNAcβ1→R 2↑ 3↑ Fucα1 Fucα1	AH6; C14/1/46/10	Abe et al. (1983), Brown et al. (1983), Lloyd et al. (1983)

(c) Monoclonal Antibodies Blood Group A and B Determinants and Carrier Carbohydrates. As the ultimate reagent for typing blood groups A and B, monoclonal antibodies directed to blood group A erythrocytes have been prepared by the hybridoma technique. The antibody is highly specific to A erythrocytes, although the exact specificity has not been determined (Voak *et al.*, 1980). Similarly, a monoclonal anti-B reagent was isolated (Sacks and Lennox, 1981). More recently, a monoclonal antibody specific to type 1 chain A but which does not cross-react with type 2 chain A was established (Abe *et al.*, 1984). The antibody does not agglutinate A erythrocytes, supporting the notion that the determinants of A erythrocytes are all type 2 chains (see Table X). Many antibodies which show tumor-associated specificity have been characterized as being directed to various fucosylated derivatives of type 1 or type 2 carbohydrate chains. The structures defined by these antibodies are listed in Table XIX.

IV. Applications and Prospects

Monoclonal anticarbohydrate antibodies directed to various cell surface glycolipids and oligosaccharides linked to proteins are extremely useful reagents for (1) qualitative and quantitative analysis of specific carbohydrates at the cell surface, (2) determination of carbohydrate structure in combination with enzymatic degradation, (3) isolation of glycoproteins by affinity chromatography (although this approach has not been successfully applied to glycolipids), (4) modification of cellular function through the use of cell surface carbohydrates, (5) immunological suppression of tumor cells through the use of specific antibodies directed to tumor-associated glycolipids and glycoproteins, (6) targeting and delivery of drugs to specific types of cells by using antibody–drug conjugates, and (7) detection and monitoring of tumor cells through the use of antibody labeled with radioactive tracers.

Anticarbohydrate antibodies have several advantages compared to the plant lectins that have been widely used for probing cell surface carbohydrates (Goldstein and Hayes, 1978). These advantages include better definition of specificity, relative lack of cytotoxicity, and ease of preparing monovalent forms (Fab). Application of monoclonal anticarbohydrate antibodies will supplement, if not replace, the use of various plant lectins in studies of the structure and function of cell surface carbohydrates. Glycolipid antigens at the cell surface, as compared to protein antigens, have not been appreciated or well characterized until recently because of their weak immunogenicity, which makes it difficult to evaluate their function. The immunogenicity of glycolipids at the cell surface has been clearly demonstrated by the monoclonal antibody approach.

Tumor-associated antigens have been identified as glycolipids through the use of monoclonal antibodies, although small quantities of these same glycolipids can be chemically detected in normal tissue as well. An accumulation of a large quantity of a specific glycolipid in some tumors has been observed by chemical analysis (Hakomori and Young, 1978). An important feature exhibited by glycolipid tumor antigens is that each one is shared among a given type of tumor and may not be a "private" tumor antigen. Therefore, a given monoclonal antibody directed to a specific tumor-associated glycolipid will be useful in the diagnosis and treatment of tumors of the same type, such as melanoma, adenocarcinoma of the colon, or lung carcinoma. A number of recent attempts to establish hybridomas producing "tumor-specific" antibodies have been stimulated by the optimistic view that these antibodies will be useful in the diagnosis and treatment of human cancer. In a model experiment, mouse lymphomas (L5178) and mouse sarcoma (KiMSV tumor) were suppressed by IgG3 monoclonal antibody or polyclonal rabbit antibodies. These tumors have a shared antigen whose structure is identical to ganglio-N-triaosylceramide (asialo-GM$_2$). This glycolipid is present in very high quantities in these tumors as compared to normal cells or tissues (Rosenfelder et al., 1977; Young et al., 1981). Two monoclonal antibodies, IgG3 and IgM, directed to this glycolipid have been prepared (Young et al., 1979). The specificity and properties of these antibodies are described in Figure 2 and Tables VII and VIII of this chapter. Growth of the mouse lymphoma L5178Y in DBA-2 mice was suppressed by passive immunization with monoclonal IgG3 antibodies to this glycolipid, but not by IgM antibodies, with or without added complement. The tumor growth was completely suppressed when purified IgG3 antibody was administered in high doses. In contrast, animals developed tumors when they were treated with small doses of IgG3 antibodies. The tumors that appeared in treated animals had a much lower quantity of ganglio-N-triaosylceramide than the original cells used for inoculation, indicating that a passive immunization with IgG3 either prevented growth of lymphoma or caused selection of a variant with a lower quantity of the antigen glycolipid (Young and Hakomori, 1981). These experiments clearly support a certain optimism for this type of approach. On the other hand, the experiments indicate a drawback of this approach in that immunotherapy directed to a glycolipid antigen may modulate the tumor cell surface, resulting in an altered antigen composition. The inability of IgM antibody to suppress tumor growth has also been supported by other experiments (Bernstein et al., 1980).

On the other hand, the old idea of directing drugs specifically to tumor cells to avoid toxic effects on normal tissues has been revived by the availability of monoclonal antibodies. More than 70 years ago, Ehrlich (1910) envisioned "the use of antibodies possessing a particular affinity for a certain organ by which to bring therapeutic active group to the organ." Numerous attempts utilizing this approach have been published in recent years, involving the conjugation of drugs and toxins to monoclonal antibodies. Because of antibody inactivation by drug conjugation, a new targeting system has been developed in which administration of biotinyl antiglycolipid antibodies was followed by the addition of avidin and biotinyl drug (e.g., neocarzinostatin). Successful targeting and killing of tumor cells expressing ganglio-N-triaosylceramide was observed in this system (Urdal and Hakomori, 1980). This system, which was initially developed for *in vitro* work, was recently applied *in vivo* and resulted in a successful suppression of tumor growth (presented at the Abel Symposium for Monoclonal Antibodies; Hakomori et al., 1982). As the method of coupling monovalent or divalent Fab to toxins and drugs continues to progress (Masuho and Hara, 1980; Raso and Griffin, 1980; Gilliland et al., 1980; Raso et al., 1982), the targeting of drugs with antiglycolipid antibodies will become increasingly useful. The drawback of antigen modulation caused by whole antibodies may well be eliminated in this approach.

Microanalysis of glycolipids and glycoproteins will be greatly facilitated by the application of monoclonal antibodies whose specificity to specific carbohydrate sequences and structures is well established, as described in this chapter. The number of established antibodies will increase, and eventually we will have a great number of antibodies with which to define many kinds of carbohydrate structures. Structural analysis of carbohydrate chains by enzymatic degradation, methylation, and mass spectrometry will eventually be supplemented or replaced by analysis of the pattern of reactivity with many sets of monoclonal anticarbohydrate antibodies because this method will be more sensitive and more specific than chemical analysis. The pattern of cell surface carbohydrates can also be determined with increasing accuracy by sets of monoclonal antibodies. This approach and the resulting knowledge will provide an important basis for understanding various aspects of cell biology and immunology.

Notes in proof: (1) The specificity of antibody A2B5 described by Eisenbarth *et al.* (see p. 92, Section B.3.b) was recently characterized to be highly specific to ganglioside GQ_{1c} (Kasai, N., and Yu, R., 1983, *Brain Res.* **277**:155–158) while the antibody also binds to GQ_{1b}, GD_3, and GD_2 and may not be a specific reagent to tetrasialogangliosides (Kundu, S. K., Pleatman, M. A., Redwine, W. A., Boyd, A. E., and Marcus, D. M., 1983, *Biochem. Biophys. Res. Commun.* **116**:836–842). (2) The antigen of human pancreatic adenocarcinoma defined by the monoclonal antibody DU-PAN-2 (Metzgar, R. S., Gaillard, M. T., Levine, S. J., Tuck, F. L., Bossen, E. H., and Borowitz, M. J., 1982, *Cancer Res.* **42**:601–608) was recently identified as a mucine type glycoprotein. The antibody specificity is directed to sialic acid as Ca 1 antibody (Entry IV, Table X, p. 81) (personal communication from Richard S. Metzgar).

ACKNOWLEDGMENT

The author's work described in this chapter has been supported by National Institutes of Health Research Grants GM23100, CA20020, and CA19224.

References

Abe, K., McKibbin, J. M., and Hakomori, S., 1983, The monoclonal antibody directed to difucosylated type 2 chain (Fucα1→2Galβ1→4[Fucα1→3]GlcNAcβ1→R; Y determinant), *J. Biol. Chem.* **258**:11793–11797.

Abe, K., Levery, S. B., and Hakomori, S., 1984, The antibody specific to type 1 chain blood group A determinant, *J. Immunol.*, April 1984 (in press).

Alving, C. R., Joseph, K. C., and Wistar, R., 1974, Influence of membrane composition on the interaction of a human monoclonal "anti-Forssman" immunoglobulin with liposomes, *Biochemistry* **13**:4818–4824.

Andrews, R. G., Torok-Storb, B., and Bernstein, I. D., 1983, Myeloid associated differentiation antigens on stem cells and their progeny identified by monoclonal antibodies, *Blood* **62**:124–132.

Anger, B. R., Lloyd, K. O., Oettgen, H. F., and Old, L. J., 1982, Mouse monoclonal IgM antibody against human lung cancer line SK-LC-3 with specificity for H(O) blood-group antigen, *Hybridoma* **1**:139–147.

Ashall, F., Bramwell, M. E., and Harris, H., 1982, A new marker for human cancer cells. 1. The Ca antigen and the Ca1 antibody, *Lancet* **1982**(July 3):1–6.

Bergsagel, D. E., 1977, Macroglobulinemia, in: *Hematology* (W. S. Williams, E. Beatler, A. J. Erslev, and R. W. Rundles, eds.), McGraw-Hill, New York, pp. 1126–1134.

Bernstein, I., Tam, M., and Nowinski, R. C., 1980, Mouse leukemia: Therapy with monoclonal antibodies against a thymus differentiation antigen, *Science* **207**:68–71.

Bramwell, M. E., Bhavanandan, V. P., Wiseman, G., and Harris, H., 1983, Structure and function of the Ca antigen, *Brit. J. Cancer* **48**:177–183.

Brockhaus, M., Magnani, J. L., Blaszczyk, M., Steplewski, Z., Koprowski, H., Karlsson, K.-A., Larson, G., and Ginsburg, V., 1981, Monoclonal antibodies directed against the human Le^b blood group antigen, *J. Biol. Chem.* **256**:13223–13225.

Brockhaus, M., Magnani, J. L., Herlyn, M., Blaszczyk, M., Steplewski, Z., Koprowski, H., and Ginsburg, V., 1982, Monoclonal antibodies directed against the sugar sequence of lacto-*N*-fucopentaose III are obtained from mice immunized with human tumors, *Arch. Biochem. Biophys.* **217**:647–651.

Brown, A., Feizi, T., Gooi, H. C., Embleton, M. J., Picard, J. K., and Baldwin, R. W., 1983, A monoclonal antibody against human colonic adenocarcinoma recognizes difucosylated type 2 blood group chain, *Biosci. Rep.* **3**:163–170.

Brunngraber, E. G., 1979, *Neurochemistry of Aminosugars,* Thomas, Springfield, Illinois.

Cahan, L. D., Irie, R. I., Singh, R., Cassidenti, A., and Paulsen, J. C., 1982, Identification of human neuroectodermal tumor antigen (IA-I-2) as ganglioside GD₂, *Proc. Natl. Acad. Sci. USA* **79**:7629–7633.

Civin, C. I., Mirro, J., and Banquerigo, M. L., 1981, My-1, A new myeloid-specific antigen identified by a mouse monoclonal antibody, *Blood* **57**:842–845.

Cuttitta, F., Rosen, S., Gazdar, A. F., and Minna, J. D., 1981, Monoclonal antibodies that demonstrate specificity for several types of human lung cancer, *Proc. Natl. Acad. Sci. USA* **78**:4591–4595.

Dippold, W. G., Lloyd, K. O., Li, L. T. C., Ikeda, H., Oettgen, H. F., and Old, L. J., 1980, Cell surface antigens of human malignant melanoma: Definition of six antigenic systems with mouse monoclonal antibodies, *Proc. Natl. Acad. Sci. USA* **77**:6114–6118.

Ehrlich, P., (1910) 1956, A general review of the recent work in immunity, in: *Collected Papers of Paul Ehrlich,* Vol. 2, *Immunology and Cancer Research,* London, Pergamon Press, pp. 442–447.

Eisenbarth, G. S., Walsh, F. S., and Nirenberg, M., 1979, Monoclonal antibody to a plasma membrane antigen of neurons, *Proc. Natl. Acad. Sci. USA* **76**:4913–4917.

Feizi, T., 1981, Blood group Ii system: A carbohydrate antigen system defined by naturally monoclonal or oligoclonal autoantibodies of man, *Immunol. Commun.* **10**:127–156.

Feizi, T., Kabat, E. A., Vicari, G., Anderson, B., and Marsh, W. L., 1971a, Immunochemical studies on blood groups. XLVII. The I antigen complex precursors in A, B, H, Le^a, and Le^b blood group system, *J. Exp. Med.* **133**:39–52.

Feizi, T., Kabat, E. A., Vicari, G., Anderson, B., and Marsh, W. L., 1971b, Immunochemical studies on blood groups. XLIX. The I antigen complex: Specificity differences among anti-I sera revealed by quantitative precipitin studies, *J. Immunol.* **106**:1578–1592.

Feizi, T., Childs, R. A., Watanabe, K., and Hakomori, S., 1979, Three types of blood group I specificity among monoclonal anti-I autoantibodies revealed by analogues of a branched erythrocyte glycolipid, *J. Exp. Med.* **149**:975–980.

Fishman, P. H., and Brady, R. O., 1976, Biosynthesis and function of gangliosides, *Science* **194**:906–915.

Fredman, P., Richer, N. D., Magnani, J. L., Willingham, M. C., Pastan, I., and Ginsburg, V., 1983, A monoclonal antibody that precipitates the glycoprotein receptor for epidermal growth factor is directed against the human blood group H type 1 antigen, *J. Biol. Chem.* **258**:11206–11210.

Fukuda, M. N., Fukuda, M., and Hakomori, S., 1979, Cell surface modification by endo-β-galactosidase. Change of blood group activities and release of oligosaccharides from glycoproteins and sphingoglycolipids of human erythrocytes, *J. Biol. Chem.* **254**:5458–5465.

Fukushi, Y., Hakomori, S., Nudelman, E., and Cochran, N., 1984, Novel fucolipids accumulating in human adenocarcinoma. II. Selective isolation of hybridoma antibodies that differentially recognize mono-, di-, and trifucosylated type 2 chain, *J. Biol. Chem.,* May 1984 (in press).

Gilliland, D. G., Steplewski, Z., Collier, R. J., Mitchell, K. F., Chang, T. H., and Koprowski, H., 1980, Antibody-directed cytotoxic agents: Use of monoclonal antibody to direct the action of toxin A chains to colorectal carcinoma cells, *Proc. Natl. Acad. Sci. USA* **77**:4539–4543.

Goldstein, I. J., and Hayes, C. E., 1978, The lectins: Carbohydrate-binding proteins of plants and animals, *Adv. Carbohydr. Chem. Biochem.* **35**:127–360.

Gooi, H. C., Feizi, T., Kapadia, A., Knowles, B. B., Solter, D., and Evans, J. M., 1981, Stage-specific embryonic antigen involves $\alpha1\rightarrow3$ fucosylated type 2 blood group chains, *Nature* **292**:156–158.

Gooi, H. C., Thorpe, S. J., Hounsell, E. F., Rumpold, H., Kraft, D., Forster, O., and Feizi, T., 1983a, Marker of peripheral blood granulocytes and monocytes of man recognized by two monoclonal antibodies VEP8 and VEP9 involves the trisaccharide 3-fucosyl-N-acetyllactosamine, *Eur. J. Immunol.* **13**:306–312.

Gooi, H. C., Williams, L. K., Uemura, K., Hounsell, E. F., McIlhinney, R. A. J., and Feizi, T., 1983b, A marker of human foetal endoderm defined by a monoclonal antibody involves type 1 blood group chain. *Mol. Immunol.* **20**:607–613.

Hakomori, S., 1972, Preparation of antisera against glycolipids, in: *Methods in Enzymology*, Vol. 28 (V. Ginsburg, ed.), Academic Press, New York, pp. 232–236.

Hakomori, S., 1981a, Blood group ABH and Ii antigens of human erythrocytes: Chemistry, poly-morphism, and their developmental change, *Semin. Hematol.* **18**:39–62.

Hakomori, S., 1981b, Glycosphingolipids in cellular interaction, differentiation, and oncogenesis, *Annu. Rev. Biochem.* **50**:733–764.

Hakomori, S., and Andrews, H. D., 1970, Sphingoglycolipids with Le^b activity and the co-presence of Le^a and Le^b glycolipids in human tumor tissue, *Biochim. Biophys. Acta* **202**:225–228.

Hakomori, S., and Kannagi, R., 1983, Glycosphingolipids as tumor-associated and differentiation markers, *J. Natl. Cancer Inst.* **71**:231–251.

Hakomori, S., and Kijimoto, S., 1972, Forssman reactivity and cell contacts in cultured hamster cells, *Nature* **239**:87–88.

Hakomori, S., and Young, W. W., Jr., 1978, Tumor associated glycolipid antigens and modified blood group antigens, *Scand. J. Immunol.* **7**:7–117.

Hakomori, S., Teather, C., and Andrews, H. D., 1968, Organizational difference of cell surface hematoside in normal and virally transformed cells, *Biochem. Biophys. Res. Commun.* **33**:563–568.

Hakomori, S., Nudelman, E., Levery, S., Solter, D., and Knowles, B. B., 1981, The hapten structure of a developmentally regulated glycolipid antigen (SSEA-1) isolated from human erythrocytes and adenocarcinoma: A preliminary note, *Biochem. Biophys. Res. Commun.* **100**(4):1578–1586.

Hakomori, S., Nudelman, E., Kannagi, R., and Levery, S. B., 1982, The common structure in fucosyllactosaminolipids accumulating in human adenocarcinomas, and its possible absence in normal tissue, *Biochem. Biophys. Res. Commun.* **109**:36–44.

Hakomori, S., Nudelman, E., Levery, S. B., and Patterson, C. M., 1983a, Cancer-associated gang-liosides defined by a monoclonal antibody (IB9) directed to sialosyl$\alpha2\rightarrow6$galactosyl residue: A preliminary note, *Biochem. Biophys. Res. Commun.* **113**:791–798.

Hakomori, S., Patterson, C. M., Nudelman, E., and Sekiguchi, K., 1983b, A monoclonal antibody directed to N-acetyl-neuroaminosyl$\alpha2\rightarrow6$galactosyl residue in gangliosides and glycoproteins, *J. Biol. Chem.* May 1984 (in press).

Hirszfeld, L., Halber, W., and Laskowski, J., 1929, Untersuchungen uber die serologischen Eigenschaften der gewebe. II. Uber serologische Eigenschaften der Neubildungen, *Z. Immu-nitatsforsch.* **64**:81–113.

Holm, M., Månsson, J.-E., Vanier, M.-T., and Svennerholm, L., 1972, Gangliosides of human, bovine, and rabbit retina, *Biochim. Biophys. Acta* **280**:356–364.

Huang, L. C., Brockhaus, M., Magnani, J. L., Cuttitta, F., Rosen, S., Minna, J. D., and Ginsburg, V., 1983a, Many monoclonal antibodies with an apparent specificity for certain lung cancers are directed against a sugar sequence found in lacto-N-fucopentaose III, *Arch. Biochem. Biophys.* **220**:318–320.

Huang, L. C., Civin, C. I., Magnani, J. L., Shaper, J. H., and Ginsburg, V., 1983b, My-1, the human myeloid-specific antigen detected by mouse monoclonal antibodies, is a sugar sequence found in lacto-N-fucopentaose III, *Blood* **61**:1020–1023.

Irie, R. F., Sze, L. L., and Saxton, R. E., 1982, Human antibody to OFA-I, a tumor antigen, produced *in vitro* by Epstein–Barr virus-transformed human β-lymphoid cell lines, *Proc. Natl. Acad. Sci. USA* **79:**5666–5670.

Järnefelt, F., Finne, J., Krusius, T., and Rauvala, H., 1978, Protein-bound oligosaccharides of cell membranes, *Trends Biochem. Sci.* **3:**110–114.

Joseph, K. C., Alving, C. R., and Wistar, R., 1974, Forssman-containing liposomes: Complement-dependent damage due to interaction with a monoclonal IgM, *J. Immunol.* **112:**1949–1951.

Kabat, E. A., Liao, J., Shyong, J., and Osserman, E. F., 1982, A monoclonal IgM macroglobulin with specificity for lacto-*N*-tetraose in a patient with bronchogenic carcinoma, *J. Immunol.* **128:**540–544.

Kannagi, R., Nudelman, E., and Hakomori, S., 1982a, The possible role of ceramide in defining the structure and function of membrane glycolipids, *Proc. Natl. Acad. Sci. USA* **79:**3470–3474.

Kannagi, R., Nudelman, E., Levery, S. B., and Hakomori, S., 1982b, A series of human erythrocyte glycosphingolipids reacting to the monoclonal antibody directed to a developmentally regulated antigen, SSEA-1, *J. Biol. Chem.* **257:**14865–14874.

Kannagi, R., Levery, S. B., Ishigami, F., Hakomori, S., Shevinsky, L. H., Knowles, B. B., and Solter, D., 1983a, New globo-series glycosphingolipids in human teratocarcinoma reactive with the monoclonal antibody directed to a developmentally regulated antigen, SSEA-3, *J. Biol. Chem.* **258:**8934–8942.

Kannagi, R., Stroup, R., Cochran, N. A., Urdal, D. L., Young, W. W., Jr., and Hakomori, S., 1983b, Factors affecting expression of glycolipid tumor antigens: Influence of ceramide composition and coexisting glycolipids on the antigenicity of gangliotriaosylceramide in murine lymphoma cells, *Cancer Res.* **43:**4997–5005.

Kannagi, R., Roelcke, D., Peterson, K. A., Okada, Y., Levery, S. B., and Hakomori, S., 1983c, Characterization of epitope structure in a developmentally regulated glycolipid antigen defined by a cold agglutinin F1: Recognition of α-sialosyl and α-L-fucosyl groups in a branched structure, *Carbohydr. Res.* **120:**143–157.

Kannagi, R., Cochran, N. A., Ishigami, F., Hakomori, S., Andrews, P. W., Knowles, B. B., and Solter, D., 1983d, Monoclonal antibodies defining stage specific embryonic antigens (SSEA-3 and 4) recognize epitopes of a unique globo-series ganglioside isolated from human teratocarcinoma, *EMBO J.* **2:**2355–2361.

Klein, G., Manneborg-Sandlund, A., Ehlin-Henriksson, B., Godal, T., Wiels, J., and Tursz, T., 1983, Expression of the BLA antigen, defined by the monoclonal 38.13 antibody, on Burkitt lymphoma lines, lymphoblastoid cell lines, their hybrids and other B-cell lymphomas and leukemias, *Int. J. Cancer* **31:**535–542.

Köhler, G., and Milstein, C., 1975, Continuous cultures of fused cells secreting antibody of predefined specificity, *Nature* **256:**495–497.

Köhler, G., and Milstein, C., 1976, Derivation of specific antibody-producing tissue culture and tumor lines by cell fusion, *Eur. J. Immunol.* **6:**511.

Koprowski, H., Steplewski, Z., Mitchell, K., Herlyn, M., Herlyn, D., and Fuhrer, P., 1979, Colorectal carcinoma antigens detected by hybridoma antibodies, *Somat. Cell Genet.* **5:**957–972.

Koprowski, H., Herlyn, M., Steplewski, Z., and Sears, H. F., 1981, Specific antigen in serum of patients with colon carcinoma, *Science* **212:**53–54.

Koscielak, J., Hakomori, S., and Jeanloz, R. W., 1968, Glycolipid antigen and its antibody, *Immunochemistry* **5:**441–455.

Kundu, S. K., Roelcke, D., and Marcus, D. M., 1982, Glycosphingolipid receptors for anti-Gd and anti-p cold agglutinin, *Immunol. Lett.* **4:**263–268.

Laine, R. A., Yogeeswaran, G., and Hakomori, S., 1974, Glycosphingolipids covalently linked to agarose gel on glass beads, *J. Biol. Chem.* **249:**4460–4466.

Lingwood, C., and Hakomori, S., 1977, Selective inhibition of cell growth and associated changes in glycolipid metabolism induced by monovalent antibody to glycolipids, *Exp. Cell Res.* **108:**385–391.

Lingwood, C. A., Ng, A., and Hakomori, S., 1978, Monovalent antibodies directed to transformation-sensitive membrane components inhibit the process of oncogenic transformation, *Proc. Natl. Acad. Sci. USA* **75:**6049–6053.

Lloyd, K. O., Larson, G., Strömberg, N., Thurin, J., and Karlsson, K.-A., 1983, Mouse monoclonal antibody F-3 recognized difucosyl type 2 blood group structure, *Immunogenetics* **17**:537–541.

Magnani, J. L., Brockhaus, M., Smith, D. F., Ginsburg, V., Blaszczyk, M., Mitchell, K. F., Steplewski, Z., and Koprowski, H., 1981, A monosialoganglioside is a monoclonal antibody-defined antigen of colon carcinoma, *Science* **212**:55–56.

Magnani, J., Nilsson, B., Brockhaus, M., Zopf, D., Steplewski, Z., Koprowski, H., and Ginsburg, V., 1982, The antigen of a tumor-specific monoclonal antibody is a ganglioside containing sialyated lacto-*N*-fucopentaose II, *Fed. Proc.* **41**:898.

Mandal, C., and Karush, F., 1981, Restrictions in IgM expression. III. Affinity analysis of monoclonal antilactose antibodies, *J. Immunol.* **127**:1240–1244.

Marcus, D. M., and Janis, R., 1970, Localization of glycosphingolipids in human tissues by immunofluorescence, *J. Immunol.* **104**:1530–1539.

Marcus, D. M., and Schwarting, G. A., 1976, Immunochemical properties of glycolipids and phospholipids, *Adv. Immunol.* **23**:203–240.

Marcus, D. M., Kabat, E. A., and Rosenfield, R. E., 1963, The action of enzymes from *Clostridium tertium* on the I antigenic determinant of human erythrocytes, *J. Exp. Med.* **118**:175–194.

Marcus, D. M., Naiki, M., and Kundu, S. K., 1976, Abnormalities in the glycosphingolipid content of human P^k and p erythrocytes, *Proc. Natl. Acad. Sci. USA* **73**:3263–3267.

Marcus, D. M., Kundu, S. K., and Suzuki, A., 1981, The P blood group system: Recent progress in immunochemistry and genetics, *Semin. Hematol.* **18**:63–71.

Masuho, Y., and Hara, T., 1980, Target-cell cytotoxicity of a hybrid of Fab or immunoglobulin and A-chain of ricin, *Gann* **71**:759–765.

Nagai, Y., and Ohsawa, T., 1974, Production of high titer antisera against sialoglycosphingolipids and their characterization using sensitized liposome, *Jpn. J. Exp. Med.* **44**:451–464.

Naiki, M., and Marcus, D. M., 1977, Binding of *N*-acetylgalactosamine-containing compounds by a human IgM paraprotein, *J. Immunol.* **119**:537–539.

Naiki, M., Marcus, D. M., and Ledeen, R. W., 1974, Properties of antisera to ganglioside GM$_1$ and asialo GM$_1$, *J. Immunol.* **113**:84–93.

Niemann, H., Watanabe, K., Hakomori, S., Childs, R. A., and Feizi, T., 1978, Blood group i and I activities of "lacto-*N*-nor-hexaosylceramide" and its analogies: The structural requirements for i-specificities, *Biochem. Biophys. Res. Commun.* **81**:1286–1293.

Nowinski, R., Berglund, C., Lane, J., Lostrom, M., Bernstein, I., Young, W., and Hakomori, S., 1980, Human monoclonal antibody against Forssman antigen, *Science* **210**:537–539.

Nudelman, E., Hakomori, S., Knowles, B. B., Solter, D., Nowinski, R. C., Tam, M. R., and Young, W. W., Jr., 1980, Monoclonal antibody directed to the stage-specific embryonic antigen (SSEA-1) reacts with a branched glycosphingolipid similar in structure to Ii antigen, *Biochem. Biophys. Res. Commun.* **97**:443–451.

Nudelman, E., Hakomori, S., Kannagi, R., Levery, S., Yeh, M.-Y., Hellström, K. E., and Hellström, I., 1982, Characterization of a human melanoma-associated ganglioside antigen defined by a monoclonal antibody, 4.2, *J. Biol. Chem.* **257**:12752–12756.

Nudelman, E., Kannagi, R., Hakomori, S., Parsons, M., Lipinski, M., Wiels, J., Fellous, M., and Tursz, T., 1983, A glycolipid antigen associated with Burkitt lymphoma defined by a monoclonal antibody, *Science* **220**:509–511.

Prokop, O., and Uhlenbruck, G., 1965, *Human Blood and Serum Groups*, McClaren, London, pp. 302–305.

Pukel, C. S., Lloyd, K. O., Trabassos, L. R., Dippold, W. G., Oettgen, H. F., and Old, L. J., 1982, GD$_3$, a prominent ganglioside of human melanoma: Detection and characterization by mouse monoclonal antibody, *J. Exp. Med.* **155**:1133–1147.

Race, R. R., and Sanger, R., 1975, *Blood Groups in Man*, 6th ed., Scientific Publisher, Oxford, pp. 447–458.

Rahman, A. F. B., and Longenecker, B. M., 1982, A monoclonal antibody specific for the Thomsen–Friedenreich cryptic T-antigen, *J. Immunol.* **129**:2021–2024.

Rapport, M. M., and Graf, L., 1961, Cancer antigens: How specific should they be?, *Cancer Res.* **21**:1225–1237.

Rapport, M. M., and Graf, L., 1969, Immunochemical reactions of lipids, *Progr. Allergy* **13:**273–331.

Raso, V., and Griffin, T., 1980, Specific cytotoxicity of a human immunoglobulin-directed Fab–ricin chain conjugate, *J. Immunol.* **125**(6):2610–2616.

Raso, V., Ritz, J., Basala, M., Schlossman, S. F., 1982, Monoclonal antibody–ricin A chain conjugate selectively cytotoxic for cells bearing the common acute lymphoblastic leukemia antigen, *Cancer Res.* **42:**457–464.

Rauvala, H., 1976, Gangliosides of human kidney, *J. Biol. Chem.* **251:**7517–7520.

Richert, N. D., Willingham, M. C., and Pastan, I. H., 1983, Epidermal growth factor receptor: Characterization of a monoclonal antibody specific for the receptor of A431 cells, *J. Biol. Chem.* **258:**8902–8907.

Roelcke, D., 1973, Specificity of IgA cold agglutinins: Anti Pr₁, *Eur. J. Immunol.* **3:**206–212.

Roelcke, D., 1974, Cold agglutination. Antibodies and antigens, *Clin. Immunol. Immunopathol.* **2:**226–280.

Roelcke, D., 1981, A further cold agglutinin, F1, recognizing a N-acetylneuraminic acid-determined antigen, *Vox Sang.* **41:**98–101.

Roelcke, D., Ebert, W., and Anstee, D. J., 1974, Demonstration of low-titer and anti-Pr cold agglutinins, *Vox Sang.* **27:**429–441.

Roelcke, D., Riesen, W., Geisen, H. P., and Ebert, W., 1977, Serological identification of the new cold agglutinin specificity anti-Gd, *Vox Sang.* **33:**304–306.

Roelcke, D., Pruzanski, W., Ebert, W., Romer, W., Fischer, R., Lenhard, V., and Rauterberg, E., 1980, A new human monoclonal cold agglutinin Sa recognizing terminal N-acetylneuraminyl groups on the cell surface, *Blood* **55:**677–681.

Rosenfelder, G., Young, W. W., Jr., and Hakomori, S., 1977, Association of the glycolipid pattern with antigenic alterations in mouse fibroblasts transformed by murine sarcoma virus, *Cancer Res.* **37:**1333–1339.

Sacks, S. H., and Lennox, E. S., 1981, Monoclonal anti-B as a new blood-typing reagent, *Vox Sang.* **40:**99–104.

Shevinsky, L. H., Knowles, B. B., Damjanov, I., and Solter, D., 1982, A stage-specific embryonic antigen (SSEA-3) defined by monoclonal antibody to murine embryos, expressed on mouse embryos and on human teratocarcinoma cells, *Cell* **30:**697–705.

Solter, D., and Knowles, B. B., 1978, Monoclonal antibody defining a stage-specific mouse embryonic antigen (SSEA-1), *Proc. Natl. Acad. Sci. USA* **75:**5565–5569.

Stern, P. L., Willison, K. R., Lennox, E., Galfre, G., Milstein, C., Secher, D., and Ziegler, A., 1978, Monoclonal antibodies as probes for differentiation and tumor-associated antigens: A Forssman specificity on teratocarcinoma stem cells, *Cell* **14:**775–783.

Sundsmo, J., and Hakomori, S., 1976, Lacto-N-neotetraosylceramide ("Paragloboside") as a possible tumor-associated surface antigen of hamster NILpy tumor, *Biochem. Biophys. Res. Commun.* **68:**799–806.

Suzuki, A., and Yamakawa, T., 1981, The different distribution of asialo GM₁ and Forssman antigen in the small intestine of mouse demonstrated by immunofluorescence staining, *J. Biochem.* **90:**1541–1544.

Symington, F. W., Bernstein, I. D., and Hakomori, S., 1984, Monoclonal antibody specific for lactosylceramide (LacCer), *J. Biol. Chem.*, submitted.

Tai, T., Paulson, J. C., Cahan, L. D., and Irie, R. F., 1983, Ganglioside GM₂ as a human tumor antigen (OFA-I-1), *Proc. Natl. Acad. Sci. USA* **80:**5392–5396.

Terashima, M., Kato, K., Osawa, T., Chiba, T., and Tejima, S., 1982, An antibody to lacto-N-biose I, *Carbohydr. Res.* **110:**345–350.

Tonegawa, Y., and Hakomori, S., 1977, "Ganglioprotein and globoprotein": The glycoproteins reacting with anti-ganglioside and anti-globoside antibodies and the ganglioprotein change associated with transformation, *Biochem. Biophys. Res. Commun.* **76:**9–17.

Tsai, C.-M., Zopf, D. A., Yu, R. K., Wistar, R., Jr., and Ginsburg, V., 1977, A Waldenstrom macroglobulin that is both a cold agglutinin and a cryoglobulin because it binds N-acetylneuraminosyl residues, *Proc. Natl. Acad. Sci. USA* **74:**4591–4594.

Urdal, D. L., and Hakomori, S., 1980, Tumor-associated ganglio-N-triaosylceramide, *J. Biol. Chem.* **255:**10509–10516.

Urdal, D. L., Kawase, I., and Henny, C. S., 1982, NK cells target interaction: Approach towards definition of recognition structure, *Cancer Metastasis Rev.* **1**:65–81.

Urdal, D. L., Brentnall, T. A., Bernstein, I. D., and Hakomori, S., 1983, A granulocyte reactive monoclonal antibody, 1G10, identifies X determinant expressed in HL60 cells on both glycolipid and glycoprotein, *Blood* **62**:1022–1026.

Voak, D., Sacks, S., Alderson, T., Takei, F., Lennox, E., Jarvis, J., Milstein, C., and Darnborough, J., 1980, Monoclonal anti-A from a hybrid myeloma: Evaluation as a blood grouping reagent, *Vox. Sang.* **39**:134–140.

Watanabe, K., Laine, R. A., and Hakomori, S., 1975, On neutral fucoglycolipids having long, branched carbohydrate chains: H-active and I-active glycosphingolipids of human erythrocyte membranes, *Biochemistry* **14**:2725–2733.

Watanabe, K., Hakomori, S., Childs, R. A., and Feizi, T., 1979, Characterization of a blood group I-active ganglioside. Structural requirements for I and i specificities, *J. Biol. Chem.* **254**:3221–3228.

Watkins, W. M., 1980, Biochemistry and genetics of the ABO, Lewis, and P blood group systems, in: *Advances in Human Genetics*, Vol. 10 (H. Harris and K. Hirschorn, eds.), Plenum Press, New York, pp. 1–136.

Wiels, J., Fellous, M., and Tursz, T., 1981, Monoclonal antibody against a Burkitt lymphoma-associated antigen, *Proc. Natl. Acad. Sci. USA* **78**:6485–6488.

Williams, L. K., Sullivan, A., McIlhinney, R. A. J., and Neville, A. M., 1982, A monoclonal antibody markers of human primitive endoderm, *Int. J. Cancer* **30**:731–738.

Willison, K. R., and Stern, P. L., 1978, Expression of a Forssman antigenic specificity in the pre-implantation mouse embryo, *Cell* **14**:785–793.

Willison, K. R., Karol, R. A., Suzuki, A., Kundu, S. K., and Marcus, D. M., 1982, Neutral glycolipid antigens as developmental markers of mouse teratocarcinoma and early embryos: An immunological and chemical analysis, *J. Immunol.* **129**:603–609.

Witebsky, E., 1929, Disponibilitat und Spezifitat alkoholloslicher Strukturen von Organen und bosartigen Geschwulsten, *Z. Immunitatsforsch. Exp. Ther.* **62**:35–73.

Wolf, B. A., and Robbins, P. W., 1974, Cell mitotic cycle synthesis of NIL hamster glycolipids including the Forssman antigen, *J. Cell Biol.* **61**:676–687.

Yang, H.-J., and Hakomori, S., 1971, A sphingolipid having a novel type of ceramide and lacto-*N*-pentaose III, *J. Biol. Chem.* **246**:1192–1200.

Yeh, M.-Y., Hellström, I., Abe, K., Hakomori, S., and Hellström, K. E., 1982, A cell-surface antigen which is present in the ganglioside fraction and shared by human melanomas, *Int. J. Cancer* **29**:269–275.

Young, W. W., Jr., and Hakomori, S., 1981, Therapy of mouse lymphoma with monoclonal antibodies to glycolipid: Selection of low antigenic variants *in vivo*, *Science* **211**:487–489.

Young, W. W., Jr., MacDonald, E. M. S., Nowinski, R. C., and Hakomori, S., 1979, Production of monoclonal antibodies specific for distinct portions of the glycolipid asialo GM_2 (gangliotriaosyl-ceramide), *J. Exp. Med.* **150**:1008–1019.

Young, W. W., Jr., Portoukalian, J., and Hakomori, S., 1981, Two monoclonal anticarbohydrate antibodies directed to glycosphingolipids with a lacto-*N*-glycosyl type II chain, *J. Biol. Chem.* **256**:10967–10972.

Young, W. W., Jr., Johnson, H. S., Tamura, Y., Karlsson, K.-A., Larson, G., Parker, J. M. R., Khare, D. P., Sophr, U., Baker, D. A., Hindsgaul, O., and Lemieux, R. U., 1983, Characterization of monoclonal antibodies specific for the Lewis human blood group determinant, *J. Biol. Chem.* **258**:4890–4894.

Zopf, D. A., and Ginsburg, V., 1975, Preparation of precipitating antigens by coupling oligosaccharides to polylysine, *Arch. Biochem. Biophys.* **167**:345–350.

Zopf, D. A., Ginsburg, A., and Ginsburg, V., 1975, Goat antibody directed against a human Le^b blood group hapten, lacto-*N*-difucohexaose I, *J. Immunol.* **115**:1525–1529.

PART III
DETECTION AND ISOLATION OF ANTIGENS IN COMPLEX BIOLOGICAL SYSTEMS

5

Adhesion-Related Integral Membrane Glycoproteins Identified by Monoclonal Antibodies

ALAN F. HORWITZ, KAREN A. KNUDSEN,
CAROLINE H. DAMSKY, CINDI DECKER,
CLAYTON A. BUCK, AND NICOLA T. NEFF

I. Monoclonal Antibodies as Reagents for the Identification and Purification of Adhesion-Related Membrane Molecules

The isolation of integral surface membrane molecules participating in adhesive phenomena is an important but elusive goal of developmental and cell biology. Adhesion-inhibiting polyclonal antibodies were first used by Gerisch (1977) to identify glycoproteins responsible for *Dictyostelium* aggregation. This immunological approach has been used subsequently by several groups for the study of cell–cell and cell–substratum adhesion in mammalian systems. In this paradigm, a broad-spectrum polyclonal antiserum is raised that interferes with the adhesion process. Relevant cell surface molecules are then detected and subsequently purified by monitoring their ability to block antibody-induced alterations in adhesion. This approach has resulted in the identification and isolation of membrane glycoproteins involved in adhesive phenomena in several systems

ALAN F. HORWITZ, CINDI DECKER, AND NICOLA T. NEFF • Department of Biochemistry and Biophysics, University of Pennsylvania School of Medicine, Philadelphia, Pennsylvania 19104.   KAREN A. KNUDSEN, CAROLINE H. DAMSKY, AND CLAYTON A. BUCK • The Wistar Institute of Anatomy and Biology, Philadelphia, Pennsylvania 19104.

(Thiery *et al.*, 1977; Bertolotti *et al.*, 1980; Edelman, 1983; Damsky *et al.*, 1981, 1983; Knudsen *et al.*, 1981; Kemler *et al.*, 1977; Johnson *et al.*, 1979; Ducibella, 1980; Takiechi *et al.*, 1981; Hyafil *et al.*, 1981). Although this approach has been fruitful, it has limitations. First, with a broad-spectrum serum that perturbs adhesion, it is not possible to use affinity chromatography to purify the antigen. Therefore purification schemes must be developed using an antiserum inhibition assay to monitor progress. Second, if more than one polypeptide is present in the purified blocking activity, the relation of each to adhesion must be established. Adhesion-perturbing monoclonal antibodies can circumvent these problems and have rapidly become the reagents of choice for identifying and isolating surface molecules involved in adhesion. One of the most attractive features of this approach is that small amounts of heterogeneous material can be used for immunization. Once hybridomas of interest are identified and their antibodies purified, the relevant antigen can often be purified rapidly by immunoaffinity chromatography. However, some assumptions are implicit in this approach. First, and most important, there must be suitable methods for detecting hybridomas of interest. Second, that portion of the antigen directly involved in the adhesive process, i.e., "the active determinant," must be immunogenic and accessible to added antibody under the conditions of the assay. In addition, the adhesive interaction should be inhibited by a single monoclonal antibody species. Finally, criteria must be available to distinguish between a direct inhibition of adhesion and indirect mechanisms: an extreme example of the latter is cell toxicity.

The use of monoclonal antibodies to study cell adhesion is a recent development. However, papers utilizing them are appearing rapidly. The most thoroughly studied component isolated using a monoclonal antibody is the neural cell adhesion molecule (N-CAM), which is involved in cell–cell interactions manifested in nerve fasiculation and histogenesis in the nervous system. The antigen was first identified and partially purified by its ability to neutralize the effect of a polyclonal adhesion-disrupting antiserum. Hybridomas were produced following immunization with this partially purified material (Hoffman *et al.*, 1982). Twelve hundred clones were tested for N-CAM binding. Nine of them produced antibodies that bound to N-CAM, and of these, six partially inhibited neuronal cell aggregation in a suspension aggregation assay. One of these antibodies appears to be directed against a sialic acid-containing oligosaccharide on N-CAM as judged by the inhibition of antibody binding by neuraminidase and sialic acid. This antibody was used as an immunoaffinity absorbent to prepare a more highly purified N-CAM. Iodinated immunoaffinity-purified N-CAM ran on sodium dodecyl sulfate–polyacrylamide gel electrophoresis (SDS–PAGE) as a continuous broad band in the molecular weight region of 200,000–250,000 daltons. This antigen is unusual in that it is rich in sialic acid, the content of which differs in embryos and adults (Rothbard *et al.*, 1982). The embryonic form has 26–35% carbohydrate, 80% of which is sialic acid. The adult form has roughly one-third the amount of sialic acid of the embryonic form. Neuraminidase treatment removes essentially all of the sialic acid and leaves a 140,000-dalton polypeptide that appears similar in both the embryo and the adult. The transition from the embryonic to the adult form of the antigen appears to be required for normal neurological development (Edelman and Chuong, 1982).

Hyafil *et al.* (1981) have described a monoclonal antibody, DE-1, that reacts with a glycoprotein on the surface of teratocarcinoma cells and early mouse embryos. This antigen, called uvomorulin, is involved in the compaction of eight-cell embryos that precedes blastocyst formation. It was first identified by the ability of its 84,000-dalton tryptic fragment to block the inhibition of compaction caused by a polyclonal antiserum raised against embryonal carcinoma cells. Rats were immunized with this partially purified material and their spleen cells fused with the Y3-Ag1.2.3. myeloma. The hybridoma clones were screened for their ability to immunoprecipitate an iodinated 84,000-dalton tryptic fragment of uvomorulin. This antigen is interesting in that it undergoes a calcium-dependent transition. The presence of calcium renders it refractory to further trypsin degradation and is essential for immunoprecipitation by DE-1. Calcium is also required for maintenance of compaction in the early embryo.

The cell adhesion molecule (L-CAM), first identified in 14-day embryonic chick liver by Bertolotti *et al.* (1980), is also a calcium-dependent cell adhesion molecule (Brackenbury *et al.*, 1981). Recently, Gallin *et al.* (1983) have reported isolation of a monoclonal antibody against chick liver L-CAM which recognizes a 124,000-dalton molecule in whole-cell lysates and an 81,000-dalton fragment generated from liver cell membranes by trypsinization in the presence of calcium. This molecule and uvomorulin appear similar with respect to their sensitivity to trypsin, calcium dependence, and molecular weight of the major trypsin-generated fragments.

Recently, Cohen *et al.* (1983) have described several monoclonal antibodies directed against bovine desmosomal glycoproteins. Of the 12 desmosomal peptides resolved by SDS–PAGE, the monoclonal antibodies reveal three antigenically distinct groups. Immunoelectron microscopy suggests that the proteins occupy the intercellular region of the desmosome and thus may be involved in desmosomal-mediated cell–cell adhesion.

Oesch and Birchmeier (1982) have described a monoclonal antibody (anti-FC-1) that delays the adhesion of trypsinized fibroblasts to tissue culture dishes. Several hybridomas were obtained following an immunization with trypsinized chick embryo fibroblasts. Two out of the 250 clones tested produced this delayed adhesion. When well-spread cultured chick fibroblasts were stained by immunofluorescence, the distribution of the FC-1 antigen was coincident with that of vinculin and with adhesion plaques visualized by interference reflection microscopy. Adhesion plaques are regions of very close (≤ 10 nm) contact between the ventral cell surface and the substratum. Vinculin appears to be involved in the organization of microfilament bundles at their sites of termination at adhesion plaques. Thus the FC-1 antigen is present in sites where it could act to mediate the interaction of the matrix and cytoskeleton-associated components at sites of cell–substratum attachment. The antigen was identified by immunoprecipitation, and it migrates at 60,000 daltons on SDS–PAGE. This same group has identified seven monoclonal antibodies that block adhesion of B 16 mouse melanoma cells to culture dishes (Vollmers and Birchmeier, 1983). The antigens recognized by these antibodies do not appear to be on normal cells, but they do seem to be involved in the metastatic behavior of the B 16 melanoma cells.

The monoclonal antibody CSAT causes myogenic cells to detach from and inhibits their attachment to extracellular matrices. A description of studies with CSAT and a similar monoclonal antibody, JG22 (Greve and Gottlieb, 1982), will be given in detail in the following sections. Accounts of the initial observations on CSAT have appeared elsewhere (Horwitz et al., 1982; Neff et al., 1982).

II. Isolation of CSAT: An Adhesion-Perturbing Monoclonal Antibody

CSAT was obtained from a hybridoma derived from the fusion between mouse plasmacytoma (SP2/0-Ag14) and spleen cells from an immunized 8-week-old male BALB/c mouse (Kohler and Milstein, 1975). Chick embryo myoblast plasma membrane vesicles produced by the method of Scott (1976) were used as the antigen. The vesicles produced by this method are the result of chemically induced blebbing of plasma membrane from tissue culture cells (Scott, 1976). This procedure is simple, rapid, and enriches for antigens present on the cell surface. The mice were immunized by three weekly intraperitoneal injections of vesicles, the first in complete Freund's adjuvant and the second in incomplete Freund's; these were followed by three daily intravenous injections initiated 1 week after the last intraperitoneal injection. The day following the last intravenous injection, the mice were sacrificed and their spleens excised.

This combination of immunization schedule and vesicle membrane preparation produces a large number of hybridomas secreting a broad spectrum of antibodies directed against plasma membrane components (Horwitz et al., 1982). In recent experiments, for example, over 1000 positive clones were obtained per immunization. Several thousand of these clones were screened using an enzyme-linked immunoassay. In screening hybridomas, binding to both myoblasts and fibroblasts was measured. Following normalization of the values to positive and negative control supernatants, the ratio of myoblast to fibroblast binding is then computed. This allows comparison of assays done on different days. We find a broad spectrum of myoblast-to-fibroblast binding ratios. Most antibodies bind equally well to both cell types. Although a small fraction (12%) of antibodies appear directed against antigens enriched on myogenic cells, very few (2%) appear directed toward antigens absolutely specific to these cells. For some fusions, we used myoblast vesicles coated with an antifibroblast antiserum as an immunogen in order to increase the percentage of hybridomas secreting antibodies against antigens enriched on myogenic cells. This procedure succeeded in raising the percentage of such antibodies (28% versus 12%); however, too high a concentration of the coating antiserum suppressed the fraction of positive hybridomas markedly.

CSAT was selected by screening hybridoma supernatants for morphological effects on myogenic cell cultures, i.e., rounding or detachment (Figure 1). In the

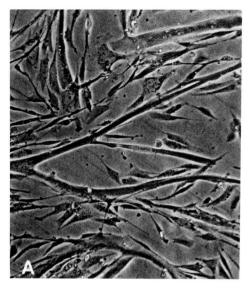
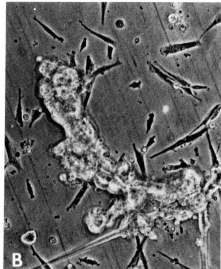

FIGURE 1. Seventy-two hour cultures of chick pectoral muscle grown on gelatin-coated dishes. (A) Control culture displaying myoblasts, fibroblasts, and multinucleate myotubes. (B) Culture treated for 1 hr with 10 μg/ml CSAT at 37°C. Most cells have rounded and detached. Cells remaining on the dish have a fibroblastic morphology and will continue to proliferate.

particular fusion from which CSAT was obtained, it was unique among the 102 clones tested in that it completely detached the myogenic cells. We have subsequently obtained a number of other putative adhesion-modulating antibodies and at present have seven recloned as stable lines. None of them has as marked an effect on myoblast adhesion as that of CSAT.

In a recent publication, Greve and Gottlieb (1982) described two antibodies with effects similar to CSAT. Although the two antibodies affect myoblast adhesion slightly differently, they compete with one another in binding assays and appear directed against a common antigen. We find that CSAT competes with one of these antibodies (JG22) and thus all three appear to be directed against a common antigen, although not necessarily the same determinant.

III. Characterization of the CSAT Antigen

CSAT is an antibody of the IgG2b class and therefore is readily purified by affinity chromatography using protein A–Sepharose. Furthermore, since CSAT has a high affinity for its antigen, immunoaffinity chromatography on CSAT–Sepharose proved very effective in obtaining sufficient purified antigen for biochemical characterization. Fibroblasts rather than myoblasts were chosen as the source of antigen, since very large quantities of metabolically labeled fibroblasts are more readily obtained. Although the CSAT antibody does not round and detach fibroblasts, it does perturb their morphology in a characteristic manner (see below). The antigenic binding site on the two cell types has a comparable affinity for CSAT; the antigen is present on the two cells in similar quantities, and detergent extracts of fibroblasts are able to block the CSAT-induced detachment of myoblasts. Thus the antigens recognized by CSAT on fibroblasts and myoblast are similar if not identical.

To purify the CSAT antigen from NP40 extracts, two differential precipitation steps are employed prior to immunoaffinity chromatography. The [^{35}S]methionine-labeled NP40 extract is first treated with 0.02 M acetic acid, which precipitates about 50% of the protein, leaving the CSAT antigen soluble. The neutralized supernatant from this step is precipitated overnight with a sixfold excess of cold acetone. Resuspension of the precipitate in NP40-containing buffer solubilizes the antigen but leaves about 50% of the protein as an insoluble pellet. The acetone precipitation step not only provides some purification but also permits concentration of the antigen as well as removal or exchange of detergents. The partially purified antigen is then applied to an affinity column, prepared by conjugating the CSAT antibody to cyanogen bromide (CNBr)–Sepharose, and eluted with 0.05 M diethylamine, pH 11.5. Approximately 1% of the [^{35}]methionine counts applied are bound by and eluted from CSAT. Roughly 80% of this affinity-purified material rebinds to immobilized CSAT. Other elution procedures, including low pH (0.2 M acetic acid) or 3 M NaSCN, result in a less efficient rebinding of the eluted antigen to the CSAT–Sepharose. The SDS PAGE profiles of the released antigen, however, are identical for each of the elution methods. The eluted antigen inhibits the CSAT-mediated rounding and detachment of myoblasts, thus confirming the presence of antigen in the affinity-purified eluate.

SDS–PAGE analysis of mercaptoethanol-treated, affinity-purified antigen on a 7% separating gel reveals one to three poorly resolved bands in the molecule weight region of 120,000–160,000 (Neff et al., 1982). On the other hand, unreduced samples display three distinct polypeptides of apparent molecular weights of 160,000 (band 1), 135,000 (band 2), and 110,000 (band 3) (Figure 2). When each band from the nonreduced gel is excised, reduced, and then re-electrophoresed on SDS–PAGE, the 160,000- and 135,000-mol. wt. bands exhibit lower apparent molecular weights of 140,000 and 115,000, respectively, while the 110,000-mol. wt. band migrates in the region of 125,000 (Knudsen et al., 1982). Neither coomassie blue staining nor iodination with ^{125}I reveals any components other than those seen by metabolic labeling with [^{35}S]methionine or [^{14}C]glucosamine. For analytical studies requiring labeled antigen, a typical preparation requires one or two T150 flasks. [^{35}S]Methionine is the label of choice for these studies. When larger quantities of antigen are required, 40 roller bottles of fibroblasts will generate about 300 μg of purified antigen. Recently we have turned to pectoral muscle explants and decapitated, eviscerated 11-day chick embryos as antigen sources. Using ~30 embryos, we obtain at least 500 μg of purified antigen.

The ready availability of pure antigen has allowed us to begin to charac-

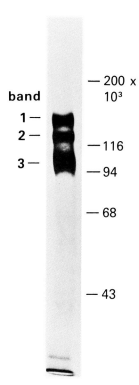

FIGURE 2. Nonreduced SDS–PAGE profile of CSAT affinity-purified antigen. Cells were grown in [^{35}S]methionine, harvested with EDTA, and extracted with 0.5% NP40. The extract was subjected to differential precipitation and applied to immobilized CSAT antibody (see text). Bound material was eluted with diethylamine (pH 11.5), neutralized, and analyzed by SDS–PAGE. The sample was boiled for 2 min in 2% SDS but was not exposed to mercaptoethanol or dithiothreitol prior to running it on a 7% acrylamide gel. Three bands, designated bands 1, 2, and 3, were resolved by this procedure.

terize its structure. Several lines of evidence suggest that the three bands are glycosylated. (1) All three bands are labeled metabolically with [^{14}C]glucosamine. (2) Treatment of purified antigen with mixed glycosidases reduces the apparent molecular weight of all three bands. (3) The purified antigen binds to *Lens culinaris* lectin. Further characterization of the solubilized, affinity-purified antigen shows that it is sensitive to trypsin but is unaltered by chondroitinase *abc*, hyaluronidase, and collagenase. Thus the antigen appears to be a glycoprotein. Since the antigen still binds to CSAT following glycosidase treatment, the antigenic determinant is likely protein rather than carbohydrate in nature. Treatment of fibroblasts with 1 M urea, 3 M KCl, or hypotonic shock prior to solubilization and purification of the antigen does not alter the SDS–PAGE profiles. This points to an integral rather than peripheral membrane association for the three bands. It is not yet clear whether the CSAT antibody recognizes a determinant on each of the bands, whether the antibody recognizes a determinant unique to one of the components and the other two copurify because they are part of an oligomeric complex, or whether the antibody recognizes a unique conformation present in a complex of the three molecules. Our efforts to understand these relationships have been hampered by the fact that CSAT antibody does not bind to any of the bands following SDS–PAGE in the immunoblotting (Western) procedures.

The affinity-purified antigen from fibroblasts was used to prepare a polyclonal antiserum in rabbits. Immunization with approximately 40 µg of protein in each of four injections produced an antiserum that rounds and detaches myoblasts at a dilution of 1 : 20,000. It also rounds fibroblasts, though a dilution of 1 : 40 is required. When protein A-purified antibody from this rabbit serum is immobilized and used to affinity-purify the antigen, all three bands are bound and eluted from the column. However, in the Western immunoblotting procedure, the rabbit antiserum stains only band 3 in NP40 extracts of pectoral muscle explant, chick embryo fibroblasts, and myoblasts. It is possible that antibodies to bands 1 and 2 are present in the serum but that the determinants do not survive the conditions of SDS–PAGE. Alternatively, bands 1 and 2 might not have elicited a sufficient immune response.

IV. *Effect of CSAT on Cell Morphology*

The addition of hybridoma supernatant or purified antibody to cultures derived from avian 10–12-day embryonic pectoral muscle explants (Figure 1) induces a rapid rounding and detachment of the majority of cells. If the rounded cells are washed free of antibody and replated, the resulting cultures are highly enriched in myogenic cells as judged both by the large percentage of multinucleate myotubes and by creatine kinase assays. The cells remaining on the dish after antibody treatment continue to proliferate and appear to be fibroblasts as judged by their morphology and by the above assays. The antibody action on myogenic tissue cultures is paralleled in organ culture; treatment of whole pectoral explants with antibody releases a subpopulation of cells that is not released by nonrelated, control antibodies.

CSAT induces morphological changes in myogenic cultures during their differentiation *in vitro*. In young cultures (24–48 hr), nearly all of the cells are rounded within 15–30 min by a saturating dose of antibody (5 µg/ml). Older cultures (3–11 days), in which extensive fusion has occurred, are also affected by the antibody; however, higher concentrations of antibody and/or longer incubation times are required. Rounding of 4-day cultures requires a 2-hr exposure to 5 µg/ml antibody.Myotubes cultured for 11 days require a 40-fold higher concentration of antibody for detachment. The effects of CSAT on myogenic cells from other species were explored. Quail skeletal muscle cultures are similarly affected; in contrast, CSAT has no effect on cultures of human, mouse, and rat muscle.

The effects of CSAT on myogenic and fibroblastic cells were observed more closely by time-lapse cinematography. When CSAT is applied to 48-hr myoblast cultures growing on collagen in the presence of calcium, myoblasts and small myotubes retract sharply from their ends as they round and detach from the substratum. Larger myotubes first change from a flat ribbonlike to a more tubular morphology. Subsequently, one or both of the ends detach and the

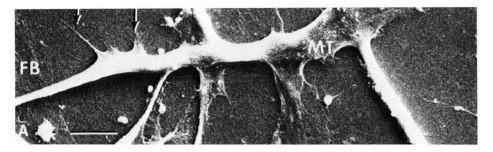

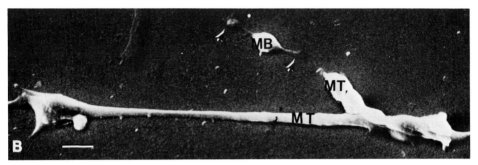

FIGURE 3. Seventy-two hour myoblast culture. (A) Untreated. Myotubes (MT) display lateral lamellae (arrows), which are attached to the substrate, as well as flattened ends (not present in this photograph). The very flat spread cells are fibroblasts (FB). (B) Treated with 20 μg/ml CSAT for 45 min at 37°C. Putative myoblast (MB) and small myotubes (MT) have rounded. The myoblast ends are still attached to the substrate (arrowheads). The large MT appears cylindrical and the lateral lamellae present in (A) have retracted. The myotube ends have become rounded. With further exposure, one or both ends of the large myotube will detach and the myotube will form a ball. Line indicates 10 μm.

myotubes appear to round up. Scanning electron microscopy (SEM) was used in conjunction with the time-lapse studies to obtain higher resolution of these processes. SEM revealed the presence of thin lateral lamellae of cytoplasm in myoblasts and myotubes (Figure 3A). These probably play a role in myoblast adhesion or motility since they, as well as the myotube ends, stain with CSAT antibody and appear dark by interference reflection microscopy. These lamellae retract quickly upon addition of CSAT prior to the detachment of the myotube ends (Figure 3B).

The effects of CSAT on fibroblasts are more subtle. In general these cells do not detach, but time-lapse cinematography using Hoffman contrast modulation optics reveals that increased surface ruffling and a less well-spread morphology are induced by the antibody. The differential effects on myogenic and fibrogenic cells prompted a broader survey of the antibody's effects on other cell types. Thus far, we have studied cardiac cells, skeletal fibroblasts, bromouracil deoxyriboside (BudR)-treated skeletal myoblasts (putative replicating myogenic precursors), mature myotubes, and chondrocytes. The CSAT antigen is present on all of these cells, as determined by immunofluorescent staining. A quantitative analysis of antibody binding reveals that the number of sites per cell and their affinities are similar within a factor of two to four for myoblasts and fibroblasts. Fluorescence staining intensity suggests that the other cell types fall within this range as well. Each cell type appears to respond characteristically to CSAT treatment. The myoblast, which is quickly rounded and detached by the antibody, lies at one extreme. The skeletal fibroblast lies at the other extreme, displaying only a slight ruffling and retraction of edges. Intermediate morphologies are seen when BudR-treated skeletal myoblasts and cardiac myoblasts are exposed to CSAT. The latter stand out strikingly in Hoffman modulation contrast optics as less well-spread islands of synchronously contracting cardiac myocytes surrounded by the flatter fibroblasts.

V. Effects of Cytochalasin B and Calcium on the Action of CSAT

The different responses of various cell types were explored further by exposing cells to CSAT along with other agents or culture conditions known to affect adhesion and morphology (Decker and Horwitz, 1982). Cytochalasin B (CB) affects cellular morphology presumably via its direct interaction with microfilaments. The action of CB appears to complement that of CSAT; i.e., when added together they produce an enhanced effect. Under our assay conditions, the antibody alone rounds and detaches myoblasts. Both CSAT and CB are required to round myoblasts exposed to BudR for 72–96 hr. Neither reagent is able to do so by itself. Fibroblasts, which are arborized in the presence of CB, undergo a further retraction of the lamellae that lie between the CB-resistant attachment sites when CSAT is also present. However, these cells are not detached.

Both calcium levels in the growth medium and time in culture also appear to modulate the effect of CSAT antibody on cells. In low-calcium medium (0.4 mM), myoblasts and BudR-treated myoblasts that have been in culture for up to 96 hr are rapidly detached. At higher calcium concentrations (approximately 2 mM), increased antibody concentrations and longer incubation with the antibody are required to round and detach myotubes. In the presence of 2 mM calcium, myoblasts grown in BudR for 72 to 96 hr are no longer rounded by CSAT alone, but do display a less well-spread morphology. If CB is also included, these cells will round and detach.

VI. Effect of CSAT on Matrix Adhesion

These morphological observations are paralleled in quantitative estimates of cell–matrix adhesion in the presence of CSAT antibody. In one assay, the cells are plated onto gelatin-coated tissue culture dishes and the number of adherent cells scored after 2–24 hr. The attachment of myoblasts is inhibited by CSAT, whereas that of the skeletal fibroblast is not. Another assay estimates the relative adhesive strength subsequent to antibody treatment of older cultures. In this assay, 24- to 72-hr cultures are treated with CSAT antibody and the weakly adherent cells removed by pipetting. In myoblast cultures, the majority of cells are removed, while fibroblast cultures resemble the untreated controls. In BudR–myoblast cultures treated with CSAT, an intermediate fraction of the cells remains. Thus the morphological observations of adhesion in the presence of antibody are paralleled by this latter assay. Assays such as the one developed by McClay *et al.* (1980), which can discriminate between initial attachment to a specific ligand and later events, such as spreading and migration, can also be very useful. Through the use of such an assay, it has been found that CSAT inhibits the initial attachment of myoblasts either to fibronectin-coated culture dishes in serum-free medium or to collagen-coated dishes in fibroblast-conditioned medium. This suggests that the CSAT antigen is involved in an early event in myoblast adhesion.

In contrast to its effects on cell–matrix interactions, CSAT has no detectable effect on two intimate cell–cell interactions, i.e., myoblast fusion and synchronous contraction of cardiac cells. Myoblast fusion, a key event in the production of skeletal muscle fibers, is a complex phenomenon (Horwitz *et al.*, 1982). It is initiated by a specific adhesive interaction that leads ultimately to membrane continuity. Using the most sensitive assay of fusion described thus far, we were unable to detect any effect of CSAT on this process (Neff *et al.*, 1982). Cardiac myoblasts interact via intercalated discs and gap junctions to form spontaneous, synchronously beating collections of cells. The presence of antibody has no detectable effect on the spontaneous, synchronous beating of these cells, showing that these interactions are also not detectably perturbed.

VII. Localization of CSAT Antigen

Some clues to the function of the CSAT antigen can be obtained from determining its localization on the cell surface using immunofluorescence. The primary question is whether the location of this antigen coincides with sites of cell–substrate adhesion as identified either by morphological criteria (i.e., interference reflection microscopy or electron microscopy) or by co-localization with other putative adhesion-related molecules. Although the adhesion of most cell types to extracellular matrix has not been well studied, the *in vitro* adhesion of fibroblasts has received intense investigation over the past few years. The emerging picture is that adhesion sites consist of highly organized supramolecular assemblies of at least two morphologically distinguishable types. Microfilament bundles or stress fibers, along with their associated proteins α-actinin and vinculin as well as the *src* gene product (Rorschneider *et al.*, 1981), are enriched at the cytosolic side of the membrane, whereas matrix molecules such as fibronectin occupy the extracellular aspect of these complexes (reviewed by Hynes, 1981; Geiger, 1981; Chen and Singer, 1982). Presumably, the adhesion of myogenic

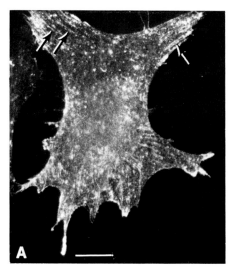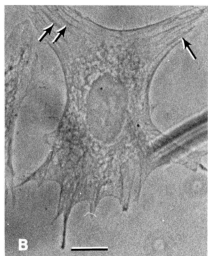

FIGURE 4. Distribution of CSAT antigen on chick embryo fibroblasts. Fibroblast incubated with 20 μg/ml CSAT in serum-free medium for 20 min at room temperature. Following fixation with 3% paraformaldehyde and permeabilization with acetone at −20°C, cells were stained with rhodamine-conjugated goat anti-mouse IgG (Cappel) for 1 hr at a dilution of 1:64. (A) Fluorescence pattern indicating the distribution of CSAT antigen. Staining is enriched at the cell periphery and at portions of stress fibers (arrows) visible by phase microscopy (B). Line indicates 10 μm.

and other cell types has some features in common with the adhesion of fibroblasts, although these systems have been less well studied.

CSAT is localized primarily at the periphery of myoblasts and myotubes. It is not restricted to the ends of these cells, but is present all around the cell at the level of the substratum. Some antigen is also present on the dorsal surface of the myoblasts and myotubes. In fibroblasts the CSAT antigen has a punctate distribution, is present primarily at the cell periphery, and can also be found colinear with portions of stress fibers (microfilament bundles) at the ventral surface of cells and at the termini of stress fibers at the cell periphery (Figure 4; Neff *et al.*, 1982). The fluorescence pattern is reminiscent of but not coincident with that of vinculin, which has been shown to localize primarily at focal contact sites (adhesion plaques). When the immunofluorescence patterns of vinculin and CSAT are compared, both appear to be localized in the vicinity of focal contact sites. However, CSAT staining appears enriched at the periphery of focal contact sites stained by vinculin. CSAT is also localized at the cell periphery in regions where vinculin staining is not found and, to a lesser extent, on the dorsal surface of the cell.

Using the greater resolution provided by double immunoelectron microscopy, Chen and Singer (1982) have reported that the antigen recognized by the monoclonal antibody JG22 (Greve and Gottlieb, 1982), which probably recognizes the same antigen as CSAT (see above), also has a punctate distribution at the cell periphery in fibroblasts. They report that at the EM level of resolution, JG22 antigen is localized in close contact sites along with fibronectin and α-actinin and not in the adjacent focal contact sites, which contain vinculin. Thus, the localization studies carried out so far for both CSAT and JG22 suggest that the antigen is localized at one of the classes of putative adhesion sites where transmembrane associations between cytoskeleton and matrix occur.

VIII. Hypothesis for the Role of the CSAT Antigen in Adhesion and Morphology

The use of a highly selective screening procedure has allowed us to isolate an adhesion-perturbing monoclonal antibody, CSAT, despite the use of a very heterogeneous immunogen. Although the antibody affects principally the adhesive interactions of myogenic cells, antibody binding studies show that the antigenic determinant is on all cell types tested. In immunoaffinity chromatography experiments, the CSAT antibody binds three glycoproteins from fibroblasts with apparent molecular weights of approximately 120,000–160,000 daltons. Whether CSAT recognizes a determinant common to all three components, a region unique to one, or a conformational determinant dependent on the interaction of all three remains to be determined. CSAT does appear to recognize a conformational determinant rather than a sequence determinant, as suggested by the sensitivity of antigen–antibody binding to the conditions of SDS PAGE.

Several observations suggest that the mechanism by which CSAT disrupts the adhesion of myogenic cells to extracellular matrices appears to be direct, via an element of an adhesion complex, rather than indirect, via a general structural, metabolic, or proteolytic perturbation of the myoblast membrane. (1) The effect of the antibody is specific for cell–matrix-related events, having no detectable effect on cell–cell interactions, such as skeletal myoblast fusion and differentiation, or on the coordinated association and synchronous contraction of cardiac cells; (2) the selectivity of the effect of CSAT on different cell types argues for a specific interaction; (3) the antigen to which CSAT binds is enriched in areas of cell–matrix adhesion, i.e., along portions of stress fibers and at the cell periphery; (4) the antibody appears to affect an early event in the adhesion process rather than cell spreading.

Several direct roles for the CSAT antigen in cell–matrix adhesion can be postulated. It might act (1) as a receptor for a matrix-associated molecule such as fibronectin, (2) as an organizer of the cytoskeleton at adhesion sites, (3) as the direct transmembrane link accomplishing both of the above roles, or (4) as an organizer of a transmembrane assembly linking the cytoskeleton and the extracellular matrix. Our working hypothesis is that the CSAT antigen is a glycoprotein complex that spans the membrane and thus can interact with both cytoskeletal and extracellular molecules.

The characteristic, differential effects of the antibody on various cell types demonstrate an intimate interrelation between adhesion and morphology and suggest the existence of an adhesive hierarchy among different cell types. The CSAT antigen, present on many cell types, plays a dominant role in the adhesion of myoblasts since they are readily rounded and detached by CSAT antibody.

The adhesive interactions of other cell types are affected less, the fibroblast being the most refractory. In addition, cell–cell interactions do not appear to require participation of the CSAT antigen. This separation of cell–cell and cell–matrix adhesion is suggested not only by these studies but also by studies on epithelial cells using antisera that selectively perturb either cell–substrate adhesion or cell–cell adhesion (Damsky *et al.*, 1981) and by the studies of neuronal cell adhesion by Edelman and co-workers (reviewed recently by Edelman, 1983).

We interpret the differential responses by various cell types to CSAT as reflecting a differential complexity in the cell–matrix adhesive mechanisms of these cell types. CSAT antigen is present in roughly comparable amounts on all cell types so far studied, and thus an adhesive hierarchy arising solely from differences in CSAT antigen concentration seems unlikely. Adhesive complexes with different organizations of common adhesive molecules could account for our observations. Alternatively, fibroblasts may have distinct classes of adhesive complexes, some containing molecules not recognized by CSAT, that are absent or expressed to a much lower degree in myoblasts. Cells with intermediate sensitivities to CSAT, such as cardiac cells or BudR-treated myoblasts, may express more of these complexes than myoblasts but fewer than fibroblasts. Thus a cell type would be sensitive to CSAT antibody only to the extent that it relies on the class of adhesive complex containing CSAT antigen for its attachment to the matrix. In this context, the choice of the myoblast for our adhesive screen was fortuitous. The postulated complexity of fibroblast adhesion renders less likely the isolation of a single monoclonal antibody capable of rounding and detaching fibroblasts.

This notion of multiple strategies for cell–matrix adhesion in fibroblasts is supported by several different kinds of evidence. First, at least two and likely more morphologically distinguishable adhesive sites have been observed in fibroblasts (Izzard and Lochner, 1976; Heath and Dunn, 1978; Chen and Singer, 1982). Second, Harper and Juliano (1980, 1981), using adhesion variants, have reported that CHO cells have both fibronectin-dependent and -independent adhesion mechanisms. Third, Oesch and Birchmeier (1982) have recently reported isolation of a monoclonal antibody (anti-FC-1) which inhibits the attachment of fibroblasts to artificial substrata in the presence of serum. In contrast to JG22 (Greve and Gottlieb, 1982; Chen, 1982) and CSAT, anti-FC-1 is localized primarily at focal contacts along with vinculin and recognizes a membrane-associated 60,000-dalton component in detergent extracts of fibroblasts. Thus two membrane components, one recognized by CSAT and JG22 monoclonal antibodies and the other by the anti-FC-1 monoclonal antibody, appear to mediate cell–matrix adhesion at distinct classes of adhesive sites in fibroblasts.

In addition to the insights CSAT has provided into adhesion, its ability to selectively round myogenic cells provides a useful and simple method for preparing fibroblast-free myogenic cultures. This allows both the growth of long-term muscle cultures without fibroblast overgrowth and a study of the fibroblast contribution to myogenesis. CSAT has been similarly useful in preparing cultures of highly purified myogenic and chondrogenic cells from limb buds (J. Sasse, H. Holtzer, and A. Horwitz, submitted).

ACKNOWLEDGMENTS

These studies were supported by U. S. Public Health Service Grants GM-23244, CA-32311, CA-19144, HD-15663, CA-27909, and CA-10815, and by the H. M. Watts Jr. Neuromuscular Disease Research Center. AFH thanks his colleagues R. Kennett and K. Bechtol for their overwhelming generosity.

References

Bertolotti, R., Rutishauser, U., and Edelman, G. M., 1980, A cell surface molecule involved in aggregation of embryonic liver cells, *Proc. Natl. Acad. Sci. USA* **77:**4831–4835.

Brackenbury, R., Thiery, J.-P., Rutishauser, U., and Edelman, G. M., 1977, Adhesion among neural cells of the chick embryo. I. An immunological assay for molecules involved in cell–cell binding, *J. Biol. Chem.* **252:**6835–6840.

Brackenbury, R., Rutishauser, U., and Edelman, G. M., 1981, Distinct calcium-independent and calcium-dependent adhesion systems of chicken embryo cells, *Proc. Natl. Acad. Sci. USA* **78:**387–391.

Chen, W.-T., 1982, Development of the attachment sites between the cell surface and the extracellular matrix in cultured fibroblasts, *J. Cell Biol.* **95:**100a (abstract).

Chen, W.-T., and Singer, J., 1982, Immunoelectron microscopic studies of the sites of cell substratum and cell–cell contact in cultured fibroblasts, *J. Cell Biol.* **95:**205–233.

Cohen, S. M., Gorbsky, G., and Steinberg, M., 1983, Immunochemical characterization of related families of glycoproteins in desmosomes, *J. Biol. Chem.* **34:**455–466.

Damsky, C. H., Knudsen, K. A., Dorio, R. J., and Buck, C. A., 1981, Manipulation of cell–cell and cell–substratum interactions in mouse mammary tumor epithelial cells using broad spectrum antisera, *J. Cell Biol.* **89:**173–184.

Damsky, C. H., Richa, J., Solter, D., Knudsen, K. A., and Buck, C. A., 1983, Identification and purification of a cell surface glycoprotein mediating intercellular adhesion in embryonic and adult tissue, *Cell* **34:**455–466.

Decker, C., and Horwitz, A. F., 1982, Adhesive and morphologic hierarchies determined using a monoclonal antibody, *J. Cell Biol.* **95:**111a (abstract).

Ducibella, T., 1980, Divalent antibodies to mouse embryonal carcinoma cells inhibit compaction in the mouse embryo, *Dev. Biol.* **79:**356–366.

Edelman, G. M., 1983, Cell adhesion molecules, *Science* **219:**450–457.

Edelman, G. M., and Chuong, C.-M., 1982, Embryonic to adult conversion of neural cell adhesion molecules in normal and staggerer mice, *Proc. Natl. Acad. Sci. USA* **79:**7036–7040.

Gallin, W. J., Edelman, G. M., and Cunningham, B. A., 1983, Characterization of L-CAM, a major cell adhesion molecule from embryonic liver cells, *Proc. Natl. Acad. Sci. USA* **80:**1083–1042.

Geiger, B., 1981, Involvement of vinculin in contact-induced cytoskeletal interactions, *Cold Spring Harbor Symp. Quant. Biol.* **XLVI:**671–682.

Gerisch, G., 1977, Univalent antibody fragments as tools for the analysis of cell interactions in *Dictyostelium*, *Curr. Top. Dev. Biol.* **14:**243–270.

Greve, J. M., and Gottlieb, D. I., 1982, Monoclonal antibodies which alter the morphology of cultured chick myogenic cells, *J. Cell Biochem.* **18:**221–230.

Harper, P. A., and Juliano, R. L., 1980, Isolation and characterization of Chinese hamster ovary cell variants defective in adhesion to fibronectin coated collagen, *J. Cell Biol.* **87:**755–763.

Harper, P. A., and Juliano, R. L., 1981, Fibronectin independent adhesion of fibroblasts to the extracellular matrix: Mediation by a high molecular weight membrane glycoprotein, *J. Cell Biol.* **91:**647–653.

Heath, J. P., and Dunn, G. A., 1978, Cell to substratum contacts of chick fibroblasts and their relation to the microfilament system. A correlated interference–reflection and high-voltage electron microscope study, *J. Cell Sci.* **29:**197–212.

Hoffman, S., Sorkin, B. C., White, P. C., Brackenbury, R., Mailhammer, R., Rutishauser, U., Cunningham, R. A., and Edelman, G. M., 1982, Chemical characterization of a neural cell adhesion molecule purified from embryonic brain membranes, *J. Biol. Chem.* **257**:7720–7729.

Horwitz, A., Neff, N., Sessions, A., and Decker, C., 1982, Cellular interactions in myogenesis, in: *Muscle Development: Molecular and Cellular Control* (H. Epstein and M. Pearson, eds.), Cold Spring Harbor Press, Cold Spring Harbor, New York, pp. 291–300.

Hyafil, F., Babinet, C., and Jacob, F., 1981, Cell–cell interaction in early embryogenesis: A molecular approach to the role of calcium, *Cell* **26**:447–454.

Hynes, R. O., 1981, Relationships between fibronectin and the cytoskeleton, in: *Cytoskeletal Elements and Plasma Membrane Organization* (G. Poste and G. L. Nicolson, eds.), Elsevier/North-Holland Biomedical Press, pp. 100–137.

Izzard, C., and Lochner, L. R., 1976, Cell to substrate contacts in lung fibroblasts. An interference reflection study with an evaluation of the technique, *J. Cell Sci.* **21**:129–159.

Johnson, M. H., Chakraborty, J., Handyside, A. H., Willison, K., and Stern, P., 1979, Effect of prolonged decompaction on one development of the preimplantation mouse embryo, *J. Embryol. Exp. Morphol.* **54**:241–261.

Kemler, R., Babinet, C., Eisen, H., and Jacob, F., 1977, Surface antigens in early differentiation, *Proc. Natl. Acad. Sci. USA* **74**:4449–4452.

Knudsen, K. A., Rao, P. E., Damsky, C. H., and Buck, C. A., 1981, Membrane glycoproteins involved in cell substratum adhesion, *Proc. Natl. Acad. Sci. USA* **78**:6071–6075.

Knudsen, K. A., Buck, C. A., Damsky, C. H., and Horwitz, A. F., 1982, Adhesion-related glycoproteins isolated using a monoclonal antibody, *J. Cell Biol.* **95**:111a. (abstract).

Kohler, G., and Milstein, G., 1975, Continuous cultures of fused cells secreting antibody of pre-defined specificity, *Nature* **256**:495–497.

McClay, D. R., Wessel, G. M., and Marchase, R. B., 1980, Intercellular recognition: Quantitation of initial binding events, *Proc. Natl. Acad. Sci. USA* **78**:4975–4979.

Neff, N. T., Lowrey, C., Decker, C., Tovar, A., Damsky, C., Buck, C., and Horwitz, A. F., 1982, A monoclonal antibody detaches embryonic skeletal muscle from extracellular matrices, *J. Cell Biol.* **95**:654–666.

Oesch, B., and Birchmeier, W., 1982, New surface components of fibroblast's focal contacts identified by a monoclonal antibody, *Cell* **31**:671–679.

Rorschneider, L., Rosok, M., and Shriver, K., 1981, Mechanism of transformation by Rous sarcoma virus. Events within adhesion plaques, *Cold Spring Harbor Symp. Quant. Biol.* **56**:953–967.

Rothbard, J. B., Brackenbury, R., Cunningham, B., and Edelman, G. M., 1982, Differences in the carbohydrate structure of neural cell adhesion molecule from adult and embryonic chicken brain, *J. Biol. Chem.* **257**:11064–11069.

Scott, R. E., 1976, Plasma membrane vesiculation: A new technique for isolation of plasma membranes, *Science* **194**:743–745.

Takeichi, M., Atsumi, J., Yoshida, K. U., and Okada, T. S., 1981, Selective adhesion of embryonal carcinoma cells and differentiated cells by Ca^{2+}-dependent sites, *Dev. Biol.* **87**:340–350.

Thiery, J.-P., Brackenbury, R., Rutishauser, U., and Edelman, G. M., 1977, Adhesion among neural cells of the chick embryo. II. Purification and characterization of a cell adhesion molecule from neural retina, *J. Biol. Chem.* **252**:6841–6845.

Vollmers, H. P., and Birchmeier, W., 1983, Monoclonal antibodies inhibit the adhesion of mouse B 16 melanoma cells *in vitro* and block lung metastases *in vivo*, *Proc. Natl. Acad. Sci. USA* **80**:3729–3733.

6
Monoclonal Antibodies to Cytoskeletal Proteins

J. J. C. Lin, J. R. Feramisco, S. H. Blose, and
F. Matsumura

I. Introduction

Cytoskeletal proteins are found, as a general rule, in highly organized arrays within the cytoplasm of higher eukaryotic cells. The three filamentous networks that comprise the cytoskeleton are the microfilaments, composed of actin and many accessory proteins; the microtubules, composed of tubulin and several accessory proteins; and the intermediate filaments, composed of vimentin (or one of four other related proteins) and at least two accessory proteins. These networks have been the objects of intense study over the past 10 years in terms of cell motility, structure, and adhesion, and have proven to be most amenable to immunofluorescence and immunoelectron microscopic examination [e.g., R. Goldman *et al.*, 1976)]. Because of the numerous applications of immunological techniques to investigate the structure and function of the cellular cytoskeleton systems, it is easily understood why many researchers in the field have begun utilizing the lymphocyte hybridoma method (Kohler and Milstein, 1975) as a source of antibodies. Studying something as complex as the cytoskeleton requires the use of the purest immunological reagents available, i.e., monoclonal antibodies.

Within the past 2 years, numerous cell systems and cytoskeleton antigens have been used as targets for research with monoclonal antibodies. Listed in Table I are some of these studies. Thus, in the brief 2-year period, monoclonal antibodies have been used to study the components of the cytoskeleton and their

J. J. C. Lin, J. R. Feramisco, S. H. Blose, and F. Matsumura • Cold Spring Harbor Laboratory, Cold Spring Harbor, New York 11724. Present address for J. J. C. L.: Department of Zoology, University of Iowa, Iowa City, Iowa 52242.

TABLE I

Some Monoclonal Antibodies to Cytoskeleton Proteins

Experimental system	Antigen	Reference
Immunofluorescence with neuroblastoma cells	Microtubule-associated protein (MAP-2)	Izant and McIntosh (1980)
Immunofluorescence with mammalian nonmuscle and muscle cells	Intermediate filament proteins	Lin (1981)
Microinjection of antibodies into fibroblasts	Intermediate filament proteins	Lin and Feramisco (1981)
Microinjection of antibodies into fibroblasts	Vimentin	Klymkowski (1981)
Functional mapping of proteins	Fibronectin	Atherton and Hynes (1981)
Cross-reactivity of monoclonal antibodies	Thy-1 and an intermediate filament protein	Dulbecco *et al.* (1981)
Cross-reactivity of monoclonal antibodies	Intermediate filament proteins	Pruss *et al.* (1981)
Myogenesis in *C. elegans*	Myosin isozymes	Miller *et al.* (1981)
Myogenesis in chicken	Myosin isozymes	Bader *et al.* (1981)
Mammalian cell compartments	Golgi-associated protein	Lin and Queally (1982)
Epithelial cells	Tonofilament proteins	Lane (1982)
Ultrastructure of intermediate filaments	Vimentin	Blose *et al.* (1982)
Ultrastructure of smooth muscle thin filaments	Tropomyosin	Matsumura and Lin (1982)
Fibroblasts	Various cytoskeleton proteins	Lin (1982)

intracellular location, changes in the expression of these elements during differentiation, and the function of the cytoskeleton in living cells by microinjection of the antibodies.

The major advantage of the use of monoclonal antibodies over conventional antisera in these types of experiments clearly is the great specificity of the monoclonal antibodies. For example, in studies designed to determine the intracellular location of cytoskeleton proteins, one can be fairly confident of immunofluorescence or immunoelectron microscopy data once the specificity of the antibody has been documented. The work of Izant and McIntosh (1980), Lin (1981), Lin and Queally (1982), and E. B. Lane (1982) has demonstrated the utility of monoclonal antibodies applied to cytoskeleton systems by showing the intracellular localization of microtubule-associated proteins (MAP-2) in neuronal cells, two novel intermediate filament proteins of 95,000 and 220,000 daltons, a Golgi-associated protein of 100,000 daltons, and cytokeratin proteins, respectively. Others have shown their use in high-resolution analysis of the ultrastructure of the intermediate filaments and smooth muscle thin filaments (Blose *et al.*, 1982; Matsumura and Lin, 1982). The images obtained in these experiments, both fluorescent and electron microscopic, are of exceptional quality and clarity when compared to those generally obtained with conventional antisera. More-over, new perspectives of the ultrastructure of the cytoskeleton can be gained through the use of monoclonal antibodies (see Section VII). The high degree of specificity of monoclonal antibodies also makes them ideally suited for experiments involving microinjection of antibodies into living cells (Lin and Feramisco, 1981; Klymkowski, 1981) and isolation of proteins or supramolecular structures (Matsumura and Lin, 1982). Both of these applications are discussed in this chapter.

At least three groups (Dulbecco *et al.*, 1981; Blose *et al.*, 1982; Pruss *et al.*, 1981) have encountered a rather interesting (but predictable) problem while examining the specificities of several monoclonal antibodies: the cross-reaction of monoclonal antibodies with two or more proteins that are seemingly unrelated. This undoubtedly occurs because of the high degree of specificity of the monoclonal antibody for only one antigenic site (as little as a few amino acids, for example); thus, with a finite number of amino acids (or carbohydrates and lipids) giving rise to virtually all of the antigenic sites on the entire spectrum of proteins in the cell, it is not unexpected to find such a cross-reaction between seemingly unrelated proteins. Conventional antisera usually do not show a total cross-reactivity for "unrelated" proteins because these antisera contain many antibodies that recognize numerous antigenic sites on a given protein, making the cross-reaction of only one of the component antibodies at one antigenic site a minor problem. Cross-reactions of this nature can cause great confusion in experiments using monoclonal antibodies; hence, great care must be taken to determine all of the antigenic proteins that are recognized by the antibody in every cell system in which they are used. This and other work from our laboratory will be discussed in detail in this chapter.

II. Monoclonal Antibodies Specific for Cytoskeletal Proteins

We have utilized both crude antigen fractions and pure ones for the immunization of mice for the generation of monoclonal antibodies to cytoskeleton proteins. We will present the results of both types of procedures here. As discussed in the next section, however, great care must be taken to document the specificity of the antibodies in either case.

Hybridoma clones secreting monospecific antibodies to various cytoskeletal proteins that we have made are listed in Table II (see also Lin, 1982). These were obtained from polyethylene glycol-induced fusions between NS-1 myeloma cells and spleen cells from BALB/c mice previously immunized with various cytoskeletal proteins or preparations. Indirect immunofluorescence was chosen to screen positive hybrids, for the following reasons: (1) Unlike enzyme-linked immunoabsorbent assay (ELISA), purified antigens are not needed for screening. (2) One can simultaneously obtain information about the localization of antigens within cells during screening by immunofluorescence. (3) As will be discussed in a later section, this method may also aid in detecting new proteins

TABLE II
List of Monoclonal Antibodies Used in This Chapter

Clones	Immunogen	Specific antigen	Species specificity	Reference
JLA20	Chicken gizzard cytoskeleton	Actin	Broad species specific	Lin (1981, 1982), Lin *et al.* (1982)
JLA8	Chicken gizzard cytoskeleton	Filamin	Chicken specific	Lin *et al.* (1982), Lin (1982)
JLN21	Chicken gizzard α-actinin fraction	Filamin	Chicken specific	Lin (1982)
JLN20	Chicken gizzard α-actinin fraction	Skeletal muscle α-actinin and fibroblast α-actinin	Chicken specific	Lin (1982)
JLF15	Rabbit skeletal muscle actin	Tropomyosin	Broad species specific	Blose *et al.* (1982), Lin (1982), Matsumura and Lin (1982)
LCK16	Chicken gizzard tropomyosin-enriched fraction	Tropomyosin and vimentin	Broad species specific	Blose *et al.* (1982), Lin (1982), Matsumura and Lin (1982)
JLK6	Chicken gizzard vinculin	Vinculin	Chicken specific	Lin (1982)
JLK3	Chicken gizzard vinculin	350K protein	Chicken specific	Lin (1982)
JLB7	Rat skeletal muscle myofibrils	95K intermediate filament associated protein	Broad species specific	Lin (1981), Lin and Feramisco (1981)
JLT7	Rabbit skeletal muscle troponin T	Troponin T	?	Unpublished results
JLT12	Rabbit skeletal muscle troponin T	Troponin T	Broad species specific	Unpublished results
JLT36	Rabbit skeletal muscle troponin T	Troponin T	?	Unpublished results
FM10	Rabbit skeletal muscle myosin	C-protein	Rabbit, rat skeletal muscle	Unpublished results
FM20	Rabbit skeletal muscle myosin	C-protein	Rabbit, rat skeletal muscle	Unpublished results
FM28	Rabbit skeletal muscle myosin	Myosin heavy chain	Rabbit, rat skeletal muscle	Unpublished results

that are present in trace amounts within the antigen preparation. All positive hybrids described here were cloned two to three times in semisoft agarose in order to obtain stable clones.

As can be seen in Table II (see also Lin, 1982), many hybridoma clones have been obtained from fusion experiments with crude protein fractions as immunogens. These results demonstrate one of the major advantages of the hybridoma technique of Kohler and Milstein (1975), in that from a single immunization, hybridomas specific for several proteins can be made. The purification of individual antibodies can be achieved by the agarose cloning of the hybridoma cells. In using crude protein mixtures, usually those proteins with strong antigenicity will be the major hybridoma clones obtained. Since the hybridoma technique itself is extremely sensitive, even small amounts of contaminants in the antigen preparation can give rise to antibody-secreting clones. For example, we have found that filamin clones were the major hybridomas isolated from fusion experiments with crude chicken gizzard cytoskeletal proteins or with a gizzard α-actinin fraction contaminated with trace amounts of filamin as the immunogen of mice (Table II and Lin, 1982). Other examples in this aspect are JLF15 and JLK3 clones, which were obtained from fusion experiments with skeletal muscle actin and chicken gizzard vinculin fractions, respectively, as the immunogen. Trace contamination of tropomyosin and a protein of 350,000 daltons in the respective antigen preparations gave rise to the clones JLF15 and JLK3, which recognize these proteins, respectively. Likewise, clones FM10 and FM20, which secrete antibodies to C-protein, were obtained from the fusion experiment involving rabbit skeletal muscle myosin as the antigen. In this case, the myosin preparation contained only 5% C-protein. Interestingly, conventional antisera against myosin usually contain C-protein antibodies (Pepe, 1973) as well.

III. Identification of Antigens

As discussed in the previous section, either crude protein mixture or purified proteins can be used as the immunogen to make monoclonal antibodies to cytoskeleton proteins and monoclonal antibodies can be often derived from trace amounts of contaminants in the purified protein fractions. Therefore, the identification of the specific antigens recognized by the monoclonal antibodies is an essential step prior to the use of the antibodies. Some factors that affect feasibility in identification of specific antigen are the following: (1) the solubility and stability of the antigen; (2) the titer of monoclonal antibody; (3) the stability of antigen–antibody complex; and (4) the class of antibody. We have applied the following methods to identify the specific antigens recognized by monoclonal antibodies.

A. Immunoautoradiography

Indirect immunoautoradiography on SDS polyacrylamide gels can be performed as described by Burridge (1978). This method is particularly suitable for IgG monoclonal antibodies, although it is time-consuming. Some examples of the use of this method with monoclonal antibodies have been published elsewhere (Lin et al., 1982; Lin, 1982; Izant and McIntosh, 1980). Since the same gel slice used for incubation with the monoclonal antibody can be subjected to coomassie blue stain, this method provides an easy and accurate alignment of the specific antigen band with coomassie blue staining band. However, proteins with antigenic determinants denatured by SDS and/or the electrophoretic field cannot be detected by this method. Also, IgM antibodies apparently cannot enter the acrylamide gel with ease, thereby making this technique of little use for the relatively large IgM antibodies.

B. *Immunoprecipitation*

Immunoprecipitation provides an alternative method to immunoautoradiography in the sense that SDS can be avoided, and a variety of antigen solubilizations can be utilized. Generally, immunoprecipitation reactions are performed with formalin-fixed *Staphylococcus aureus* with a modified (Lin, 1981) version of the original method (Kessler, 1975; Goding, 1978). Briefly, the antigen in the protein mixture or cell lysate is first incubated with the monoclonal antibody, followed by the addition of a second antibody that reacts with the mouse immunoglobulins (i.e., a rabbit antiserum against mouse immunoglobulins). The antigen–monoclonal antibody–second antibody complexes are then precipitated with *S. aureus*. The reason for using second antibody (from rabbit or goat) is that protein A molecules on *S. aureus* react well with all classes of rabbit or goat IgG but only with some classes of mouse IgG (i.e., IgG2a, IgG2b, IgG3, and some IgG1) (Goding, 1978; Ey *et al.*, 1978; Medgyesi *et al.*, 1978).

The choice of buffer conditions for immunoprecipitation usually depends upon the solubility and nature of the antigen, the stability of monoclonal antibody itself, and the stability of the antigen–antibody complex. From our experience and that of others (Herrman and Mescher, 1979) immunoprecipitations by some monoclonal antibodies work well in relatively low salt buffer conditions (e.g., 15 mM sodium phosphate buffer pH 7.0, 1 mM EGTA, 1 mM phenylmethylsulfonylfluoride, and 0.5% Triton X-100) as opposed to physiological salt buffers. Figure 1 shows a two-dimensional gel analysis of an immunoprecipitate from a total cell extract in low salt buffer by the JLB7 monoclonal antibody. A protein spot with apparent molecular weight of 95,000 daltons was identified as the antigen recognized by JLB7 monoclonal antibody. This protein was characterized as a new intermediate-filament-associated protein in gerbil fibroma cells (Lin, 1981).

Other buffers of physiological salt concentration (0.5% Triton X-100, 1 mM phenylmethylsulfonylfluoride in phosphate-buffered saline) can also be used for immunoprecipitation with monoclonal antibodies (e.g., JLK3; Lin, 1982). In this case the specific antigen identified from immunoprecipitates is a high-molecular-weight protein (350,000 daltons) (Figure 2). This protein is not solubilized in low salt buffer even though both buffers contain 0.5% Triton X-100. For some proteins insoluble in these low- and physiological salt buffers, such as vimentin, various amounts of SDS or other detergents can be added in the buffer for immunoprecipitation. One such example has been described previously for the LCK16 monoclonal antibody to immunoprecipitate vimentin (Blose *et al.*, 1982).

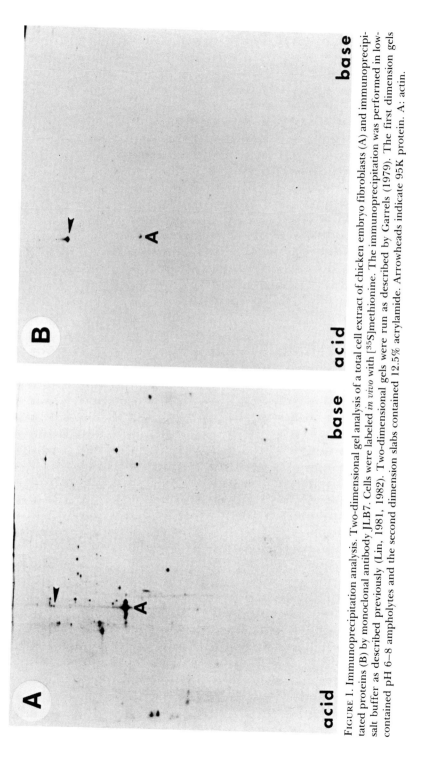

FIGURE 1. Immunoprecipitation analysis. Two-dimensional gel analysis of a total cell extract of chicken embryo fibroblasts (A) and immunoprecipitated proteins (B) by monoclonal antibody JLB7. Cells were labeled *in vivo* with [³⁵S]methionine. The immunoprecipitation was performed in low-salt buffer as described previously (Lin, 1981, 1982). Two-dimensional gels were run as described by Garrels (1979). The first dimension gels contained pH 6–8 ampholytes and the second dimension slabs contained 12.5% acrylamide. Arrowheads indicate 95K protein. A: actin.

◄ IEF

SDS ▼

acid   base

FIGURE 2. Immunoprecipitation analysis. Two-dimensional gel analysis of immunoprecipitated proteins by monoclonal antibody JLK3 from a total cell extract of chicken embryo fibroblasts. The immunoprecipitation was performed in physiological salt buffer (or lysis buffer) as described previously (Lin, 1982). The first dimension gel contained pH 6–8 ampholytes and the second dimension slab contained 7.5% acrylamide.

C. Solid Phase Radioimmunoassay

This technique can be used with either pure antigens or antigens separated by SDS polyacrylamide gels to identify the specificity of the monoclonal antibody. Total proteins of cultured cells are first separated on an SDS polyacrylamide gel. After electrophoresis, gel tracks are sliced into 1-mm fractions. Each slice is then put into the microtiter well and soaked with 100 μl of coating buffer (0.1 M sodium bicarbonate buffer pH 9.6, 0.02% NaN$_3$) for 2 days at 4°C in order to extract the separated proteins out of the gel and to bind them to the surface of the microtiter wells. The monoclonal antibody is then added to the well; after a suitable incubation time, unbound antibody is washed away. Then I^{125}-labeled goat anti-mouse IgG (heavy and light chains) is added to the wells as a second antibody to detect the bound mouse monoclonal antibody. After washing three times, the radioactivity remaining in each well is measured. One example of this type of analysis has been described elsewhere (Lin, 1982).

Similarly, purified proteins (1–5 µg), if available, can be used instead of gel slices to coat onto microtiter wells. Such examples are shown in Figure 3. Both FM10 (IgG1) and FM20 (IgG1) antibodies specifically recognize C-protein from skeletal muscle (Figure 3A), whereas FM28 (IgG1) antibody recognizes column-purified myosin (Figure 3B). It should be mentioned that in the case of the FM20 antibody only the technique of solid phase radioimmunoassay has been successful in the determination of its specificity. The FM20 antibody failed to detect the C-protein from skeletal myofibrils after SDS polyacrylamide gel electrophoresis and transfer to nitrocellulose paper in the Western blot method (see Section IIID). Therefore, it is likely that the antigenic determinant on the C-protein molecule recognized by the FM20 antibody is rather unstable and easily destroyed by SDS and/or electrophoretic field.

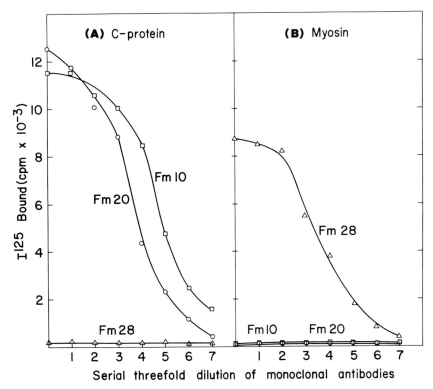

FIGURE 3. Solid-phase radioimmunoassay. An amount of 2.5 µg of the purified proteins, C-protein or myosin, in 50 µl of coating buffer was pipetted onto microtiter wells. After incubation overnight at 4°C, wells were washed three times with PBS containing 0.05% Tween 80 and 0.01% NaN₃ (washing buffer). The remaining protein film on the surface of the microtiter well was used as solid-phase antigen for incubation with monoclonal antibodies (FM10, FM20, and FM28). Iodine-125-labeled goat anti-mouse IgG (heavy and light chains) was used to detect the bound monoclonal antibody. After extensive washing, wells were sliced off and the radioactivities were measured by a counter. (A) C-protein used as the antigen; (B) column-purified myosin used as the antigen.

D. Western Blot Method

The Western blot method for identification of antigens is carried out according to the method of Towbin *et al.* (1979). Total protein mixtures are first separated on SDS polyacrylamide gels and then electrophoretically transferred onto nitrocellulose paper. The paper is soaked in 3% bovine serum albumin to block the excess binding sites and incubated with the monoclonal antibody. After extensive washing, the bound monoclonal antibody is detected by I^{125}-labeled goat anti-mouse IgG (heavy and light chains). Such examples are shown in Figure 4. The JLT7, JLT36, and JLT12 antibodies recognize troponin T from

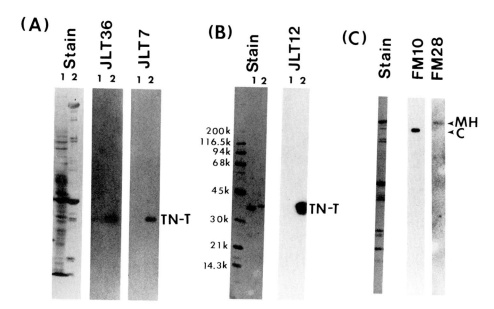

FIGURE 4. Western blotting method. (A) Total proteins of gerbil fibroma cells (lane 1) and rabbit skeletal myofibrils (lane 2) were resolved on a 12.5% SDS–polyacrylamide gel and transferred onto nitrocellulose paper. The papers were first incubated with monoclonal antibody (JLT7 or JLT36) and then with ^{125}I-labeled goat anti-mouse IgG (heavy and light chains). The bound antibodies were detected by autoradiography on X-ray films (JLT36 and JLT7). An identical transfer was stained with amido black (stain). TN-T: troponin T. (B) Purified tropomyosin (lane 1) and troponin T (lane 2) from rabbit skeletal muscle were resolved on a 12.5% SDS polyacrylamide gel and transferred onto nitrocellulose paper. The papers were first reacted with monoclonal antibody JLT12 and then with ^{125}I-labeled goat anti-mouse IgG (heavy and light chains). The bound radioactivity was detected by autoradiography on X-ray film (JLT12). An identical transfer, including molecular weight standard proteins, was stained with amido black (stain). TN-T: troponin T. (C) Total proteins of rabbit skeletal myofibrils were resolved on a 12.5% SDS polyacrylamide gel and transferred onto nitrocellulose paper. The papers were first incubated with monoclonal antibody (FM10 or FM28) and then with ^{125}I-labeled goat anti-mouse IgG (heavy and light chains). The bound radioactivity was detected by autoradiography on X-ray film (FM10 and FM28). An identical transfer was stained with amido black (stain). MH: myosin heavy chain; C: C-protein.

skeletal muscle myofibrils (Figures 4A and 4B). In the case of the JLT12 antibody, it is difficult to determine whether JLT12 antibody recognizes only troponin T or both tropomyosin and troponin T. This is so because troponin T and tropomyosin from skeletal muscle run close to each other in 12.5% SDS polyacrylamide gels and because it is difficult to align the amido black-stained transfer with X-ray film derived from the parallel antibody-stained paper. For this purpose, we have purified tropomyosin and troponin T from preparative gels and applied them in different lanes of gel. Western blotting was performed on these lanes containing α-tropomyosin (lane 1 of Figure 4B) and troponin T (lane 2 of Figure 4B). This analysis shows that the JLT12 antibody reacts only with troponin T. The same result is also obtained by performing Western blotting on SDS–urea polyacrylamide gels, in which tropomyosin and troponin T separate very well (data not shown).

Figure 4C also shows that the FM10 and FM28 antibodies recognize C-protein and myosin heavy chain, respectively, from rabbit skeletal muscle myofibrils, while the FM20 antibody fails to detect any protein band (data not shown). As can be seen in Figure 3A, it can be concluded that FM20 antibody does bind to C-protein under conditions that are free of SDS or electrophoresis. Therefore, the failure to detect C-protein by the FM20 antibody in Western blotting experiments may be due to the instability of the antigenic site in C-protein recognized by FM20 in SDS and/or the electrophoretic field.

IV. Monoclonal Antibodies That Cross-React with Different Molecules

In several different cases, proteins that are seemingly unrelated have been shown to have small stretches of homologous amino acid sequence. C1q, a subcomponent of the first component of the complement pathway, contains a region of approximately 78 residues with a collagenlike sequence (Porter and Reid, 1978; Reid, 1974, 1979); and a collagenlike sequence has been found in the tail portion of the 16S form of acetylcholinesterase (Lwebuga-Mukasa et al., 1976). Two cytoskeletal proteins, desmin (an intermediate filament protein) and tropomyosin (a regulatory protein bound to F-actin) and kerateine-A (a proteolytic fragment of sheep merino wool), contain a homologous region of nine amino acids (Geisler and Weber, 1981; Osborn et al., 1982). From these emerging examples it is very plausible that monoclonal antibodies could identify these common regions on apparently different molecules. Although the amino acid sequences of the binding sites have yet to be determined, several cross-reacting monoclonal antibodies to the cytoskeleton proteins have been described as well as monoclonals that cross-react with viral proteins and cell surface proteins (for review see Lane and Koprowski, 1982). Dulbecco et al. (1981) have reported a monoclonal antibody that cross-reacts with Thy-1 antigen and the cytoskeletal intermediate filament protein, and Pruss et al. (1981) and Dellagi et al. (1982) have monoclonal antibodies that recognize several discrete biochemical and immunological classes of intermediate filaments. Recently, we have described a mouse monoclonal IgM, LCK16, that cross-reacts with vimentin and tropomyosin (Blose *et al.*, 1982). LCK16 will be used to (1) illustrate how one deals with the possibility that a monoclonal may cross-react with more than one molecule and (2) show in subsequent sections (Sections VI and VII) that cross-reacting monoclonals can be useful probes of molecular and cellular structure.

We initially observed by immunofluorescence screening (Lin, 1982) that LCK16 stained cultured cells with an intermediate filament pattern and a microfilament-tropomyosin pattern (Figure 5). Both of these staining patterns were abolished when either purified tropomyosin or vimentin was used to absorb LCK16. This preabsorption gave early confirmation that LCK16 recognizes two different antigens.

To eliminate the possibility that LCK16 was contaminated with a second hybridoma clone or that the IgM was an anomalous hybrid molecule that contained two or more dissimilar antibody-binding regions, secreting clones of LCK16 were metabolically labeled with [^{35}S]methionine. The recovered LCK16 antibody was subjected to two-dimensional gel electrophoresis (O'Farrell, 1975) and gel fluorography (Bonner and Laskey, 1974). This molecule was found to have only one light chain, indicating LCK16 had homologous binding sites.

To determine the cellular proteins to which LCK16 binds, several SDS–gel chromatographic techniques were employed to present the total cellular protein to LCK16. We found that surface staining of acrylamide gels (Burridge, 1978) or Western (nitrocellulose) blots (Towbin *et al.*, 1979) did not work with LCK16. This was not surprising since in our experience surface staining does not work very well with IgM molecules. Therefore, we resorted to immunoprecipitation with *S. aureus* (Kessler, 1975). Since vimentin is very insoluble, total cell extracts were made by boiling (5 min at 100°C) [^{35}S]methionine-labeled cells in 2% SDS, 100 mM DTT, 15% glycerol, 80 mM Tris-HCl, pH 6.8, then diluting the total extract to 0.05% SDS in 0.5% Triton X-100. After centrifugal clarification (130,000 x*g*, 2 hr) the extract was immunoprecipitated with LCK16 (Blose *et al.*, 1982). As observed in Figure 6, LCK16 immunoprecipitated vimentin but did not precipitate tropomyosin under these conditions. In pilot experiments we determined that precipitation of tropomyosin would not occur in the presence of SDS. Figure 7 shows that partially purified tropomyosin would precipitate in the presence of 0.5% Triton X-100. The different conditions required to precipitate the two different proteins by LCK16 are related to the solubility of the antigen, ionic strength, and the degree of denaturation of antigen still permissible for antibody recognition. Unfortunately, there is no universal "cocktail" for immunoprecipitation; therefore, we routinely use several different preparations of cell lysates and purified candidate antigens in which different detergent mixtures are used. The detergent concentrations, especially SDS, are varied over a hundredfold dilution, from 1% to 0.01% (in suggested increments of 1%, 0.5%, 0.1%, 0.05%, and 0.01%). As a rule, we screen with our monoclonal antibodies by immunoprecipitation, "Burridge gels," and nitrocellulose blots. These procedures are especially necessary when a monoclonal antibody is suspected to recognize two different antigens.

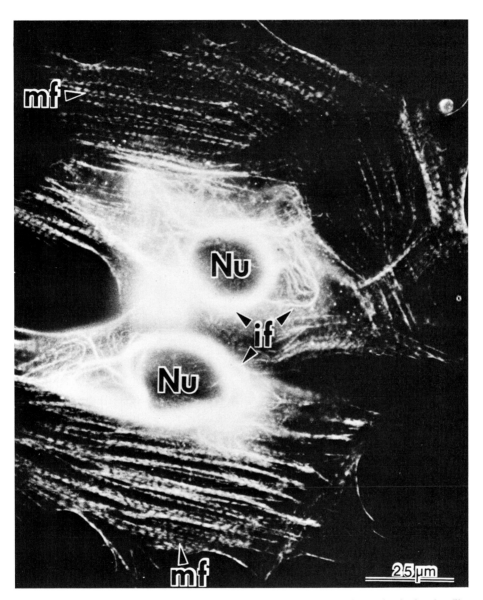

FIGURE 5. Immunofluorescence with a monoclonal antibody (LCK16) that stains both microfilaments and intermediate filaments. An immunofluorescence micrograph of two gerbil fibroma cells treated with 1 μM colcemid for 24 hr, then fixed and stained with the monoclonal antibody LCK16 is shown. Two patterns of staining are observed: (1) the striated or interrupted pattern on the microfilaments (mf), typical of the tropomyosin pattern found in interphase cells (Lazarides, 1975; Feramisco and Blose, 1980); and (2) the 10-nm filaments (if) found collapsed near the nucleus (Nu). Colcemid was employed to collapse the 10-nm filaments to the juxtanuclear region to allow distinction between the two staining patterns.

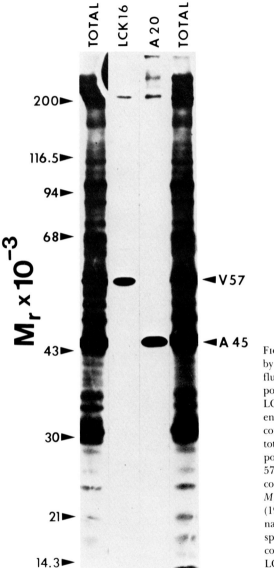

FIGURE 6. Multiple antigens recognized by the monoclonal antibody LCK16. A fluorograph of [35S]methionine-labeled polypeptides immunoprecipitated by LCK16 and JLA20 (antiactin) in the presence of 0.05% SDS is given. Under these conditions, LCK16 precipitated from the total cell lysate (TOTAL) and vimentin polypeptide (V57) with an apparent M_r of 57,000 (Blose and Meltzer, 1981). In the control, JLA20 precipitated actin (A45), M_r 45,000, as previously shown by Lin (1981). JLA20 is a mouse IgM monoclonal which also serves as a control for nonspecific binding to mouse IgMs. Under conditions of low SDS concentration, LCK16 did not optimally bind and precipitate tropomyosin (see Figure 7).

As will be shown later with LCK16 (Sections VI and VII), monoclonal antibodies that cross-react with different proteins are very useful probes of molecular structure and function. Therefore, investigators that generate these cross-reacting species should not discard them. These antibodies will undoubtedly continue to show us that cells can utilize common molecular building blocks to construct different proteins.

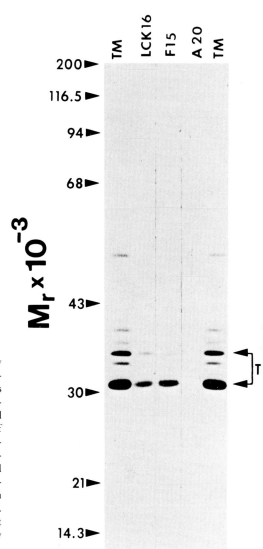

FIGURE 7. Multiple antigens recognized by the monoclonal antibody LCK16. A fluorograph of immunoprecipitated proteins from a [³⁵S]methionine-labeled, tropomyosin-enriched fraction prepared from gerbil fibroma cells is shown. Under conditions of low salt and no SDS, LCK16 immunoprecipitated the tropomyosin polypeptides (T) from the tropomyosin-enriched fraction (TM). JLF15 is a mouse monoclonal IgM directed against tropomyosin (Lin, 1982) was included as a control. JLA20, a mouse monoclonal IgM against actin (Lin, 1981), did not precipitate any proteins in this fraction.

V. Immunofluorescent Localization of Cytoskeletal Proteins

One of the conventional approaches to study the localization of cytoskeletal proteins within cells is to purify proteins to homogeneity and to immunize animals with the pure protein in order to obtain specific antibodies. The intracellular localization of cytoskeletal proteins can then be studied by immunofluorescence microscopy and/or immunoelectron microscopy.

The first problem associated with this type of approach is that the proteins being studied need to be present in relatively large amounts so that they can be easily purified. Thus, for the minor but presumably important proteins in the cytoskeleton, this approach is difficult or, as yet, impossible. The second problem is that conventional antisera often contain autoimmune antibodies, which raise the background of staining or contribute significant cytoskeleton staining (Gordon *et al.*, 1977; Osborn *et al.*, 1977; Kurki *et al.*, 1977). These sera may also contain a high titer of antibodies against minor contaminants present in the "pure" protein immunogen (Pepe, 1966, 1973). Monoclonal antibodies produced by hybridoma clones certainly reduce both of these problems.

We have used monoclonal antibodies to study intracellular localization of various cytoskeletal proteins. As can be seen in Figure 8A, JLA20 monoclonal antibodies against actin give stress fiber and some diffuse staining throughout the gerbil fibroma cell. Polygonal microfilament networks can be seen around the nucleus, and fluorescent staining at ruffle regions of the cell is visible. These results are in agreement with reports by other investigators (Lazarides and Weber, 1974; Lazarides, 1976). It should be noted that immunofluorescence of cultured cells with monoclonal antibodies often shows only a weak background stain. This is probably due to the homogeneous, monospecific nature of monoclonal antibody.

Figure 8B shows the immunofluorescence pattern of gerbil fibroma cell stained with the monoclonal antibody JLF15 against tropomyosin. The staining is confined to the stress fibers with the characteristic periodicity. In addition, the staining is also found in the connecting fibers of polygonal microfilament networks but not in the foci of the networks.

Figure 8C shows the periodic stress-fiber staining and the staining at the focal adhesion plaques of chicken embryo fibroblasts produced by the monoclonal antibody JLN20 against α-actinin. It is known that the α-actinin and tropomyosin staining units are arranged alternately along the stress fibers (Lazarides and Burridge, 1975; Feramisco and Blose, 1980; Gordon and Blose, 1979; R. D. Goldman *et al.*, 1979).

Figure 8D shows the staining pattern on chicken embryo fibroblasts revealed by immunofluorescence with monoclonal antibody against filamin (JLA8). The staining pattern, unlike that for actin, tropomyosin, or α-actinin, is less structured and somewhat diffuse.

Figure 8E shows the staining pattern on chicken embryo fibroblasts given by immunofluoescence with a monoclonal antibody (JLK6) against vinculin. The staining in focal adhesion plaques and a fibrillar staining throughout the cytoplasm are apparent as described previously by Geiger (1979) and Burridge and Feramisco (1980).

Figure 8F shows the typical intermediate filament staining pattern on gerbil fibroma cells seen by the use of a monoclonal antibody (JLB7) against a 95K protein component of these filaments. The intermediate filaments are concentrated around the nucleus, from which they appear to extend into the cell periphery.

Some of the monoclonal antibodies against components of microfilaments have been used to isolate native microfilaments from cultured cells by immunoprecipitation. Some experiments of this nature will be discussed in the next

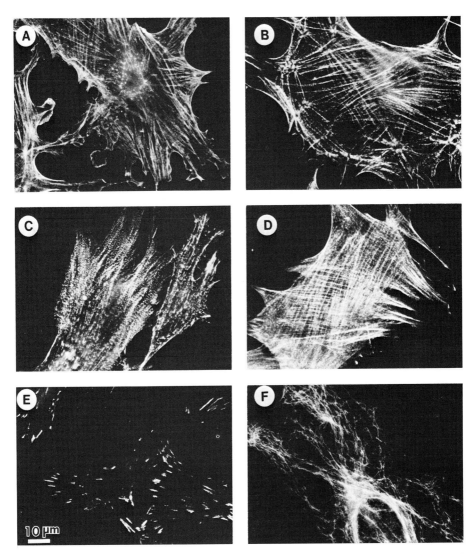

FIGURE 8. Immunofluorescence analysis of cytoskeletal proteins. Indirect immunofluorescence with monoclonal antibodies was used to show the distributions of several cytoskeletal proteins in gerbil fibroma cells (A, B, and F) or chicken embryo fibroblasts (C–E). (A) A monoclonal antibody JLA20 against actin; (B) a monoclonal antibody JLF15 against tropomyosin; (C) a monoclonal antibody JLN20 against α-actinin; (D) a monoclonal antibody JLA8 against filamin; (E) a monoclonal antibody JLK6 against vinculin; and (F) a monoclonal antibody JLB7 against 95 K intermediate-filament-associated protein.

section. The monoclonal antibody JLB7 has been used in conjunction with microinjection technique to disrupt specifically the *in vivo* distribution of the intermediate filaments (Lin and Feramisco, 1981) and to assess the physiological functions of the intermediate filaments (see Section VIII).

VI. Use of Monoclonal Antibodies to Isolate and Characterize Microfilaments from Tissue Culture Cells

Monoclonal antibodies provide an essentially unlimited reagent with constant specificity to a particular antigen. Secher and Burke (1980) have recently reported that monoclonal antibodies against human leukocyte interferon can be used to purify biologically active interferon by immunoadsorption chromatography. Sarnow *et al.* (1982) have also used a monoclonal antibody against a cellular 54,000-dalton protein that precipitates a complex of T antigen (54,000 dalton) from SV40-transformed cells and a complex of an adenovirus EIb protein (58,000 daltons) with the same 54,000-dalton protein from adenovirus-infected cells. We have used antitropomyosin monoclonal antibody to precipitate apparently native thin filaments from smooth muscle cells and to directly observe, for the first time, the organization of tropomyosin molecules along the thin filaments (Matsumura and Lin, 1982). As will be discussed in the following paragraphs, a similar method is now being applied to isolate microfilaments from cultured nonmuscle cells.

Microfilaments appear to play central roles in cell motility and cell shape changes in nonmuscle cells. One of our goals in studying the function of microfilaments is to determine the protein composition or ultrastructural organization of the microfilaments concomitant with changes in biological activities such as spreading, mitosis, movement, and transformation, for example. For this purpose, it is necessary to isolate microfilaments in intact form from cultured cells. We have chosen to use several antitropomyosin monoclonal antibodies (JLF15, LCK16) to isolate intact microfilaments, for the following reasons: (1) tropomyosin is one of the most abundant components of microfilaments, making it suitable as an antigen for immunoprecipitation of the microfilaments; and (2) monoclonal antibodies to tropomyosin cause the aggregation of microfilaments into ordered bundles, which can be easily collected by low-speed centrifugation.

The procedure to isolate microfilaments is simple and rapid. Briefly, monolayer cells are first extracted with Triton X-100/glycerol solution to stabilize the cytoskeleton and then homogenized in the presence of Mg-ATP. After centrifugation, the supernatant is incubated with monoclonal antibodies against tropomyosin. Microfilaments present in the supernatant become aggregated into ordered bundles by the antibodies (see below, Figure 12A), and the resultant bundles are collected by low-speed centrifugation. The bundles can be analyzed by a variety of methods, including electron microscopy, biochemical methods such as SDS polyacrylamide gel analysis, and enzymatically by their actin-activated myosin ATPase activity. The isolated microfilaments appear to be native with respect to the following criteria: (1) they have the typical filament

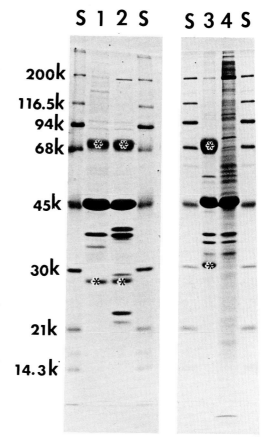

FIGURE 9. Immunoprecipitation of thin filaments. A 12.5% polyacrylamide gel analysis of thin filament fractions isolated from 18-day-old chicken embryo smooth muscle (gizzard, lane 1) and skeletal muscle (leg, lane 2), and microfilament fraction isolated from secondary culture of chicken embryo fibroblasts (lane 3) prepared by immunoprecipitation with monoclonal antibody JLF15 (lanes 1 and 2) or LCK16 (lane 3) against tropomyosin is shown. In lane 4, the supernatant of total cytoskeletal proteins from chicken embryo fibroblasts after low-speed centrifugation (12,800 × g, 15 min) is displayed. This supernatant fraction was incubated with the monoclonal antibody LCK16 for 30 min at room temperature. Microfilaments in the supernatant became aggregated into bundles and were collected by low-speed centrifugation (12,800 × g, 5 min). After three washes, the microfilaments were analyzed by SDS gels (lane 3). Lane S shows molecular weight standard proteins. Asterisks on lanes 1–3 indicate the heavy and light chains of monoclonal antibody. Different isoforms of tropomyosin (protein bands between the 45 K and 30 K standard proteins) exist among smooth muscle, skeletal muscle, and nonmuscle cells.

morphology of a double helical structure with a periodic arrangement of tropomyosin on the actin filaments; and (2) the microfilament fraction can activate the myosin ATPase activity to nearly the same extent as skeletal muscle F-actin can activate the ATPase. Figure 9 shows SDS polyacrylamide gel analysis of the isolated microfilament fraction from chick embryo skeletal muscle (leg), smooth muscle (gizzard), and fibroblasts.

One potential problem with the isolation of microfilaments by this method is that we do not yet know if the microfilaments are altered in any way during the Triton–glycerol extraction or the immunoprecipitation. However, by using antibodies directed against different components of the microfilaments, and by using cells of varying biological states as the source of microfilaments, we hope to resolve this problem. To date, we have been able to isolate microfilaments from various cell types, such as rat embryo fibroblasts and their SV40-transformed counterparts, gerbil fibroma, chicken embryo fibroblasts, BHK-21 cells, L6 myoblasts and myotubes, and chicken embryo myoblasts and myotubes. We have not been able to isolate microfilaments as yet from HeLa cells and HL-60 cells (round cells). A comparison of these microfilament fractions as well as the use of other monoclonal antibodies (such as antifilamin, anti-α-actinin, and antivinculin) to isolate microfilament fractions is in progress in our laboratory.

VII. Monoclonal Antibody Decoration of the Cytoskeleton at the Ultrastructural Level

Conventional immunoelectron microscopy has employed monospecific polyclonal antibodies, which have been visualized in several ways. The simplest method has been used by Pepe (1973, 1975), in which permeabilized muscle strips are stained with antibody, thin-sectioned, and examined in the electron microscope. When compared to controls the periodic distribution of antibody could be observed. This method has been used to decorate intermediate filaments, which were then examined by negative staining with uranyl acetate (Willard and Simon, 1981; Schlaepfer, 1977) or by deep etching of decorated cytoskeletons (Heuser and Kirschner, 1980). Willard and Simon (1981) probed the molecular structure of neurofilaments with an anti-195K antibody. They found the antibody decorated the filaments in a helical fashion with a 140-nm repeat. Monoclonal antibodies have the advantage over conventional antibodies in recognizing only one antigenic determinant. Therefore, one can expect to obtain high resolution in localizing that single determinant within cytoskeletal filament systems by electron microscopy. We have used three different monoclonal antibodies against tropomyosin to localize this antigen along smooth muscle thin filaments (Matsumura and Lin, 1982) and microfilaments from nonmuscle cells.

We have decorated cytoskeletal microfilaments and intermediate (10-nm-diameter) filaments with a monoclonal antibody, LCK16 (Blose *et al.*, 1982), as seen in Figures 10–12. LCK16, an IgM, was found to be easily visualized because of its large size (~30 nm diameter; $M_r \approx 900,000$). In cytoskeletons decorated with LCK16 and thin-sectioned, the antibody can be observed more easily by including tannic acid in the staining protocol (Figures 10 and 11). Tannic acid acts primarily as a mordant between osmium-treated structures and the lead stain (Mizuhira and Futaesaku, 1971; Simionescu and Simionescu, 1976). As Figure 12A shows, monoclonal antibodies caused the aggregation of microfilaments from REF52 rat embryo fibroblasts into ordered bundles that displayed cross-striations with a periodicity of 36 ± 1 nm. In contrast, conventional rabbit antiserum to tropomyosin distorted and aggregated the thin filaments without generating cross-striations (Figure 12B). Thus, monoclonal antibodies to tropomyosin allow us for the first time to observe directly the distribution of tropomyosin molecules along microfilaments of cultured cells. A similar approach with the use of other monoclonal antibodies that we have prepared will be applied to show the ultrastructural arrangement of other cytoskeletal proteins, such as α-actinin, filamin, and vinculin, along microfilaments.

These simple methods of staining with an unmodified antibody lend themselves to well-ordered structures of the cytoskeleton. However, if antigens are

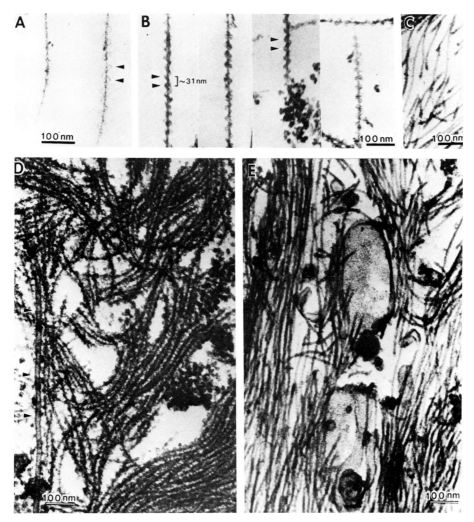

FIGURE 10. Ultrastructure of antibody-decorated cytoskeletons. Electron micrographs of 10-nm filaments in gerbil fibroma cells decorated with mouse monoclonal antibody LCK16 are given. All micrographs are of thin-sectioned (60- to 80-nm thick) specimens. (A) Two examples of single 10-nm filaments decorated with LCK16 in which tannic acid was excluded from the fixation protocol. The filaments decorate with a very fine lace of antibody, and in some regions a helix or period can be seen (arrowheads). (B) Several examples of single 10-nm filaments decorated with LCK16 and fixed with tannic acid. The antibody decorates the filaments in a periodic-helical fashion (arrowheads) that is more clearly observed by the inclusion of the tannic acid stain (compare B to A). The antibody decorates the filaments with a period of ~31 nm. (C) A control in which 10-nm filaments were incubated with JLA20 monoclonal against actin and stained with tannic acid. As expected, the 10-nm filaments did not decorate with the actin antibody. (D) An aggregate of 10-nm filaments (produced by colcemid treatment) decorated with LCK16 antibody and stained with tannic acid. All of the 10-nm filaments are coated with the antibody in a helical-periodic fashion. A single microtubule (arrowheads) can be seen in this section, which is not decorated. (E) A control to that in (D), showing aggregated 10-nm filaments after incubation with JLA20 antiactin and staining with tannic acid; again, the 10-nm filaments are not decorated with JLA20.

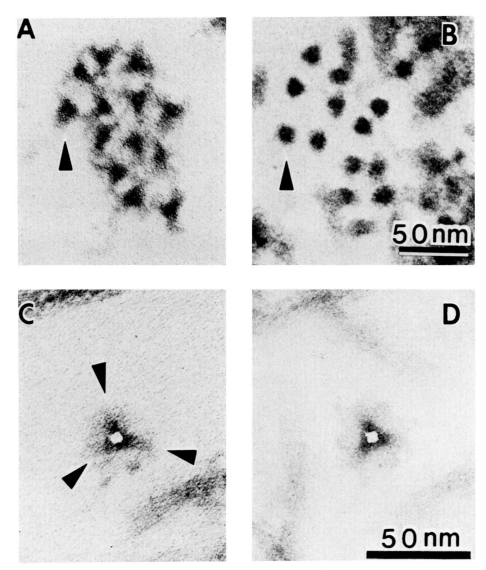

FIGURE 11. Cross sections of antibody-decorated cytoskeletons. Electron micrographs of cross-sectional profiles of 10-nm filaments in gerbil fibroma cells decorated with mouse monoclonal antibody LCK16 and stained with tannic acid are shown. (A) A cluster of 10-nm filaments decorated with LCK16, which reveals that the antibody imparts a triangular profile to the individual filaments (arrowhead) when compared to the control in (B). The antibody produces small surface projections at the "points" of the triangle that appear to link adjacent filaments. (B) A control in which 10-nm filaments were incubated with a monoclonal antibody to actin (JLA20; Lin, 1981). No decoration can be observed; instead the filament profiles remain round and individual filaments (arrowhead) measure ~10 nm in diameter (9.9 ± 2.1 nm). (C) A single 10-nm filament decorated with LCK16 showing the triangular profile. Arrowheads indicate the points of the triangle produced by antibody decoration. Each point protrudes ~12.2 nm off the surface of the 10-nm filament. The filament in (C) was used for Markham rotation (Markham et al., 1963) as indicated in (D). (D) The triangular profile of an LCK16-decorated 10-nm filament, reinforced by three 120° angle Markham rotations.

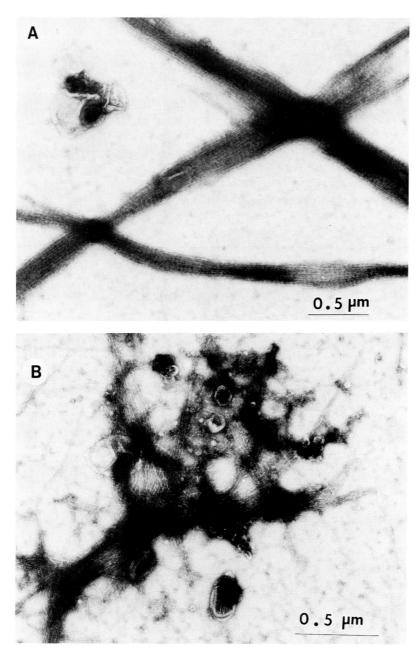

FIGURE 12. Ultrastructure of microfilaments decorated with a monoclonal antibody. Electron micrographs of rat embryo fibroblast (REF52) microfilaments incubated with monoclonal antibodies (A) or polyclonal rabbit antibody to tropomyosin (B) and negatively stained with 2% aqueous uranyl acetate are given. LCK16 causes the microfilaments to laterally aggregate into bundles. The LCK16 antibody also decorates the microfilaments with a prominent ~36-nm periodicity. The periodicity is interpreted to correspond to the length of a tropomyosin molecule on the actin filament. When the microfilaments are incubated with a polyclonal rabbit antiserum to tropomyosin, amorphous clumps of microfilaments are generated.

more diffusely distributed in the cytoplasm, in small amounts, or on membranes, more complicated methods to locate the bound antibody are necessary. For these applications, methods commonly used include: (1) ferritin-conjugated primary antibody or Fab fragments (Kishida *et al.*, 1975); (2) the ferritin bridge method (Willingham *et al.*, 1971, 1979); (3) PAP, the peroxidase–antiperoxidase technique (Sternberger *et al.*, 1970); and (4) the iron–dextran antibody conjugates of Dutton *et al.* (1979). Each of these methods produces an electron-dense product, which allows visualization of the antibody location over background staining. To improve preservation of ultrastructural morphology and fix more labile structures, and allow better antibody penetration into cellular structures, fixation and permeabilization should be conducted according to protocols of Willingham *et al.* (1978) and Willingham and Yamada (1979).

VIII. Microinjection of Monoclonal Antibodies into Living Cells

Efforts to understand the functional roles of cytoskeleton proteins in living cells require techniques that complement and even extend beyond those that utilize fixed cells (e.g., immunofluorescence or electron microscopy) or cell homogenates or purified proteins (e.g., *in vitro* biochemistry). This is so because of the difficulty in the interpretation and application of data derived from dead or disrupted cells in terms of living cell functions. As discussed here, through the microinjection of defined monoclonal antibodies into living cells with the aim of blocking the function(s) of the antigen(s) *in vivo*, it is possible to deduce the function(s) of the antigen(s) in their natural environment. It should be noted that one is not restricted to the injection of monoclonal antibodies into living cells (Lin and Feramisco, 1981; Klymkowski, 1981), as it is possible to use conventional polyclonal antibodies as well (Mabuchi and Okuno, 1977; Yamaizumi *et al.*, 1978; Antman and Livingston, 1980).

With the basic strategy being to introduce by either microneedle injection (for review, see Graessmann *et al.*, 1980; Diacumakos, 1978; Wang *et al.*, 1982) or liposome- or red cell-mediated fusion (Gregoria, 1976; Schlegel and Rechsteiner, 1975) sufficient antibody to complex with all of the target antigen in the cell, several considerations must first be taken into account. These will be discussed in light of our studies on the function of intermediate filaments through the microneedle injection of antibodies that recognize 95,000-dalton-protein (clone JLB7) and 220,000-dalton-protein (clone JLB1) components of these filaments (Lin and Feramisco, 1981).

First, the antibody to be used should be documented by some acceptable analysis as to its specificity and purity. This can be done with a variety of methods, including immunoprecipitation, immunoautoradiography of SDS polyacrylamide gels, or affinity chromatography (see Section III). We utilized, for example, immunoprecipitation and immunofluorescence to document the specificity of the two antibodies, JLB1 and JLB7, that recognize two distinct intermediate filament proteins (Lin, 1981). Second, some estimate of the amount of the antigen present in an average cell must be made. One of the ways to accomplish this is by analysis of two-dimensional gels (O'Farrell, 1975; Garrels, 1979) of total cell lysates of a known number of cells. This type of analysis indicated that in the case of the 95,000-dalton intermediate filament protein recognized by the antibody JLB7, there was about 10^5-10^6 molecules of the 95K protein in a single cell (Lin and Feramisco, 1981). Typical amounts of other proteins in cells might range from 10^3 to 10^8 molecules per cell. Other factors to be considered initially are the antibody concentration and volume to be introduced into each cell. By microneedle injection, a typical fibroblast can be injected with $10^{-13}-10^{-14}$ ml of solution (Graessmann *et al.*, 1980; Stacey and Allfrey, 1976). Using an antibody concentration of 10–20 mg/ml, it is possible to introduce up to 10^7 molecules of antibody per cell, a sufficient amount to complex with all of a given antigen in the case of many cellular proteins.

There are at least two additional parameters that are important to consider in these types of experiments but are somewhat out of the investigator's control. The first is the accessibility of the antigen in the cell to the injected antibody. If the antigenic site on the target protein is not available to the antibody because of, for example, its involvement in some other interaction, one may not observe any effect on the cell caused by the antibody. This problem must be carefully examined in the case of a negative result after injection of an antibody (e.g., Wehland *et al.*, 1981) before the data can be interpreted. The second parameter involves the effect that the antibody has on the function of the antigen by virtue of the complexation reaction. Ideally, one can determine if a given monoclonal antibody inhibits some measurable biochemical activity of the antigen and can correlate the inhibition with an observable or measurable effect on the cell after introduction of the antibody into the cell. In some cases, however, the antigen may not have a known activity; thus, it is impossible to determine the *in vitro* effect of the antibody on the antigen. Just as is the case in which the antibody does not have access to the antigen in the cell, when the antibody complexes with the antigen but does not interfere with the activity of the antigen (whatever that activity may be), the injected antibody may not have an effect on the cell.

We have examined the effects on intermediate filaments of two monoclonal antibodies directed against minor components of these filaments (Lin, 1981) by the microinjection technique (Lin and Feramisco, 1981). Immunofluorescence staining of fibroblasts by the antibodies JLB1 and JLB7 shows their distribution on the intermediate filaments (e.g., see Figure 8F for the staining by JLB7). After microinjection of JLB1 (specific for the 220,000-dalton protein), double-label immunofluorescence indicated that while the injected antibody binds to the intermediate filaments (Figure 13B), no obvious change in the typical distribution of these filaments occurs (as indicated by staining with an antivimentin antibody) (Fig. 13C). However, within minutes after injection of JLB7 (specific for the 95,000-dalton protein), a dramatic reorganization of the intermediate filaments occurs (Figure 13E). The filaments are now found in a tight aggregate near the nuclei of the injected cells. Inspection of these cells by electron microscopy (thin sections) reveals what appear to be antibody cross-links along the lengths of the filaments, in the aggregates. Similar results have been obtained by Klymkowski (1981) through the injection of a monoclonal antibody to vimentin.

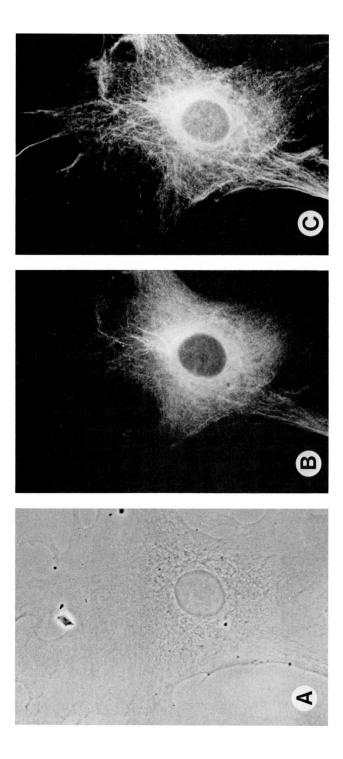

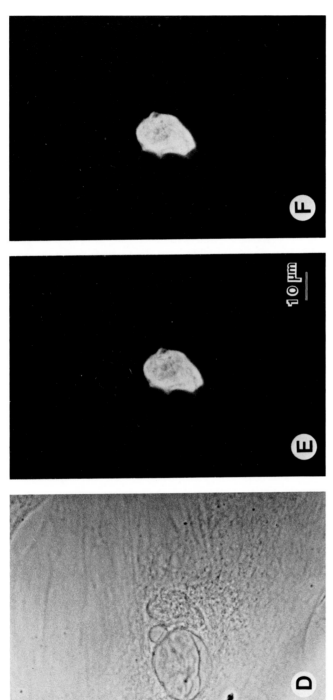

FIGURE 13. Microinjection of monoclonal antibodies to the intermediate filaments. Gerbil fibroma cells were microinjected with either JLB1 (A–C) or JLB7 (D–F) monoclonal antibody and, 3 hr after injection, counterstained with rabbit antibody against vimentin. The distributions of injected mouse antibody and vimentin were detected by double-label immunofluorescence by a mixture of second antibodies containing fluorescein-conjugated goat anti-mouse IgG and rhodamine-conjugated goat anti-rabbit IgG. (A, D) Phase-contrast micrographs. (B, E) Injected cells viewed selectively for fluorescein fluorescence to allow the microinjected mouse antibody to be visualized. (C, F) The same fields seen in (B) and (E), respectively, except viewed selectively for rhodamine fluorescence to allow the distribution of vimentin to be visualized.

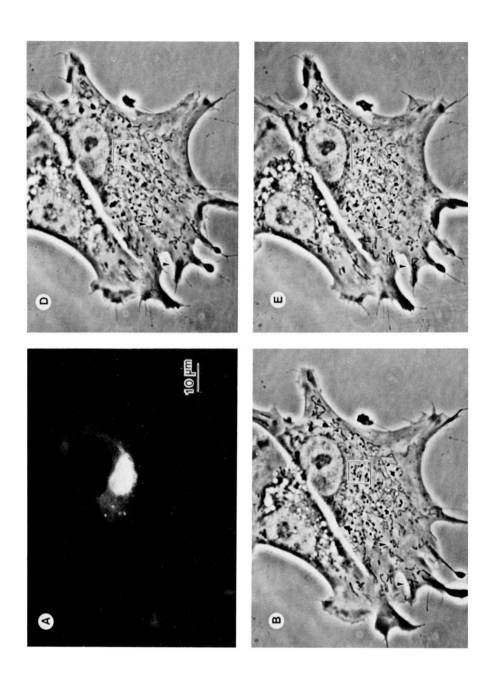

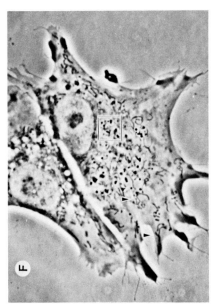

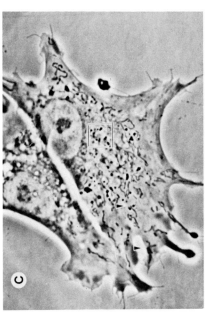

FIGURE 14. Organelle movements in cells lacking a normal intermediate filament distribution. A sequence of micrographs of the JLB7 antibody-injected and control gerbil fibroma cells is given. (A) The fluorescence micrograph, which allows for the visualization of the intermediate filaments in the living cell. (B–F) Phase-contrast micrographs of the cells in the same field as in (A). The relative time points for (B)–(F) are 0, 2, 4, 8, and 10 min, respectively. A variety of saltatory movements are apparent: dark granules and mitochondria (for example, those close to the arrowheads) can be seen to move about as in the control cell. Ruffles and blebs at the cell periphery undergo dynamic displacements, rearrangements, and extensions as in the control cell. In contrast, the granules within the indicated square boxes appeared nonmotile within this 10-min period: it is possible that these granules were trapped within the aggregates of the intermediate filaments.

Given that the injection of the monoclonal antibody JLB7 results in the essentially complete reorganization of the intermediate filaments in living cells, it is possible to search for biological effects of the reorganization of these filaments. Analysis of the distributions of the other two known filamentous networks in these cells, microfilaments and microtubules, suggests that neither of these two networks was altered by the intermediate filament reorganization (Lin and Feramisco, 1981). Organelle movements (Figure 14) (i.e., saltatory motion), cell shape and polarity, and cell respreading also seem normal in spite of the thoughts that the intermediate filaments may be involved in some or all of these phenomena (R. D. Goldman and Knipe, 1972; Wang and Goldman, 1978; Wang *et al.*, 1979). Thus, while the biological effects of the loss of the intermediate filaments from the normal cytoplasmic array are not known, it is hoped that by analysis of mitotic cells or cells that undergo differentiation (e.g., myoblasts-myotubes) the effects may become apparent.

ACKNOWLEDGMENTS

The authors wish to express their gratitude to J. D. Watson, who has supported this work with enthusiasm. We thank J. I. Garrels for running the two-dimensional gels and S. Matsumura for help in the purification of microfilaments; and S. Queally, T. Lukralle, P. Renna, N. Haffner, D. Meltzer, B. McLaughlin, and J. Leibold for expert technical assistance. The patience of M. Szadkowski in typing this manuscript is also greatly appreciated. This work was supported in part by NIH Grants GM28277 (to J. R. F.), GM31048 (to J. J. C. L.), NHLBI-HL23848-04 (to S. H. B.), by Muscular Dystrophy Association Grants (to J. J. C. L. and S. H. B.), by a grant from American Heart Association—Nassau Chapter (to S. H. B.), by a Muscular Dystrophy Association Postdoctoral Fellowship (to F. M.), and by Grant CA 13106 to the Cold Spring Harbor Laboratory from the National Cancer Institute.

References

Antman, K. H., and Livingston, D. M., 1980, Intracellular neutralization of SV40 tumor antigens following microinjection of specific antibody, *Cell* **19:**627–635.

Atherton, B. T., and Hynes, R. O., 1981, A difference between plasma and cellular fibronectins located with monoclonal antibodies, *Cell* **25:**133–141.

Bader, D., Masaki, T., and Fischman, D. A., 1981, Myosin isoform transitions during chick myogenesis, *J. Cell Biol.* **91:**352a.

Blose, S. H. and Meltzer, D. I., 1981, Visualization of the 10 nm filament-vimentin rings in vascular endothelial cells *in situ:* Close resemblance to vimentin cytoskeletons found in monolayers *in vitro*, *Exp. Cell Res.* **135:**299–309.

Blose, S. H., Matsumura, F., and Lin, J. J. C., 1982, The structure of vimentin—10 nm filaments probed with a monoclonal antibody that recognizes a common antigenic determinant on vimentin and tropomyosin, *Cold Spring Harbor Symp. Quant. Biol.* **46:**455–463.

Bonner, W. M., and Laskey, R. A., 1974, A film detection method for tritium-labelled proteins and nucleic acids in polyacrylamide gels, *Eur. J. Biochem.* **46:**83–88.

Burridge, K., 1978, Direct identification of specific glycoproteins and antigens in sodium dodecyl sulfate gels, in: *Methods in Enzymology*, Volume 50, Academic Press, New York, pp. 54–64.

Burridge, K., and Feramisco, J. R., 1980, Microinjection and localization of a 130K protein in living fibroblasts: A relationship to actin and fibronectin, *Cell* **19**:587–595.

Dellago, K., Brouet, J. C., Perreau, J., and Paulin, D., 1982, Human monoclonal IgM with autoantibody activity against intermediate filaments, *Proc. Natl. Acad. Sci. USA* **79**:446–450.

Diacumakos, E. G., 1978, Methods for micromanipulation of human somatic cells in culture, *Methods Cell Biol.* **7**:287–311.

Dulbecco, R., Unger, M., Bologna, M., Battifora, H., Syka, P., and Okada, S., 1981, Cross-reactivity between Thy-1 and a component of intermediate filaments demonstrated using a monoclonal antibody, *Nature* **292**:772–774.

Dutton, A. H., Tokuyasu, K. T., and Singer, S. J., 1979, Iron-dextran antibody conjugates: General method for simultaneous staining of two components in high-resolution immunoelectron microscopy, *Proc. Natl. Acad. Sci. USA* **76**:3392–3396.

Ey, P. L., Prowse, S. J., and Jenkin, C. R., 1978, Isolation of pure IgG$_1$, IgG$_{2a}$, and IgG$_{2b}$ immunoglobulins from mouse serum using protein A–sepharose, *Immunochemistry* **15**:429–436.

Feramisco, J. R., and Blose, S. H., 1980, Distribution of fluorescently labeled alpha-actinin in living and fixed fibroblasts, *J. Cell Biol.* **86**:608–615.

Garrels, J. I., 1979, Two-dimensional gel electrophoresis and computer analysis of proteins synthesized by clonal cell lines, *J. Biol. Chem.* **254**:7961–7977.

Geiger, B., 1979, A 130K protein from chicken gizzard: Its localization at the termini of microfilament bundles in cultured chicken cells, *Cell* **18**:193–205.

Geisler, N., and Weber, K., 1981, Comparison of the proteins of two immunologically distinct intermediate-sized filaments by amino acid sequence analysis: Desmin and vimentin, *Proc. Natl. Acad. Sci. USA* **78**:4120–4123.

Goding, J. W., 1978, Use of staphylococcal protein A as an immunological reagent, *J. Immunol. Methods* **29**: 241–253.

Goldman, R., Pollard, T., and Rosenbaum, J. (eds.), 1976, *Cold Spring Harbor Conference on Cell Proliferation*, Books A–C, Cold Spring Harbor, New York.

Goldman, R. D., and Knipe, D. M., 1972, The functions of cytoplasmic fibers in non-muscle cell motility, *Cold Spring Harbor Symp. Quant. Biol.* **37**:523–533.

Goldman, R. D., Chojnack, B., and Yerna, M.-J., 1979, Ultrastructure or microfilament bundles in baby hamster kidney (BHK-21) cells, *J. Cell Biol.* **80**:759–766.

Gordon, W. E., and Blose, S. H., 1979, Double lable immunofluorescence studies of actin, myosin, tropomyosin, alpha-actinin, and filamin in a non-muscle cell type, *J. Supramol. Struct.* **10**(Suppl.): 111.

Gordon, W. E., Bushnell, A., and Burridge, K., 1977, Characterization of the intermediate (10 nm) filaments of cultured cells using an autoimmune rabbit antiserum, *Cell* **13**:249–261.

Graessmann, A., Graessmann, M., and Mueller, C., 1980, Microinjection of early SV40 DNA fragments and T-antigen, in: *Methods in Enzymology*, Volume 65, Academic Press, New York, pp. 816–826.

Gregoria, G., 1976, The carrier potential of liposomes in biology and medicine, *N. Engl. J. Med.* **295**:704–710, 765–770.

Herrmann, S. H., and Mescher, M. F., 1979, Purification of the H-2K^k molecule of the murine major histocompatibility complex, *J. Biol. Chem.* **254**:8713–8716.

Heuser, J. E., and Kirschner, M. W., 1980, Filament organization revealed in platinum replicas of freeze-dried cytoskeletons, *J. Cell Biol.* **86**:212–234.

Izant, J. G., and McIntosh, J. R., 1980, Microtubule-associated proteins: A monoclonal antibody to MAP-2 binds to differentiated neurons, *Proc. Natl. Acad. Sci. USA* **77**:4741–4745.

Kessler, S. W., 1975, Rapid isolation of antigens from cells with a staphylococcal protein A–antibody adsorbent: Parameters of the interaction of antibody–antigen complexes with protein A, *J. Immunol.* **115**:1617–1624.

Kishida, Y., Olsen, B. R., Berg, R. A., and Prockop, D. J., 1975, Two improved methods for preparing ferritin–protein conjugates for electron microscopy, *J. Cell Biol.* **64**:331–339.

Klymkowsky, M. W., 1981, Intermediate filaments in 3T3 cells collapse after intracellular injection of a monoclonal anti-intermediate filament antibody, *Nature* **291**:249–251.

Kohler, G., and Milstein, C., 1975, Continuous cultures of fused cells secreting antibody of pre-defined specificity, *Nature* **256**:495–497.

Kurki, P., Linder, E., Virtanen, I., and Stenman, S., 1977, Human smooth muscle autoantibodies reacting with intermediate (100 Å) filaments, *Nature* **268**:240–241.

Lane, D., and Koprowski, H., 1982, Molecular recognition and the future of monoclonal antibodies, *Nature* **296**:200–202.

Lane, E. B., 1982, Monoclonal antibodies provide specific intramolecular markers for the study of epithelial tonofilament organization, *J. Cell Biol.* **92**:665–673.

Lazarides, E., 1975, Tropomyosin antibody: The specific localization of tropomyosin in nonmuscle cells, *J. Cell Biol.* **65**:549–561.

Lazarides, E., 1976, Actin, alpha-actinin, and tropomyosin interaction in the structural organization of actin filaments in nonmuscle cells, *J. Cell Biol.* **68**:202–219.

Lazarides, E., and Burridge, K., 1975, Alpha-actinin: Immunofluorescent localization of a muscle structural protein in nonmuscle cells, *Cell* **6**:289–298.

Lazarides, E., and Weber, K., 1974, Actin antibody: The specific visualization of actin filaments in non-muscle cells, *Proc. Natl. Acad. Sci. USA* **71**:2268–2272.

Lin, J. J. C., 1981, Monoclonal antibodies against myofibrillar components of rat skeletal muscle decorate the intermediate filaments of cultured cells, *Proc. Natl. Acad. Sci. USA* **78**:2335–2339.

Lin, J. J. C., 1982, Mapping structural proteins of cultured cells by monoclonal antibodies, *Cold Spring Harbor Symp. Quant. Biol.* **46**:769–783.

Lin, J. J. C., and Feramisco, J. R., 1981, Disruption of the *in vivo* distribution of the intermediate filaments in fibroblasts through the microinjection of a specific monoclonal antibody, *Cell* **24**:185–193.

Lin, J. J. C., and Queally, S. A., 1982, A monoclonal antibody that recognizes Golgi-associated protein of cultured fibroblast cells, *J. Cell Biol.* **92**:108–112.

Lin, J. J. C., Burridge, K., Blose, S. H., Bushnell, A., Queally, S. A., and Feramisco, J. R., 1982, Use of monoclonal antibodies to study cytoskeleton, in: *Cell and Muscle Motility*, Volume 2 (R. M. Dowben and J. W. Shay, eds.), Plenum Press, New York, pp. 63–71.

Lwebuga-Mukasa, J. S., Lappi, S., and Taylor, P., 1976, Molecular forms of acetylcholinesterase from *Torpedo californica:* Their relationship to synaptic membranes, *Biochemistry* **15**:1425–1434.

Mabuchi, F., and Okuno, M., 1977, The effect of myosin antibody on the division of starfish blastomeres, *J. Cell Biol.* **74**:251–264.

Markham, R., Trey, S., and Hills, G. J., 1963, Methods for the enhancement of image detail and accentuation of structure in electron microscopy, *Virology* **20**:88–102.

Matsumura, F., and Lin, J. J. C., 1982, Visualization of monoclonal antibody binding to tropomyosin on native smooth muscle thin filaments by electron microscopy, *J. Mol. Biol.* **157**:163–171.

Medgyesi, G. A., Fust, G., Gergely, J., and Bazin, H., 1978, Classes and subclasses of rat immunoglobulins: Interaction with the complement system and with staphylococcal protein A., *Immunochemistry* **15**:125–129.

Miller, D. M., Mackenzie, J. M., Bolton, L. H., and Epstein, H. F., 1981, Monoclonal antibodies to nematode myosin heavy chain isozymes, *J. Cell Biol.* **91**:346a.

Mizuhira, V., and Futaesaku, Y., 1971, On the new approach of tannic acid and digitonine to the biological fixation, in: *Procedings of the 29th Annual Meeting of the Electron Microscopy Society of America* (G. W. Bailey, eds.), Claitor's Publishing Division, Boston, pp. 494–495.

O'Farrell, P. H., 1975, High resolution two-dimensional electrophoresis of proteins, *J. Biol. Chem.* **250**:4007–4021.

Osborn, M., Franke, W. W., and Weber, K., 1977, Visualization of a system of filaments 7–10 nm thick in cultured cells of an epithelioid line (PtK2) by immunofluorescence microscopy, *Proc. Natl. Acad. Sci. USA* **74**:2490–2494.

Osborn, M., Geisler, N., Shaw, G., Sharp, G., and Weber, K., 1982, Intermediate filaments, *Cold Spring Harbor Symp. Quant. Biol.* **46**:413–429.

Pepe, F. A., 1966, Some aspects of the structural organization of myofibril as revealed by antibody staining method, *J. Cell Biol.* **28**:505–525.

Pepe, F. A., 1973, The myosin filament: Immunochemical and ultrastructural approaches to molecular organization, *Cold Spring Harbor Symp. Quant. Biol.* **37**:97–108.

Pepe, F. A., 1975, Structure of muscle filaments from immunohistochemical and ultrastructural studies, *J. Histochem. Cytochem.* **23**:543–562.

Porter, R. R., and Reid, K. B. M., 1978, The biochemistry of complement, *Nature* **275**:699–704.

Pruss, R. M., Mirsky, R., Raff, M. C., Thorpe, R., Dowding, A. M., and Anderton, B. H., 1981, All classes of intermediate filaments share a common antigenic determinant defined by a monoclonal antibody, *Cell* **27**:419–428.

Reid, K. B. M., 1974, A collagen-like amino acid sequence in a polypeptide chain of human C1q (a subcomponent of the first component of complement), *Biochem. J.* **141**:189–203.

Reid, K. B. M., 1979, Complete amino acid sequences of the three collagen-like regions present in subcomponent C1q of the first component of human complement, *Biochem. J.* **179**:367–371.

Sarnow, P., Ho, Y. S., Williams, J., and Levine, A. J., 1982, Adenovirus E1b-58kd tumor antigen and SV40 large tumor antigen are physically associated with the same 54kd cellular protein in transformed cells, *Cell* **28**:387–394.

Schlaepfer, W. W., 1977, Immunological and ultrastructural studies of neurofilaments, *J. Cell Biol.* **74**:226–240.

Schlegel, R. A., and Rechsteiner, M. C., 1975, Microinjection of thymidine kinase and bovine serum albumin into mammalian cells by fusion with red blood cells, *Cell* **5**:371–379.

Secher, D. S., and Burke, D. C., 1980, A monoclonal antibody for large-scale purification of human leukocyte interferon, *Nature* **285**:446–450.

Simionescu, N., and Simionescu, M., 1976, Galloylglucoses of low molecular weight as mordant in electron microscopy, *J. Cell Biol.* **70**:608–633.

Stacey, D. W., and Allfrey, V. G., 1977, Evidence for the autophagy of microinjected proteins in HeLa cells, *J. Cell Biol.* **75**:807–817.

Sternberger, L. A., Hardy, R. H., Cuculis, J. J., and Meyer, H. G., 1970, The unlabeled antibody enzyme method of immunohistochemistry: Preparation and properties of soluble antigen–antibody complex (horseradish peroxidase–antihorseradish peroxidase) and its use in identification of spirochetes, *J. Histochem. Cytochem.* **18**:315–333.

Towbin, H., Staehelin, T., and Gordon, J., 1979, Electrophoretic transfer of proteins from polyacrylamide gels to nitrocellulose sheets: Procedure and some applications, *Proc. Natl. Acad. Sci. USA* **76**:4350–4354.

Wang, E., and Goldman, R. D., 1978, Functions of the cytoplasmic fibers in intracellular movements in BHK21 cells, *J. Cell Biol.* **79**:708–726.

Wang, E., Cross, R. K., and Choppin, R. W., 1979, Involvement of microtubules and 10 nm filaments in the movement and positioning of nuclei in syncytia, *J. Cell Biol.* **83**:320–337.

Wang, K., Feramisco, J. R., and Ash, J. F., 1982, Fluorescent localization of contractile proteins in tissue culture cells, in: *Methods in Enzymology*, Volume 85, Academic Press, New York, pp. 514–562.

Wehland, J., Willingham, M. C., Dickson, R., and Pastan, I., 1981, Microinjection of anticlathrin antibodies into fibroblasts does not interfere with the receptor-mediated endocytosis of alpha$_2$-macroglobulin, *Cell* **25**:105–119.

Willard, M., and Simon, C., 1981, Antibody decoration of neurofilaments, *J. Cell Biol.* **89**:198–205.

Willingham, M. C., and Yamada, S. S., 1979, Development of a new primary fixative for electron microscopic immunocytochemical localization of intracellular antigens in cultured cells, *J. Histochem. Cytochem.* **27**:947–960.

Willingham, M. C., Spicer, S. S., and Graber, C. D., 1971, Immunocytologic labeling of calf and human lymphocyte surface antigens, *Lab. Invest.* **25**:211–219.

Willingham, M. C., Yamada, S. S., and Pastan, I., 1978, Ultrastructural antibody localization of alpha$_2$-macroglobulin in membrane-limited vesicles in cultured cells, *Proc. Natl. Acad. Sci. USA* **75**:4359–4363.

Willingham, M. C., Jay, G., and Pastan, I., 1979, Localization of the ASV *src* gene product to the plasma membrane of transformed cells by electron microscopic immunocytochemistry, *Cell* **18**:125–134.

Yamaizumi, M., Uchida, T., Okada, Y., and Furusawa, M., 1978, Neutralization of diphtheria toxin in living cells by microinjection of antifragment A contained within resealed erythrocyte ghosts, *Cell* **13**:222–232.

7

Molecular Bases of Neuronal Individuality

Lessons from Anatomical and Biochemical Studies with Monoclonal Antibodies

LOIS ALTERMAN LAMPSON

I. Introduction

Monoclonal antibody analysis has been particularly welcome for studies of the nervous system. The number of cell types, their delicate and often extensive processes, their dense interconnections, and the inability of mature cells to divide *in vitro* make it particularly difficult to obtain separated subpopulations for conventional immunization or antibody purification. Thus, the possibility of obtaining cell-type-specific antibodies by cloning the immune response to a mixed population is especially attractive.

A second consequence of the physical organization of neural tissue is that morphological criteria, rather than biochemical or physiological criteria, are frequently used to discriminate among different cell types. Because of this, microscopic assays have been especially important in characterizing antineuronal antibodies. Section IIA reviews experimental systems that have been particularly amenable to microscopic analysis, and discusses some generalizations that seem valid.

The necessary reliance on microscopic assays for immunological studies of the nervous system poses an important problem of interpretation. The microscopic assay is essentially a binding assay. When two cell types bind the same

LOIS ALTERMAN LAMPSON • Department of Anatomy, University of Pennsylvania School of Medicine, Philadelphia, Pennsylvania 19104.

153

antibody strongly, all that can be said is that they share a cross-reactive determinant, and, perhaps, that the determinant has the same subcellular localization in each case. This is no less a problem when one is dealing with monoclonal antibodies. The antibody combining site is small compared to the size of most proteins. Thus, molecules with very different structures, and possibly very different functions, can bind strongly to a monoclonal antibody if they share a single cross-reactive determinant. The difficulty of physically separating the different neuronal cell types that bind a single monoclonal antibody may prevent a definitive biochemical or functional comparison of the molecules expressed by each. Other aspects of this problem, and possible strategies for approaching it, are discussed in Sections IIB and IIC.

The particular interest of this laboratory is to use monoclonal antibodies to probe molecular bases of neuronal individuality: In what ways do neurons differ from other cell types, and from each other, in their biochemical composition, particularly at the cell membrane? Our experimental system for the study of human neuronal antigens is described in Section III. Our own studies of neuronal proteins are reviewed in Sections IV and V, and relevant studies from other laboratories in Sections VI and VII. This body of work is interpreted in terms of a model of cellular individuality in Section VIII.

As understanding of neuronal individuality increases, one practical development will be to apply that knowledge to the detection, classification, or treatment of neural tumors. Our approach to these clinical uses is described in Section IX.

II. Antibodies to Neural Antigens: A Review of Recent Work

A. Anatomical Studies: Lessons from Studies in Well-Characterized Systems

1. Antibodies of Predetermined Specificity

Monoclonal antibodies should be powerful tools for probing cellular individuality in the nervous system. They may be used to study one antigenic determinant at a time, and many techniques for localizing antibodies for analysis by light or electron microscopy are already well-established. Some of the most informative studies have come from experimental systems in which existing knowledge of the morphological and physiological properties of the different cells provides a framework for interpreting the antibody binding patterns. The nervous system of the leech is an example of such an experimental system in lower animals. The retina, where a few major cell types are formed into ordered layers, has served as one source of well-characterized tissue from vertebrates.

An early question that might be asked in such well-defined systems is this: To what extent is the anatomical distribution of single antigenic determinants, defined by monoclonal antibodies, consistent with principles of neuronal organization that have been established by morphological and functional criteria? Some examples of recent studies in which immunological work has supported previously established systems of neuronal classification, or given fresh evidence for widely held ideas about neuronal organization, are reviewed here.

Perhaps the broadest anatomical subdivision is that which distinguishes neurons of the central nervous system from those with their cell bodies in the periphery. Consistent with this traditional subdivision, monoclonal antibodies have been described with specificity for either central (Cohen and Selvendran, 1981) or peripheral neurons (Vulliamy et al., 1981).

The vertebrate retina provides an experimental system in which many finer neuronal subdivisions are easily recognized. Morphological and physiological criteria have been used to divide retinal neurons into five major classes (photoreceptors, horizontal cells, bipolars, amacrines, and ganglion cells), as well as many subclasses (Dowling, 1975; Kolb, 1979; Sterling, 1983). Barnstable has described a group of monoclonal antibodies to "new" antigens whose distributions fit cleanly within this scheme. The panel includes antibodies that recognize all photoreceptors or only rod photoreceptors, as well as antibodies that distinguish between neurons and glial cells (Barnstable, 1980). In a series of studies of well-defined molecules, Karten and colleagues have used both monoclonal and conventional antibodies to localize several different neuropeptides in the avian retina. They have also found distributions that fit well within the established anatomical scheme. Each of the peptides localizes to one of the major cell types, the amacrine cells, and, moreover, appears to define a characteristic subset of amacrine cells (Brecha et al., 1981; Karten and Brecha, 1980, 1981). As discussed by the authors, these findings agree in principle, and in some cases, in detail, with previous anatomical studies suggesting that the retina amacrine cells may contain as many as 20 different subclasses (reviewed in Sterling 1983).

Because of its well-ordered structure, the retina has frequently been used to explore the question of positional specificity. During development in lower vertebrates, cells from retina project onto corresponding positions of the optic tectum (reviewed in Fraser and Hunt, 1980). Although it has been difficult to define the mechanism by which this specificity is achieved, it is often suggested that molecular gradients may play a role. Trisler et al. (1981) have now described a monoclonal antibody that defines a topographic gradient in the chick retina. Besides providing fresh evidence for the existence of such gradients, the antibody should be an important probe for analyzing their biochemistry and mode of action.

In the nervous system of the leech, many neurons have been classified, not only by morphological criteria, but also according to function. The leech, therefore, provides a system in which it has been possible to ask whether functional subclasses of neurons do, as has been widely assumed, bear characteristic antigenic markers. This assumption has received striking support in the work of Zipser and McKay (1981). They have described monoclonal antibodies that are specific for small groups, or even pairs, of cells among the 400 neurons of the leech ganglion. The functions served by some of these groups or pairs had already been defined. In other cases, the particular groupings established by the antibodies have suggested additional functional relationships. The appeal of this experimental system is that the existing knowledge of the physiological connections and available techniques facilitate direct testing of the suggested functional relationships. Therefore, in the future, we may expect this system to tell us how frequently cross-reactions established by monoclonal antibodies actually have a functional basis.

An important feature of each of these examples is that knowledge of the target molecule or of the experimental system permitted a very directed screening of the antibodies. The monoclonal antibodies were originally chosen, sometimes among hundreds of others, because they were specific for a single neuropeptide, did define a gradient, or did define small subpopulations. The existing literature makes it clear that antibodies with these predetermined specificities can be found and that they can be of great help in refining our understanding of well-characterized neural tissue.

2. Newly Defined Antigens

Another application for monoclonal antibodies should be to help complete the characterization of parts of the nervous system that have not been as extensively studied by other methods. In these cases, one may not have the benefit of either predetermined target molecules (such as a specific neuropeptide) or extensive anatomical subdivisions to aid in choosing the most appropriate antibodies. This consideration led us to ask this question: Suppose one were to raise a series of antibodies to a well-defined tissue, and, without prior selection, examine their distribution. How frequently would the distribution of a single antibody map onto the existing morphological or functional classifications? In collaboration with Dr. Peter Sterling, we have used a panel of monoclonal antibodies to the cat retina to address this question.

Monoclonal antibodies were raised to a retina homogenate, and 19 that bound strongly to the retina in microscopic assays were studied, Monoclonal antibody A257 provides a striking example of the type of distribution we have seen. As illustrated in Figure 1, A257 fills cells, binding strongly in both the cytoplasm and nucleus. This makes it particularly easy to appreciate the binding pattern at the light level. Light and electron microscopic studies show that A257 cuts across the five major divisions of retinal neurons in an unanticipated way: The antibody stains ganglion cells; some, but not all, amacrine cells; and a few bipolar cells. The majority of the bipolar cells, the horizontal cells, and the photoreceptors are completely unstained, as are the Muller glial cells. The other antibodies we have analyzed, most of which are to cell membrane rather than internal antigens, display a similar kind of pattern. That is, they do discriminate between neurons and glial cells, and they also discriminate between subpopulations of neurons, but not in a way that would have been predicted from existing knowledge of the retina's organization. Existing knowledge of the cat retina can help us determine whether these reaction patterns can give new insight into functional relationships. The important point here is that the anatomical dis-

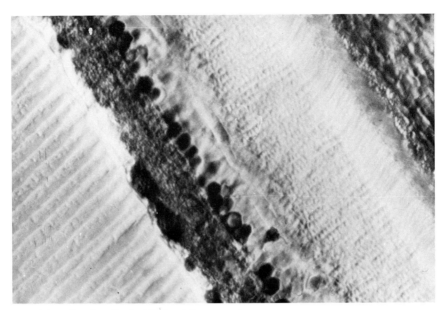

FIGURE 1. Monoclonal antibody A257 staining cat retina. The unlabeled antibody peroxidase–antiperoxidase (PAP) technique was used to stain a 50-μm section
of perfused cat retina. This antibody is able to stain
both cytoplasm and nuclei of some cell types, including
ganglion cells (examples are indicated by 1 in the drawing), amacrine cells (3), and occasional bipolar cells (4).
Staining is also seen within the processes of the inner
plexiform layer (2). At the same time, horizontal cells,
photoreceptors (5), and most bipolar cells are unstained. Electron microscopy confirms this pattern, and
shows that glial cell bodies and processes are also unstained (P. Sterling and L. Lampson, unpublished).

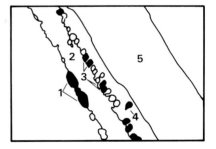

tribution of "new" antigens may frequently cut across the classifications that
would be established by more traditional criteria. Another example of this point
is seen among the anticerebellar antibodies recently described by Lagenauer *et
al.* (1980).

To summarize, recent work supports two conclusions about the use of
monoclonal antibodies in neural tissue. (1) When one has the advantage of
working with known molecules or a well-defined system, it is clearly possible to
select monoclonal antibodies that are specific for fine neuronal subpopulations
and to use these as immunological probes. (2) While monoclonal antibodies
should be important tools for clarifying less well-defined systems, great care
must be used in interpreting the binding patterns. If one does not have the
benefit of either a known molecule or a morphologically well-defined tissue to
aid in screening the antibodies, one cannot expect that the immunological classifications will necessarily coincide with independent morphological or functional
studies.

B. Biochemical Studies: Distinguishing between an Antigenic Determinant and the Molecule That Bears It

Two factors make it essential to complement anatomical studies with biochemical analysis. First, it is important to stress that a single antibody is specific for an antigenic determinant, rather than a whole molecule. Although the estimated size of an antigenic determinant may vary with the particular antigen–antibody combination and the assay, it is certainly small relative to the size of most proteins. Fewer than 10 amino acids, sugar residues, or nucleotides are sufficient to give maximal binding energy for most of the antibodies that have been studied (Kabat, 1966). This means that it is possible to obtain monoclonal antibodies to a variety of different determinants on a single molecule. Moreover, experience with molecules whose structures are well known demonstrates that different anatomical distributions may be obtained depending upon which antibody is used. The immunoglobulin molecule itself provides a very clear illustration of this point. Although immunoglobulins are the definitive marker for B lymphocytes, not every antiimmunoglobulin antibody will react with all B lymphocytes, or only B lymphocytes. An antibody to an immunoglobulin idiotype will react with at most a few clones of B lymphocytes. An antibody to the determinant on human immunoglobulin light chains that cross-reacts with β2-microglobulin (β2-m) (Gottlieb *et al.*, 1977) will react with all human cells that express β2-m, which includes most of the nucleated cells in the adult. Other examples are given in Table I. As these examples show, the anatomical distribution of a single molecule may be either broader or narrower than that observed with a particular monoclonal antibody. That is, the distribution of the immunoglobulin molecule is broader than would be seen with an antiidiotype antibody, and narrower than would be seen with an antibody to the β2-m cross-reactive determinant.

The second important point is that many molecules display tissue-specific differences in their structure. For example, Thy-1 and Ia are each expressed in the nervous system as well as in lymphoid and other tissues (Ting *et al.*, 1981; Williams and Gagnon, 1982). Each of these molecules displays tissue-specific variation in its carbohydrate composition (Barclay *et al.*, 1976; Cullen *et al.*, 1981). An antibody to the carbohydrate portion of these molecules might therefore display a narrower tissue distribution than would one to the common pro-

TABLE I

Anatomical Distributions That Would Be Observed with Different
Antiimmunoglobulin Antibodies

Antibody specificity	Anatomical distribution
Immunoglobulin	All B lymphocytes
Light chains	All B lymphocytes
κ Light chains	Sixty percent B lymphocytes
λ Light chains	Forty percent of B lymphocytes
Idiotype	One or few clones of B lymphocytes
Ig/β2-m cross-reactive determinant	Most nucleated human cells

tein portion. Examples of families of molecules that express tissue-specific differences in the protein backbone itself include isozymes (Harris, 1979) and the intermediate filament subunits (discussed in Section VI.D).

Thus, when a monoclonal antibody to a previously uncharacterized molecule shows an apparently restricted anatomical distribution, one must ask whether the molecule that bears the antigenic determinant might belong to a family of functionally-related molecules with a broader distribution. Conversely, if a monoclonal antibody displays a broad or unexpected distribution, one must ask whether the molecules that bear the antigenic determinant are the same in the different cells or tissues. Possibilities in this case are that the molecules might be identical, they might have an obvious structural relationship (tissue-specific forms of Thy-1 or Ia), or they might have a more subtle structural or evolutionary relationship (Ig and β2-m). In addition, a monoclonal antibody may react with different molecules for which no functional, structural or evolutionary relationship is currently known. The reported cross-reaction between Thy-1 and intermediate filaments is an example (Dulbecco *et al.*, 1981). In these cases, there is no *a priori* way of knowing whether the antibody has revealed an informative relationship as opposed to a "fortuitous" cross-reaction.

It is worth reiterating that the degree of homology between the members of a protein family may vary widely. At one end of the spectrum, we have the isozymes and the immunoglobulins. In these cases, members of a family may differ from each other by only a few amino acids. Approaching the other end of the spectrum, we have the intermediate filaments, which display gross differences in molecular weight and chain structure. Yet their physical properties, as well as recent amino acid sequence data, suggest a basis for the recently described immunological cross-reactivity, and strongly support thinking of the intermediate filaments as members of a family of functionally related proteins (Geisler *et al.*, 1982; Lazarides, 1980; Pruss *et al.*, 1981). Additional examples are discussed in Section VI. The point here is that the ability to recognize cross-reactions between nonidentical molecules should not be regarded as a weakness of monoclonal (or conventional) antibodies. Rather, these cross-reactions may often give very useful information about molecular relationships.

To summarize, in interpreting microscopic or other binding assays, it is essential to discriminate between the distribution of an antigenic determinant and the distribution of the molecule that bears the determinant. When a monoclonal antibody (or a conventional serum) does reveal cross-reactions between nonidentical molecules, this is not necessarily a "fortuitous" cross-reaction. Rather, the antibody may be revealing a family of functionally or evolutionarily related proteins. (This is discussed further in Section VI.)

C. Sources of Tissue for Biochemical Studies: The Potential of Cloned Cell Lines

One general impediment limits the biochemical studies: In order to compare the biochemical composition of molecules recognized by a single antibody in different cells, one must first separate the cells from each other. Although it is relatively simple to make this comparison at the level of whole tissues (brain versus peripheral nerve; brain versus retina; retina versus cortex; motor cortex versus visual cortex), it is much more difficult to achieve it for individual cell types (such as subpopulations of amacrine cells). Techniques that have been used or suggested include selective culture conditions to permit the growth of only some cell types; antibody-mediated killing of selected cells; and antibody-mediated separation of cells, such as by the fluorescence-activated cell sorter. In some cases, simple physical separations are also possible, such as isolation of large retinal ganglion cells by means of unit-gravity sedimentation (Kornguth *et al.,* 1981). Clearly, as finer subpopulations are studied, these techniques become increasingly more difficult to use.

An alternative approach is to use cloned cell lines of known origin as antigenic models of different cell types. Previous experience in the lymphoid system, in which cell lines bearing markers associated with many different lymphocyte subpopulations and stages of differentiation are available, shows the potential value of this approach. At present, cloned neural cell lines are available from only relatively few cell types and species. The most commonly used include rodent lines derived from embryonic neural tissue, and human and rodent lines derived from neural tumors. Most of these lines have been categorized as corresponding to neurons, glia, or intermediate types (Stallcup *et al.,* 1981), or to broad subdivisions within the first two categories [for example, granule cells or oligodendrocytes (Heitzmann *et al.,* 1981)]. In generating and defining cells corresponding to finer subdivisions (such as subpopulations of amacrine cells), monoclonal antibodies should be of use both for isolating selected populations for expansion and for characterizing the resulting clones. The antibodies will be particularly important for classification, since the morphological criteria that form the basis of much *in vivo* discrimination between cell types will no longer be applicable to cell lines.

Perhaps the most important technical limitation in producing new cell lines is that, unlike mature lymphoid cells, differentiated neurons do not normally divide. Thus, it is not yet clear to what extent neuronal cell lines can be matched to adult neuronal cell types. Neuronal cell lines can express some properties of differentiated cells. For example, human neuroblastoma lines, which are derived from a tumor of the sympathetic neuroblast, can express properties associated with electrically excitable membranes, as well as neurotransmitters and enzymes of neurotransmitter biosynthesis (Biedler *et al.,* 1973; Schlesinger *et al.,* 1976; Tischler *et al.,* 1977; West *et al.,* 1977). In addition, we have found that neuroblastoma lines reflect the unusually weak expression of the major histocompatibility antigens that is seen in normal brain (Section IV).

The ability of neuronal cell lines to express differentiated properties may reflect that fact that these properties were already present in the immature cell of origin. Alternatively, expression of differentiated phenotypes may result from transformation or adaptation to tissue culture, or, when the cell line has been created by fusion, interaction between the two parental cells (Minna, 1978). Additional differentiated properties may also be revealed by *in vitro* differentiation of the cell lines (Imada and Sueoka, 1980; Littauer *et al.*, 1980). It is, of course, of great interest to know whether a particular differentiated phenotype is characteristic of the cell of origin or its progeny. In addition, the cell lines can serve as expedient, homogeneous sources of large quantities of cellular components (such as neuropeptides or their receptors), and this use is independent of whether the component is normally expressed by the cell of origin.

It seems likely that, as monoclonal antibodies are used to select cells for expansion and to characterize new and existing lines (Bechtol *et al.*, 1980; Heitzmann *et al.*, 1981; Kennett *et al.*, 1980; Seeger *et al.*, 1982; Stallcup *et al.*, 1981; Trisler *et al.*, 1979; Section IV), the lines will become increasingly useful for biochemical analysis of both developmental and adult phenotypes.

III. An Experimental System for Studying Neuronal Individuality in Human Tissue

A. Human Neuroblastoma-Derived Cell Lines for Biochemical Analysis

We have sought to establish an experimental system that would allow both anatomical and biochemical studies of mammalian neural antigens. In the human lymphoid system, normal tissue, tumors, and cloned cell lines have been used very successfully as sources of tissue, with the results obtained in one system frequently reinforcing those from the others. We have sought to establish a similar interplay in the nervous system. The heart of our system is a panel of human neuroblastoma-derived cell lines. Each cell line is derived from a different neuroblastoma tumor, which in turn represents a clonal expansion of a different sympathetic neuroblast.

Several types of studies support the idea of using neuroblastoma cell lines as a biochemical model for the original tumor. The cell lines and tumor also display many properties of normal neurons. Different neuroblastoma tumors and their derivative cell lines have been shown to express individual neurotransmitters or enzymes of neurotransmitter biosynthesis. Many of the cell lines express the action potential Na^+ ionophore, suggesting that they have excitable membranes. Other proteins that are specific for, or characteristic of, the nervous system, such as the neuron-specific enolase (NSE or 14-3-2) and Thy-1, are also synthesized by these cell lines (Biedler *et al.*, 1973; Herschman and Lerner, 1973; Schlesinger *et al.*, 1976; Seeger *et al.*, 1982; West *et al.*, 1977).

In studies with monoclonal antineuroblastoma antibodies, we have observed frequent cross-reactions between the cell lines and normal brain, and this agrees with studies using both monoclonal and conventional antibodies in other laboratories. However, the biochemical basis of most of these immunological cross-reactions has not been directly studied. Thus, in most cases, it is not possible to say whether a monoclonal (or conventional) antibody is recognizing the same molecule in the cell line as in normal neural tissue. Therefore, the studies with known molecules are the best current evidence that the cell lines (and tumors) can express individual phenotypes of normal neurons.

Our approach is to use these cloned lines as "antigen factories"—sources of freshly synthesized molecules produced by individual clones of cells—for biochemical analysis. The information we gain may help characterize the neuroblastoma tumor, which is a major solid tumor of early childhood (Evans, 1980). Information we gain from the study of the cell lines may also help us to understand normal neurons. The way in which this interplay has helped us to probe the neural expression of the molecules bearing the conventional major transplantation antigens (HLA-A,B,C molecules) is described in Section IV and in Lampson *et al.* (1983) and Lampson and Whelan (1983).

B. Complementary Microscopic Studies of Primary Tumors and Normal Tissue

An essential part of our approach is that results that are obtained with the cloned cell lines must be extended to primary tumors and normal nervous tissue. Because neither of these represent homogeneous, or easily separable, populations of cells, we must rely on microscopic analysis for much of this work. Many other laboratories have shown the feasibility of using frozen human material obtained at biopsy or autopsy for immunological studies. Because of the difficulty of obtaining such material at will, we have explored two additional approaches to anatomical analysis.

1. Paraffin Sections

One approach is to exploit the extensive collections of formalin-fixed, paraffin-embedded material, taken from both normal and malignant tissue, that are maintained in many hospitals. For appropriate antigen–antibody combinations, immunocytochemical techniques, such as the peroxidase–antiperoxidase (PAP) technique, can be used for studies of such material, at least when conventional antisera are used (Sternberger, 1979).

In asking whether this material is suitable for analysis with individual monoclonal antibodies, three independent factors must to be considered. (1) Some antigens might be destroyed by the fixation (4% formaldehyde) (many of our antibodies were initially screened against cells that had been "lightly" fixed in 0.1% glutaraldehyde). (2) Some molecules might be lost during the paraffin embedding and the attendant exposure to warm wax, acids, alcohol, and xylene. (3) Some determinants on a molecule might survive these procedures, whereas others would be destroyed. Thus, only some monoclonal antibodies to a given molecule might be usable. Our initial findings may be summarized as follows:

1. To test the effects of fixation, eight antineuroblastoma antibodies were chosen for their strong binding to neural tissue in radioimmunoassays using lightly fixed material. In two assays, binding to lightly fixed tissue was compared

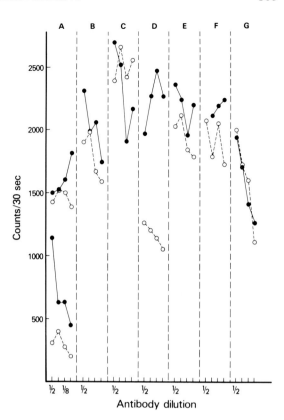

FIGURE 2. Effect of fixation upon monoclonal antibody binding. Cat cortex was fixed with 0.1% glutaraldehyde for 5 min at room temperature (open circles) or with 2% glutaraldehyde + 2% paraformaldehyde for 18 hr at 4°C (closed circles). Graph shows results of radioimmunoassays with seven different monoclonal antibodies and with spent culture medium containing plasmacytoma protein MOPC21, which was used as a negative control (lower curves in panel A). Note that, for one of the antibodies (D), there was stronger binding to the more rigorously fixed material.

to the binding to tissue that had been fixed in 4% aldehydes overnight. In seven of the cases, there was no difference in the extent of binding. In the eighth case, the binding was actually increased for the more rigorously fixed target tissue (Figure 2). Thus, for antibodies chosen at random from screenings against lightly fixed material, the more rigorous fixation did not usually destroy the antigenic determinants.

Of course, not every antigen will be unaffected or enhanced by fixation. For example, reactivity of L368, a monoclonal antibody to β2-microglobulin, was reduced when the concentration of fixative was increased from 0.1 to 4% aldehydes.

2. Four antibodies known to bind strongly to tissue that had been fixed in 4% aldehydes were tested in the PAP assay against paraffin-embedded tissue. We found that two of the antibodies bound strongly to the paraffin-embedded tissue, one bound weakly, and one did not show any detectable binding. Thus, while the paraffin embedding can cause loss of antigenic determinants over and above that resulting from the fixation procedure, many determinants can survive this treatment (J. Whelan and L. Lampson, unpublished; Sternberger *et al.*, 1982).

2. Species Cross-Reactions

A second approach to microscopic analysis, particularly for studies of normal tissue, is to exploit interspecies cross-reactions and perform microscopic studies in tissue obtained from perfused laboratory animals. We have found that many of the monoclonal antibodies we have raised to mammalian neural tissue do show cross-reactivity between humans, mice, rats, and cats. This is true whether the original immunogen was a human neuroblastoma-derived cell line or normal cat tissue (homogenized retina), and agrees with previous reports for both monoclonal and conventional antibodies.

As discussed above, we must confirm biochemically that the same molecules are being recognized in the different species. The antiretina antibody A257 provides a striking illustration of this point. In microscopic and radioimmunoassays, A257 binds strongly to the human neuroblastoma-derived cell line IMR-5 and displays the relatively uncommon intracellular distribution that had been seen in several neuronal cell types in the cat: The antibody stains the nucleus and cytoplasm, but not the outer membrane. However, when immunoblots were used to identify the polypeptide chains recognized in the different tissues, it was seen that A257 binds to human neuroblastoma and cat retina polypeptides of different apparent molecular weights (Figure 3). Presumably, closer correspondence between the sources of cat and human tissues would have increased the

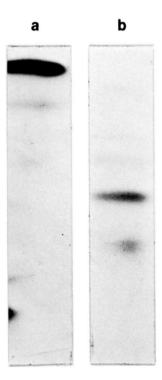

FIGURE 3. Analysis of A257 on immunoblots. Monoclonal antibody A257 (Figure 1) was allowed to bind to electrophoretically separated proteins from either (a) the neuroblastoma cell line IMR-5 or (b) normal adult cat retina. The procedure was as described in Fisher and Lampson, Appendix to this volume. Note that, although the antibody binds strongly to both tissues, in agreement with microscopic analysis, the predominant polypeptide chain that is recognized has a different apparent molecular weight in the two tissues.

likelihood of finding a similar molecule in the two species. The important point here is that even a strong cross-reaction and a similar subcellular distribution in microscopic assay do not ensure biochemical identity of the recognized molecules.

Thus, both clinical material preserved as paraffin sections, and perfused tissue of laboratory animals, may provide alternative sources of tissue for microscopic analysis with carefully selected antibodies. However, the effect of fixation and embedding and the possibility of cross-reactions between nonidentical molecules must be evaluated in each case.

3. Conclusions

As a system for study, the human nervous system offers the potential of immediate clinical applicability. Indeed, clinical interest has led to the establishment and characterization of many different cell lines from neuronal, glial, and other human cell types. By using monoclonal antibodies as probes for single molecules, the structure of individual molecules expressed by individual cells can be compared. The comparison can be made between different cell types (neurons versus glial or lymphoid cells) as well as between different cells of a single type (different neuronal cell lines). Microscopic assays can then be used to relate observations made on the cell lines to individual cells in primary tumors and in normal tissue. Existing collections of fixed material can provide one source of such tissue for appropriate antibodies. It may also be possible to exploit species cross-reactions, again for appropriate antibodies. Our laboratory is using this experimental approach to study the molecular bases of neuronal individuality, as described in Sections III.C, IV, and V.

C. Neurons versus Other Cell Types: Do Similarities or Differences Predominate?

Most mature mammalian neurons differ from other cell types in one or all of these ways: The neuron is incapable of division, it has an excitable membrane, it has a cell body in a specific place, it extends processes in specific directions, it makes specific synaptic contacts with other cells, and it recognizes and expresses characteristic neurotransmitters. One would expect that molecules serving each of these functions might serve as neuronal markers, particularly at the cell surface. At the same time, many other cellular components are very widespread or ubiquitous. In probing neuronal individuality, one might begin by asking which of these factors predominates. We have used monoclonal antibodies to ask this question at the level of the cell membrane: Are most of the molecules on the surface of a neuron widely distributed among other cell types, or do most of them serve more specific functions?

One might approach this problem by comparing neuronal membrane proteins *en masse* with membrane proteins of other cell types (reviewed in Moore,

1975). One problem with this approach is that, without knowing the function or finer structure of the proteins, it is not possible to be certain of the interpretation. For example, the Thy-1 molecule has the same protein backbone but a different carbohydrate structure in neurons and lymphocytes. If neuronal and lymphocyte membrane proteins were compared without realizing that one of the molecules was Thy-1, the different bands would be seen as different glycoproteins.

A second way of approaching this question is to examine individual major cell surface proteins one at a time. This approach has been used very successfully in the analysis of erythrocytes and lymphocytes (Branton *et al.*, 1981; Brown *et al.*, 1981), and monoclonal antibodies have now facilitated extending the approach to other cell types. Our studies of the neuronal expression of both known and newly defined molecules are described in Sections IV and V.

IV. Striking Paucity of HLA-A,B,C Molecules on Cells of Neuronal Origin

To begin our studies of the human neuronal surface, we chose the HLA-A,B,C molecules, which bear the conventional major transplantation antigens, for several reasons. The structure of the molecules has been intensively studied, their general tissue distribution is established, and well-characterized conventional and monoclonal antibodies, some of which we ourselves had raised, were already available. We expected that the study of these known molecules would help us to work out assay procedures to be used later for new molecules. In addition, two points lent this work a more theoretical interest. First, although the HLA-A,B,C molecules are generally thought to be present on most nucleated human cells, they are only poorly expressed by homogenates of whole brain. Since glial cell lines have been shown to express the molecules strongly, this suggested that neurons may express them only weakly. The second point is that the extensive structural studies of the HLA-A,B,C molecules have for the most part utilized material isolated from lymphoid cells. We were interested to know, therefore, whether there might be tissue-specific variations in the structure of the molecules.

A. HLA-A,B,C Function and Structure: Antibody Probes

The HLA-A,B,C molecules are important in several ways. As transplantation antigens, they form a principal barrier to successful organ transplantation. In addition, they are involved in cellular interactions in the immune response. A third important property is that a growing list of human diseases are associated with particular HLA phenotypes.

The clinical importance of these molecules has led to intensive study of their structure. The HLA-A,B,C molecules are a family of closely related proteins. In each case, the molecule is composed of two chains. The HLA chains, which are coded by the major histocompatibility complex on chromosome 6, are glycoproteins of 43,000 daltons apparent molecular weight. These chains are highly polymorphic. Approximately 20 alleles at the A locus, 40 at the B locus, and six at the C locus have been identified (Bodmer, 1981). For each of these molecules, the polymorphic HLA chain is linked to an invariant 12,000-dalton chain, β2-microglobulin.

Because of their clinical importance and the resulting knowledge of their structure, these molecules were among the first subjects for study with monoclonal antibodies (Barnstable et al., 1978; Lampson et al., 1978a; Parham and Bodmer, 1978). Of the many possible specificities, we have chosen two monoclonal antibodies that serve as very broad probes for these molecules. L368 recognizes β2-microglobulin, the invariant chain of all HLA-A,B,C molecules (Lampson and Levy, 1980). W6/32 recognizes a nonpolymorphic determinant on the native two-chain molecules (Barnstable et al., 1978). A conventional rabbit antiserum to β2-microglobulin (Dako Immunoglobulins), which presumably contains antibodies to more than one determinant on that chain, was also used.

B. Striking Paucity of HLA-A,B,C on Neuroblastoma Cell Lines: Results from Four Kinds of Assays

In order to be able to compare the structure of the HLA-A,B,C molecules on neurons, glia, and lymphoid cells, we used a panel of human cell lines. In part because these experiments were intended as a model for later studies with new antibodies, we compared a number of different assays, as described below.

Among assays for cell surface determinants, the most convenient is the radioimmunoassay against glutaraldehyde-fixed target cells. We had previously established that the light fixation (0.1% glutaraldehyde for 5 min at room temperature) did not destroy the determinants recognized by L368 or W6/32 on lymphoid cells. Our standard assay employs cell pellets consisting of 250,000 fixed target cells. Under these conditions, we obtained strong binding of L368 and W6/32 to glial and lymphoid cells, but no consistent specific binding to four different neuroblastoma-derived cell lines (Figure 4). By increasing the number of neuroblastoma targets, we were able to reveal some binding with L368 and even weaker binding with W6/32 against some of the neuroblastoma lines (Lampson et al., 1983).

Complement-mediated cytotoxicity is generally regarded as a potentially more sensitive assay for cell surface antigens. In collaboration with Dr. Roger Kennett, we used this assay to assess HLA-A,B,C expression on the different cell lines. In this case, the assay was not more sensitive than the binding assay. In three experiments, we detected no specific lysis of any of the neuroblastoma-derived lines, whereas the antibodies did lyse a B cell line, and a previously characterized antineuroblastoma antibody did lyse the neuroblastoma lines (Kennett et al., 1982).

In order to be able to detect internal as well as cell surface determinants, we analyzed sections of fixed cells that had been embedded in agarose. This en-

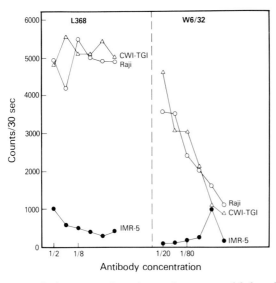

FIGURE 4. Binding of monoclonal antibodies to human cell lines. Monoclonal antibodies L368 and W6/32 were assayed against neuronal (IMR-5), glial (CW1-TG1), and lymphoid (Raji) cell lines in radioimmunoassay. Negative controls, described in Figure 2, were a few hundred counts/30 sec for the different cell lines (Lampson, 1981).

sured that cytoplasmic antigens would be directly exposed to antibody. The unlabeled antibody peroxidase–antiperoxidase (PAP) procedure was used to assess the binding of L368 and W6/32 to lymphoid, glial, and neuronal cell lines (Lampson and Whelan, 1983; Lampson *et al.*, 1983; and Lampson *et al.*, Appendix to this volume). The results of these assays are illustrated in Figure 5. Strong binding to lymphoid and glial cells was seen, with a dark rim of stain surrounding a less darkly stained cytoplasm. This characteristic pattern of stain agrees with the previously established subcellular localization of these antigens. However, even when 30-fold more concentrated antibodies were used, we detected no specific staining in the neuroblastoma lines.

The fourth assay in this series was a binding inhibition assay. In this case, detergent (Nonidet P-40) extracts of the cell lines were used to inhibit the binding of the monoclonal antibodies to a B-cell target (Lampson, Appendix to this volume). The advantages of this assay were that it had the potential to reveal both internal and cell surface antigens in unfixed tissue and that it allowed us to quantify the differences in HLA-A,B,C expression. In addition, this assay proved to be the most sensitive of the four assays in these experiments. As illustrated in Figure 6, we were able to obtain clear inhibition of both L368 and W6/32 with the neuroblastoma extracts. Yet, these extracts were clearly much less efficient inhibitors than were the glial or lymphoid extracts. In 10 experiments, the amount of B-cell extract needed to obtain 50% inhibition was compared to the amount of neuroblastoma or glial extract needed for 50% inhibition. We found that the neuroblastoma extracts were always less than 1% as efficient, per microgram of extract protein, than the B-cell extract, and the B-cell and glial cell extracts were about equally efficient (Lampson and Whelan, 1983).

Thus, in four different assays in which both internal and cell surface antigens of fixed or unfixed tissue might be revealed, neuroblastoma cell lines showed a striking paucity of HLA-A,B,C molecules as compared to glial or lymphoid lines. Indeed, our results suggest that the neuroblastoma cell lines are

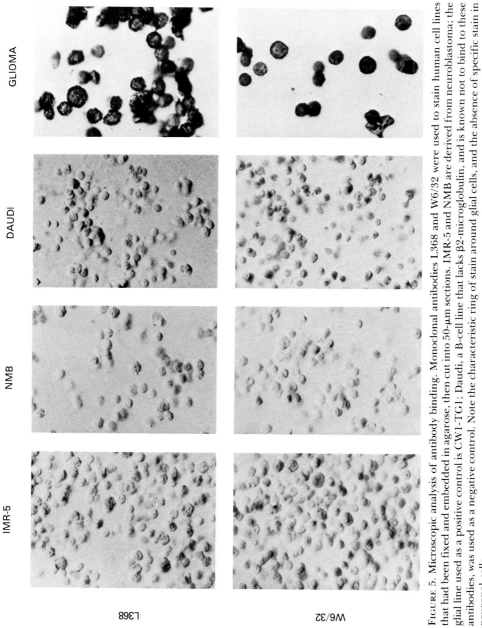

FIGURE 5. Microscopic analysis of antibody binding. Monoclonal antibodies L368 and W6/32 were used to stain human cell lines that had been fixed and embedded in agarose, then cut into 50-μm sections. IMR-5 and NMB are derived from neuroblastoma; the glial line used as a positive control is CW1-TG1; Daudi, a B-cell line that lacks β2-microglobulin, and is known not to bind to these antibodies, was used as a negative control. Note the characteristic ring of stain around glial cells, and the absence of specific stain in neuronal cells.

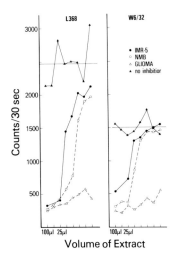

FIGURE 6. Binding inhibition assays. Diminishing volumes of cell extracts were used to inhibit the binding of a constant volume of monoclonal antibody (L368 or W6/32) to a human B-cell line. Extracts were prepared from the same starting cell concentration, and final protein concentrations varied by a factor of two or less. Solid line shows mean of values obtained with no inhibitor. Note that both neuronal (IMR-5 and NMB) and glial extracts do inhibit the antibodies, but the glial extract is much more efficient.

at the low end of the observed spectrum of HLA-A,B,C activity (Lampson *et al.*, 1983).

C. HLA-A,B,C Expression on Neuroblastoma Tumors and Normal Brain

As we continued to study HLA-A,B,C expression on neuroblastoma lines, it became of increasing interest to know whether the paucity of the molecules reflected a property of either the original tumor or normal neurons.

To study the tumor, we first used a microscopic assay to analyze metastatic neuroblastoma in bone marrow. Here, the tumor may appear as aggregates, which are readily identified by their morphology, as well as single cells. Normal bone marrow was used as a control. The results of this type of assay are illustrated in Figure 7. The majority ($\geq$ 96%) of the nucleated normal bone marrow cells were clearly stained with monoclonal antibody L368, in agreement with previous reports of HLA-A,B,C expression in this tissue (Brown *et al.*, 1979; Fitchen *et al.*, 1981). In contrast, many fewer of the single cells (< 50%) in the neuroblastoma marrow were stained. More strikingly, all tumor aggregates appeared negative. The unstained aggregates were readily distinguished from clumps or groups of cells in the normal marrow, which were clearly stained (Lampson *et al.*, 1983).

These results confirm that the paucity of HLA-A,B,C is a characteristic of at least one form of neuroblastoma tumor rather than a culture artifact. They also suggest a possible use for the antibodies in helping to discriminate between tumor cells and HLA-A,B,C-rich normal tissue, as discussed in Section IX.

Previous studies had shown that normal human and mouse brain express at best weak HLA-A,B,C or H-2,K,D activity, respectively (Berah *et al.*, 1970; Schachner and Sidman, 1973; Williams *et al.*, 1980). We have confirmed this in our laboratory, using both radioimmunobinding assays and binding inhibition assays. We are now using the microscopic assay to directly compare the HLA-A,B,C expression on normal neurons and glial cells.

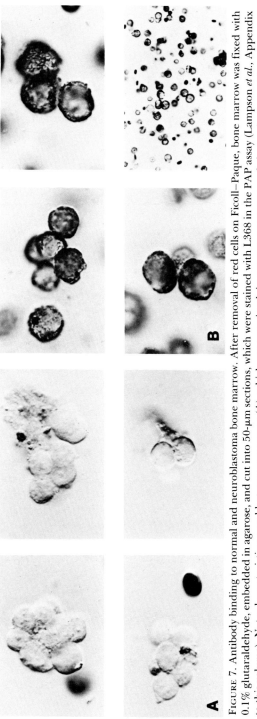

FIGURE 7. Antibody binding to normal and neuroblastoma bone marrow. After removal of red cells on Ficoll–Paque, bone marrow was fixed with 0.1% glutaraldehyde, embedded in agarose, and cut into 50-μm sections, which were stained with L368 in the PAP assay (Lampson *et al.*, Appendix to this volume). Note characteristic neuroblastoma aggregates (A), which are unstained, in contrast to groups and clumps in normal bone marrow (B), which are stained. Cells were photographed at 600× (Nomarski optics). Part (B) also shows normal bone marrow photographed at lower magnification (120×). Note frequency of stained cells, many showing characteristic ringlike stain, similar to that seen in Figure 5. (Reprinted by permission from Lampson *et al.*, 1983).

D. Possible Functional Significance of Weak HLA-A,B,C Expression on Neural Tissue and Tumors

In general, "foreign" antigens, such as viruses, must be associated with the host's own HLA-A,B,C molecules if they are to be the target of T-cell-mediated cytotoxicity (Dausset, 1981). This is relevant to our HLA results in three ways.

First, if normal neurons lack HLA-A,B,C molecules, they may be protected from T-cell-mediated cytotoxicity, even if they express viral or other inappropriate antigens. In theory, this may serve to protect postmitotic cells, such as neurons, which cannot be replaced. Second, if neurons lack HLA-A,B,C molecules, neurons in grafted neural tissue may be protected from T-cell-mediated killing, even if they come from donors expressing inappropriate HLA-A,B,C specificities, or they express other inappropriate antigens. Third, if tumor-specific antigens do not appear in conjunction with appropriate HLA-A,B,C molecules, then the tumor cells may also be protected from T-cell-mediated cytotoxicity. Thus, tumors or metastases with weak HLA-A,B,C expression may be relatively more successful in escaping host rejection (Bodmer, 1981). In this context, it is interesting to note that neuroblastoma can be a particularly aggressive tumor.

Of course, several other interpretations of weak neuronal HLA-A,B,C expression must also be considered. Low levels of HLA-A,B,C (compared to what is expressed on other cell types) may be sufficient to mediate T-cell restriction; HLA-A,B,C expression may increase under certain pathological conditions; or other molecules may serve as restriction elements in neural tissue. Direct microscopic analysis of normal and pathological neural tissue, and structural and functional studies of restriction in the T-cell-mediated killing of *neuronal* target cells are needed to test these possibilities.

E. Further Studies: Immunoprecipitation

In seeking the functional significance of the observed weak HLA-A,B,C expression on cells of neuronal origin, we have first sought to characterize the molecules that inhibit the monoclonal antibodies. First, we wish to know whether the binding inhibition assays reveal cross-reactive molecules rather than conventional HLA-A,B,C molecules. Immunoprecipitation studies have given us a partial answer to this question.

For immunoprecipitation, cell lines were labeled biosynthetically with [^{35}S]methionine or [^{3}H]-sugars, extracted with nonionic detergent (Nonidet P-40), and then incubated with antibody bound to *Staphylococcus aureus*, as described previously (Lampson, 1980). The precipitates were analyzed by SDS–polyacrylamide gel electrophoresis, on 10–20% gradient polyacrylamide slab gels, using the Laemmli buffer system. Monoclonal antibodies L368 and W6/32, as well as a conventional rabbit anti-β2-m serum, were used. The molecules precipitated from three neuroblastoma lines and one glial line were directly compared to the molecules precipitated from the B-cell line Raji.

These experiments have shown that all of the neural cell lines (neuronal and glial) do synthesize a polypeptide chain that comigrates with the β2-microglobulin precipitated from Raji (Lampson *et al.*, 1983). The experiments also

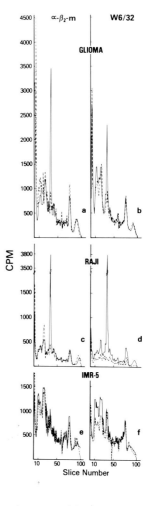

FIGURE 8. Immunoprecipitation from cell extracts. Cell lines were labeled biosynthetically with a mixture of [³H]-sugars, extracted with NP-40, and precipitated with anti-β2-m serum or with monoclonal antibody W6/32. The precipitates were analyzed by SDS–polyacrylamide gel electrophoresis on 10–20% polyacrylamide gradient slab gels. Precipitates from a glioma line (CW1-TG1) and Raji were electrophoresed on the same gel; precipitates from IMR-5 were also electrophoresed on the same gel with Raji precipitates. Individual lanes were cut into 1-μm slices and solublized in Econofluor + Protosol (New England Nuclear) for scintillation counting. Solid lines show precipitates with antibody; dashed lines show precipitates with appropriate controls (normal rabbit serum for the anti-β2-m, and normal mouse ascites for W6/32). Note that both antibodies precipitate a single specific glycopeptide from the glioma line, and this comigrates with the HLA chain from Raji. No specific HLA-like material is seen in the IMR-5 precipitates. (Reprinted by permission.)

show that the glial line synthesizes a glycoprotein that comigrates with the HLA chain from Raji (Figure 8). At the same time, we have been unable to visualize a specific HLA-like chain in the neuroblastoma extracts. This was true when either anti-β2-m serum or W6/32 was used, and whether the cells had been biosynthetically labeled with [³⁵S]methionine or [³H]-sugars. The results with extracts that had been labeled with [³H]-sugars are illustrated in Figure 8.

We are now using other strategies to characterize the molecule recognized by W6/32 on neuroblastoma cells. At present, we cannot say whether the conventional HLA chain is present in small quantities, present in an altered form, or absent. These questions are of interest in the functional context described above, and also because of the developing picture of qualitative and quantitative variations among HLA-A,B,C molecules and their analogs in other human cell types (Brown et al., 1979; Cotner et al., 1981; Law and Bodmer, 1978; Sunderland et al., 1981; Trowsdale et al., 1980; von Willebrand et al., 1980; Ziegler and Milstein, 1979).

F. Summary and Conclusions

We have used well-characterized monoclonal antibodies in a variety of assays to study the expression of HLA-A,B,C molecules on a panel of human cell lines. These studies have revealed a striking paucity of HLA-A,B,C molecules on neuroblastoma-derived cell lines as compared to glial, lymphoid, and many other cell types.

An important aspect of these results is that they do not represent a culture artifact. Rather, the paucity of HLA-A,B,C is also a property of the tumor from which the neuroblastoma cell lines were derived, as well as a property of normal adult brain. Although it is, of course, necessary to test these correspondences directly in each case, these findings do support the general plan of using the neuronal cell lines to complement studies of more complex tissue.

The paucity of HLA-A,B,C in brain and neuroblastoma tumor has been discussed in terms of the role of HLA-A,B,C molecules in T-cell-mediated cytotoxicity. Further experiments are needed to test the several possible implications of our results.

V. Tissue Distribution of Newly Defined Molecules

We have also approached the question of neuronal individuality through analysis of antigens that are newly defined by monoclonal antibodies. We have worked with panels of monoclonal antibodies to two different kinds of mammalian neural tissue, human neuroblastoma-derived cell lines and normal adult cat retina. In each case, antibodies were selected for their ability to bind strongly to the immunizing neural tissue in radioimmuno- or microscopic assays. These assays were then used to ask how many of the antibodies were specific for the immunizing tissue.

The results of these initial assays were consistent with previous work from many other laboratories: Monoclonal antibodies that define a single tissue or cell type are infrequent. In these particular experiments, each of 200 antineuroblastoma antibodies also reacted with nonneuronal human cell lines or tissue, and 19/19 of the antiretina antibodies reacted with other cat tissues. In addition, we observed frequent interspecies cross-reactions between human, rodent, and cat tissue, and this is also in agreement with previous work.

As discussed in Section IIB, even a strong immunological cross-reaction and a similar subcellular distribution need not mean that a monoclonal antibody has identified the same molecule in different cells or tissues. In order to test this, a group of antibodies showing strong tissue cross-reactions were chosen for structural analysis of their antigens.

A. Analysis of Tissue Cross-Reactions by Immunoblots

For the structural analyses, we turned first to the immunoblot technique. Here, tissue extracts are first electrophoresed on SDS–polyacrylamide gels. The separated proteins are then electrophoretically transferred to nitrocellulose sheets. The nitrocellulose sheets are exposed first to monoclonal antibody, and antigen present in an average cell must be made. One of the ways to accomplish this is by analysis of two-dimensional gels (O'Farrell, 1975; Garrels, 1979) of total cell lysates of a known number of cells. This type of analysis indicated that in the case of the 95,000-dalton intermediate filament protein recognized by the antibody JLB7, there was about 10^5-10^6 molecules of the 95K protein in a single cell (Lin and Feramisco, 1981). Typical amounts of other proteins in cells might range from 10^3 to 10^8 molecules per cell. Other factors to be considered initially are the antibody concentration and volume to be introduced into each cell. By microneedle injection, a typical fibroblast can be injected with $10^{-13}-10^{-14}$ ml of solution (Graessmann *et al.*, 1980; Stacey and Allfrey, 1976). Using an antibody concentration of 10–20 mg/ml, it is possible to introduce up to 10^7 molecules of antibody per cell, a sufficient amount to complex with all of a given antigen in the case of many cellular proteins.

There are at least two additional parameters that are important to consider in these types of experiments but are somewhat out of the investigator's control. The first is the accessibility of the antigen in the cell to the injected antibody. If the antigenic site on the target protein is not available to the antibody because of, for example, its involvement in some other interaction, one may not observe any effect on the cell caused by the antibody. This problem must be carefully examined in the case of a negative result after injection of an antibody (e.g., Wehland *et al.*, 1981) before the data can be interpreted. The second parameter involves the effect that the antibody has on the function of the antigen by virtue of the complexation reaction. Ideally, one can determine if a given monoclonal antibody inhibits some measurable biochemical activity of the antigen and can correlate the inhibition with an observable or measurable effect on the cell after introduction of the antibody into the cell. In some cases, however, the antigen may not have a known activity; thus, it is impossible to determine the *in vitro* effect of the antibody on the antigen. Just as is the case in which the antibody does not have access to the antigen in the cell, when the antibody complexes with the antigen but does not interfere with the activity of the antigen (whatever that activity may be), the injected antibody may not have an effect on the cell.

We have examined the effects on intermediate filaments of two monoclonal antibodies directed against minor components of these filaments (Lin, 1981) by the microinjection technique (Lin and Feramisco, 1981). Immunofluorescence staining of fibroblasts by the antibodies JLB1 and JLB7 shows their distribution on the intermediate filaments (e.g., see Figure 8F for the staining by JLB7). After microinjection of JLB1 (specific for the 220,000-dalton protein), double-label immunofluorescence indicated that while the injected antibody binds to the intermediate filaments (Figure 13B), no obvious change in the typical distribution of these filaments occurs (as indicated by staining with an antivimentin antibody) (Fig. 13C). However, within minutes after injection of JLB7 (specific for the 95,000-dalton protein), a dramatic reorganization of the intermediate filaments occurs (Figure 13E). The filaments are now found in a tight aggregate near the nuclei of the injected cells. Inspection of these cells by electron microscopy (thin sections) reveals what appear to be antibody cross-links along the lengths of the filaments, in the aggregates. Similar results have been obtained by Klymkowski (1981) through the injection of a monoclonal antibody to vimentin.

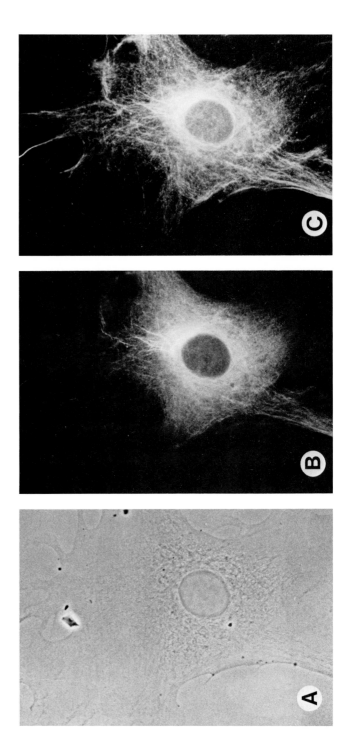

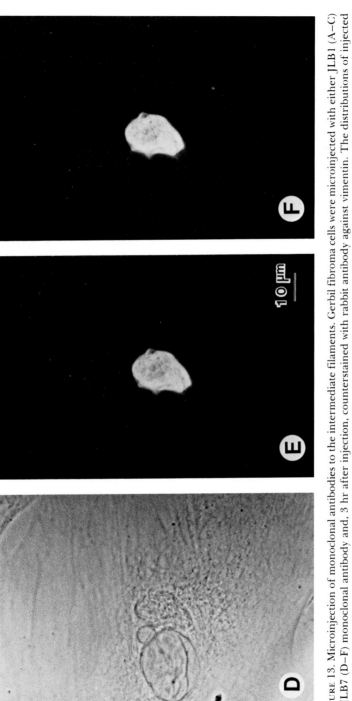

FIGURE 13. Microinjection of monoclonal antibodies to the intermediate filaments. Gerbil fibroma cells were microinjected with either JLB1 (A–C) or JLB7 (D–F) monoclonal antibody and, 3 hr after injection, counterstained with rabbit antibody against vimentin. The distributions of injected mouse antibody and vimentin were detected by double-label immunofluorescence by a mixture of second antibodies containing fluorescein-conjugated goat anti-mouse IgG and rhodamine-conjugated goat anti-rabbit IgG. (A, D) Phase-contrast micrographs. (B, E) Injected cells viewed selectively for fluorescein fluorescence to allow the microinjected mouse antibody to be visualized. (C, F) The same fields seen in (B) and (E), respectively, except viewed selectively for rhodamine fluorescence to allow the distribution of vimentin to be visualized.

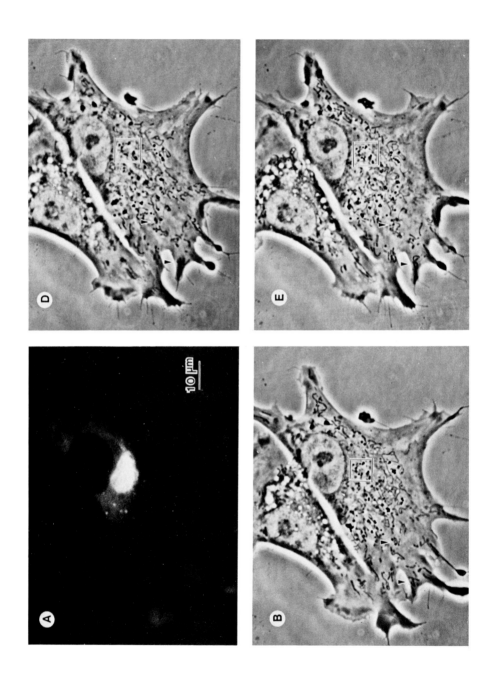

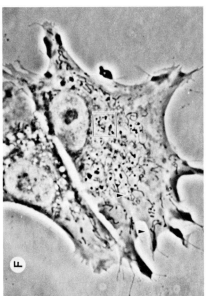

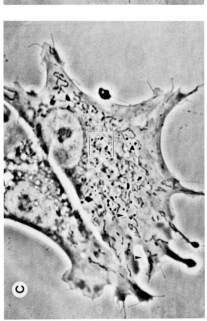

FIGURE 14. Organelle movements in cells lacking a normal intermediate filament distribution. A sequence of micrographs of the JLB7 antibody-injected and control gerbil fibroma cells is given. (A) The fluorescence micrograph, which allows for the visualization of the intermediate filaments in the living cell. (B–F) Phase-contrast micrographs of the cells in the same field as in (A). The relative time points for (B)–(F) are 0, 2, 4, 8, and 10 min, respectively. A variety of saltatory movements are apparent: dark granules and mitochondria (for example, those close to the arrowheads) can be seen to move about as in the control cell. Ruffles and blebs at the cell periphery undergo dynamic displacements, rearrangements, and extensions as in the control cell. In contrast, the granules within the indicated square boxes appeared nonmotile within this 10-min period: it is possible that these granules were trapped within the aggregates of the intermediate filaments.

Given that the injection of the monoclonal antibody JLB7 results in the essentially complete reorganization of the intermediate filaments in living cells, it is possible to search for biological effects of the reorganization of these filaments. Analysis of the distributions of the other two known filamentous networks in these cells, microfilaments and microtubules, suggests that neither of these two networks was altered by the intermediate filament reorganization (Lin and Feramisco, 1981). Organelle movements (Figure 14) (i.e., saltatory motion), cell shape and polarity, and cell respreading also seem normal in spite of the thoughts that the intermediate filaments may be involved in some or all of these phenomena (R. D. Goldman and Knipe, 1972; Wang and Goldman, 1978; Wang *et al.*, 1979). Thus, while the biological effects of the loss of the intermediate filaments from the normal cytoplasmic array are not known, it is hoped that by analysis of mitotic cells or cells that undergo differentiation (e.g., myoblasts-myotubes) the effects may become apparent.

Acknowledgments

The authors wish to express their gratitude to J. D. Watson, who has supported this work with enthusiasm. We thank J. I. Garrels for running the two-dimensional gels and S. Matsumura for help in the purification of microfilaments; and S. Queally, T. Lukralle, P. Renna, N. Haffner, D. Meltzer, B. McLaughlin, and J. Leibold for expert technical assistance. The patience of M. Szadkowski in typing this manuscript is also greatly appreciated. This work was supported in part by NIH Grants GM28277 (to J. R. F.), GM31048 (to J. J. C. L.), NHLBI-HL23848-04 (to S. H. B.), by Muscular Dystrophy Association Grants (to J. J. C. L. and S. H. B.), by a grant from American Heart Association—Nassau Chapter (to S. H. B.), by a Muscular Dystrophy Association Postdoctoral Fellowship (to F. M.), and by Grant CA 13106 to the Cold Spring Harbor Laboratory from the National Cancer Institute.

References

Antman, K. H., and Livingston, D. M., 1980, Intracellular neutralization of SV40 tumor antigens following microinjection of specific antibody, *Cell* **19**:627–635.

Atherton, B. T., and Hynes, R. O., 1981, A difference between plasma and cellular fibronectins located with monoclonal antibodies, *Cell* **25**:133–141.

Bader, D., Masaki, T., and Fischman, D. A., 1981, Myosin isoform transitions during chick myogenesis, *J. Cell Biol.* **91**:352a.

Blose, S. H. and Meltzer, D. I., 1981, Visualization of the 10 nm filament-vimentin rings in vascular endothelial cells *in situ:* Close resemblance to vimentin cytoskeletons found in monolayers *in vitro, Exp. Cell Res.* **135**:299–309.

Blose, S. H., Matsumura, F., and Lin, J. J. C., 1982, The structure of vimentin—10 nm filaments probed with a monoclonal antibody that recognizes a common antigenic determinant on vimentin and tropomyosin, *Cold Spring Harbor Symp. Quant. Biol.* **46**:455–463.

Bonner, W. M., and Laskey, R. A., 1974, A film detection method for tritium-labelled proteins and nucleic acids in polyacrylamide gels, *Eur. J. Biochem.* **46**:83–88.

Burridge, K., 1978, Direct identification of specific glycoproteins and antigens in sodium dodecyl sulfate gels, in: *Methods in Enzymology*, Volume 50, Academic Press, New York, pp. 54–64.

Burridge, K., and Feramisco, J. R., 1980, Microinjection and localization of a 130K protein in living fibroblasts: A relationship to actin and fibronectin, *Cell* **19**:587–595.

Dellago, K., Brouet, J. C., Perreau, J., and Paulin, D., 1982, Human monoclonal IgM with autoantibody activity against intermediate filaments, *Proc. Natl. Acad. Sci. USA* **79**:446–450.

Diacumakos, E. G., 1978, Methods for micromanipulation of human somatic cells in culture, *Methods Cell Biol.* **7**:287–311.

Dulbecco, R., Unger, M., Bologna, M., Battifora, H., Syka, P., and Okada, S., 1981, Cross-reactivity between Thy-1 and a component of intermediate filaments demonstrated using a monoclonal antibody, *Nature* **292**:772–774.

Dutton, A. H., Tokuyasu, K. T., and Singer, S. J., 1979, Iron-dextran antibody conjugates: General method for simultaneous staining of two components in high-resolution immunoelectron microscopy, *Proc. Natl. Acad. Sci. USA* **76**:3392–3396.

Ey, P. L., Prowse, S. J., and Jenkin, C. R., 1978, Isolation of pure IgG_1, IgG_{2a}, and IgG_{2b} immunoglobulins from mouse serum using protein A–sepharose, *Immunochemistry* **15**:429–436.

Feramisco, J. R., and Blose, S. H., 1980, Distribution of fluorescently labeled alpha-actinin in living and fixed fibroblasts, *J. Cell Biol.* **86**:608–615.

Garrels, J. I., 1979, Two-dimensional gel electrophoresis and computer analysis of proteins synthesized by clonal cell lines, *J. Biol. Chem.* **254**:7961–7977.

Geiger, B., 1979, A 130K protein from chicken gizzard: Its localization at the termini of microfilament bundles in cultured chicken cells, *Cell* **18**:193–205.

Geisler, N., and Weber, K., 1981, Comparison of the proteins of two immunologically distinct intermediate-sized filaments by amino acid sequence analysis: Desmin and vimentin, *Proc. Natl. Acad. Sci. USA* **78**:4120–4123.

Goding, J. W., 1978, Use of staphylococcal protein A as an immunological reagent, *J. Immunol. Methods* **29**: 241–253.

Goldman, R., Pollard, T., and Rosenbaum, J. (eds.), 1976, *Cold Spring Harbor Conference on Cell Proliferation*, Books A–C, Cold Spring Harbor, New York.

Goldman, R. D., and Knipe, D. M., 1972, The functions of cytoplasmic fibers in non-muscle cell motility, *Cold Spring Harbor Symp. Quant. Biol.* **37**:523–533.

Goldman, R. D., Chojnack, B., and Yerna, M.-J., 1979, Ultrastructure or microfilament bundles in baby hamster kidney (BHK-21) cells, *J. Cell Biol.* **80**:759–766.

Gordon, W. E., and Blose, S. H., 1979, Double lable immunofluorescence studies of actin, myosin, tropomyosin, alpha-actinin, and filamin in a non-muscle cell type, *J. Supramol. Struct.* **10**(Suppl.): 111.

Gordon, W. E., Bushnell, A., and Burridge, K., 1977, Characterization of the intermediate (10 nm) filaments of cultured cells using an autoimmune rabbit antiserum, *Cell* **13**:249–261.

Graessmann, A., Graessmann, M., and Mueller, C., 1980, Microinjection of early SV40 DNA fragments and T-antigen, in: *Methods in Enzymology*, Volume 65, Academic Press, New York, pp. 816–826.

Gregoria, G., 1976, The carrier potential of liposomes in biology and medicine, *N. Engl. J. Med.* **295**:704–710, 765–770.

Herrmann, S. H., and Mescher, M. F., 1979, Purification of the $H-2K^k$ molecule of the murine major histocompatibility complex, *J. Biol. Chem.* **254**:8713–8716.

Heuser, J. E., and Kirschner, M. W., 1980, Filament organization revealed in platinum replicas of freeze-dried cytoskeletons, *J. Cell Biol.* **86**:212–234.

Izant, J. G., and McIntosh, J. R., 1980, Microtubule-associated proteins: A monoclonal antibody to MAP-2 binds to differentiated neurons, *Proc. Natl. Acad. Sci. USA* **77**:4741–4745.

Kessler, S. W., 1975, Rapid isolation of antigens from cells with a staphylococcal protein A–antibody adsorbent: Parameters of the interaction of antibody–antigen complexes with protein A, *J. Immunol.* **115**:1617–1624.

Kishida, Y., Olsen, B. R., Berg, R. A., and Prockop, D. J., 1975, Two improved methods for preparing ferritin–protein conjugates for electron microscopy, *J. Cell Biol.* **64**:331–339.

Klymkowsky, M. W., 1981, Intermediate filaments in 3T3 cells collapse after intracellular injection of a monoclonal anti-intermediate filament antibody, *Nature* **291**:249–251.

Kohler, G., and Milstein, C., 1975, Continuous cultures of fused cells secreting antibody of pre-defined specificity, *Nature* **256:**495–497.

Kurki, P., Linder, E., Virtanen, I., and Stenman, S., 1977, Human smooth muscle autoantibodies reacting with intermediate (100 Å) filaments, *Nature* **268:**240–241.

Lane, D., and Koprowski, H., 1982, Molecular recognition and the future of monoclonal antibodies, *Nature* **296:**200–202.

Lane, E. B., 1982, Monoclonal antibodies provide specific intramolecular markers for the study of epithelial tonofilament organization, *J. Cell Biol.* **92:**665–673.

Lazarides, E., 1975, Tropomyosin antibody: The specific localization of tropomyosin in nonmuscle cells, *J. Cell Biol.* **65:**549–561.

Lazarides, E., 1976, Actin, alpha-actinin, and tropomyosin interaction in the structural organization of actin filaments in nonmuscle cells, *J. Cell Biol.* **68:**202–219.

Lazarides, E., and Burridge, K., 1975, Alpha-actinin: Immunofluorescent localization of a muscle structural protein in nonmuscle cells, *Cell* **6:**289–298.

Lazarides, E., and Weber, K., 1974, Actin antibody: The specific visualization of actin filaments in non-muscle cells, *Proc. Natl. Acad. Sci. USA* **71:**2268–2272.

Lin, J. J. C., 1981, Monoclonal antibodies against myofibrillar components of rat skeletal muscle decorate the intermediate filaments of cultured cells, *Proc. Natl. Acad. Sci. USA* **78:**2335–2339.

Lin, J. J. C., 1982, Mapping structural proteins of cultured cells by monoclonal antibodies, *Cold Spring Harbor Symp. Quant. Biol.* **46:**769–783.

Lin, J. J. C., and Feramisco, J. R., 1981, Disruption of the *in vivo* distribution of the intermediate filaments in fibroblasts through the microinjection of a specific monoclonal antibody, *Cell* **24:**185–193.

Lin, J. J. C., and Queally, S. A., 1982, A monoclonal antibody that recognizes Golgi-associated protein of cultured fibroblast cells, *J. Cell Biol.* **92:**108–112.

Lin, J. J. C., Burridge, K., Blose, S. H., Bushnell, A., Queally, S. A., and Feramisco, J. R., 1982, Use of monoclonal antibodies to study cytoskeleton, in: *Cell and Muscle Motility,* Volume 2 (R. M. Dowben and J. W. Shay, eds.), Plenum Press, New York, pp. 63–71.

Lwebuga-Mukasa, J. S., Lappi, S., and Taylor, P., 1976, Molecular forms of acetylcholinesterase from *Torpedo californica:* Their relationship to synaptic membranes, *Biochemistry* **15:**1425–1434.

Mabuchi, F., and Okuno, M., 1977, The effect of myosin antibody on the division of starfish blastomeres, *J. Cell Biol.* **74:**251–264.

Markham, R., Trey, S., and Hills, G. J., 1963, Methods for the enhancement of image detail and accentuation of structure in electron microscopy, *Virology* **20:**88–102.

Matsumura, F., and Lin, J. J. C., 1982, Visualization of monoclonal antibody binding to tropomyosin on native smooth muscle thin filaments by electron microscopy, *J. Mol. Biol.* **157:**163–171.

Medgyesi, G. A., Fust, G., Gergely, J., and Bazin, H., 1978, Classes and subclasses of rat immunoglobulins: Interaction with the complement system and with staphylococcal protein A., *Immunochemistry* **15:**125–129.

Miller, D. M., Mackenzie, J. M., Bolton, L. H., and Epstein, H. F., 1981, Monoclonal antibodies to nematode myosin heavy chain isozymes, *J. Cell Biol.* **91:**346a.

Mizuhira, V., and Futaesaku, Y., 1971, On the new approach of tannic acid and digitonine to the biological fixation, in: *Procedings of the 29th Annual Meeting of the Electron Microscopy Society of America* (G. W. Bailey, eds.), Claitor's Publishing Division, Boston, pp. 494–495.

O'Farrell, P. H., 1975, High resolution two-dimensional electrophoresis of proteins, *J. Biol. Chem.* **250:**4007–4021.

Osborn, M., Franke, W. W., and Weber, K., 1977, Visualization of a system of filaments 7–10 nm thick in cultured cells of an epithelioid line (PtK2) by immunofluorescence microscopy, *Proc. Natl. Acad. Sci. USA* **74:**2490–2494.

Osborn, M., Geisler, N., Shaw, G., Sharp, G., and Weber, K., 1982, Intermediate filaments, *Cold Spring Harbor Symp. Quant. Biol.* **46:**413–429.

Pepe, F. A., 1966, Some aspects of the structural organization of myofibril as revealed by antibody staining method, *J. Cell Biol.* **28:**505–525.

Pepe, F. A., 1973, The myosin filament: Immunochemical and ultrastructural approaches to molecular organization, *Cold Spring Harbor Symp. Quant. Biol.* **37:**97–108.

Pepe, F. A., 1975, Structure of muscle filaments from immunohistochemical and ultrastructural studies, *J. Histochem. Cytochem.* **23**:543–562.

Porter, R. R., and Reid, K. B. M., 1978, The biochemistry of complement, *Nature* **275**:699–704.

Pruss, R. M., Mirsky, R., Raff, M. C., Thorpe, R., Dowding, A. M., and Anderton, B. H., 1981, All classes of intermediate filaments share a common antigenic determinant defined by a monoclonal antibody, *Cell* **27**:419–428.

Reid, K. B. M., 1974, A collagen-like amino acid sequence in a polypeptide chain of human C1q (a subcomponent of the first component of complement), *Biochem. J.* **141**:189–203.

Reid, K. B. M., 1979, Complete amino acid sequences of the three collagen-like regions present in subcomponent C1q of the first component of human complement, *Biochem. J.* **179**:367–371.

Sarnow, P., Ho, Y. S., Williams, J., and Levine, A. J., 1982, Adenovirus E1b-58kd tumor antigen and SV40 large tumor antigen are physically associated with the same 54kd cellular protein in transformed cells, *Cell* **28**:387–394.

Schlaepfer, W. W., 1977, Immunological and ultrastructural studies of neurofilaments, *J. Cell Biol.* **74**:226–240.

Schlegel, R. A., and Rechsteiner, M. C., 1975, Microinjection of thymidine kinase and bovine serum albumin into mammalian cells by fusion with red blood cells, *Cell* **5**:371–379.

Secher, D. S., and Burke, D. C., 1980, A monoclonal antibody for large-scale purification of human leukocyte interferon, *Nature* **285**:446–450.

Simionescu, N., and Simionescu, M., 1976, Galloylglucoses of low molecular weight as mordant in electron microscopy, *J. Cell Biol.* **70**:608–633.

Stacey, D. W., and Allfrey, V. G., 1977, Evidence for the autophagy of microinjected proteins in HeLa cells, *J. Cell Biol.* **75**:807–817.

Sternberger, L. A., Hardy, R. H., Cuculis, J. J., and Meyer, H. G., 1970, The unlabeled antibody enzyme method of immunohistochemistry: Preparation and properties of soluble antigen–antibody complex (horseradish peroxidase–antihorseradish peroxidase) and its use in identification of spirochetes, *J. Histochem. Cytochem.* **18**:315–333.

Towbin, H., Staehelin, T., and Gordon, J., 1979, Electrophoretic transfer of proteins from polyacrylamide gels to nitrocellulose sheets: Procedure and some applications, *Proc. Natl. Acad. Sci. USA* **76**:4350–4354.

Wang, E., and Goldman, R. D., 1978, Functions of the cytoplasmic fibers in intracellular movements in BHK21 cells, *J. Cell Biol.* **79**:708–726.

Wang, E., Cross, R. K., and Choppin, R. W., 1979, Involvement of microtubules and 10 nm filaments in the movement and positioning of nuclei in syncytia, *J. Cell Biol.* **83**:320–337.

Wang, K., Feramisco, J. R., and Ash, J. F., 1982, Fluorescent localization of contractile proteins in tissue culture cells, in: *Methods in Enzymology*, Volume 85, Academic Press, New York, pp. 514–562.

Wehland, J., Willingham, M. C., Dickson, R., and Pastan, I., 1981, Microinjection of anticlathrin antibodies into fibroblasts does not interfere with the receptor-mediated endocytosis of alpha$_2$-macroglobulin, *Cell* **25**:105–119.

Willard, M., and Simon, C., 1981, Antibody decoration of neurofilaments, *J. Cell Biol.* **89**:198–205.

Willingham, M. C., and Yamada, S. S., 1979, Development of a new primary fixative for electron microscopic immunocytochemical localization of intracellular antigens in cultured cells, *J. Histochem. Cytochem.* **27**:947–960.

Willingham, M. C., Spicer, S. S., and Graber, C. D., 1971, Immunocytologic labeling of calf and human lymphocyte surface antigens, *Lab. Invest.* **25**:211–219.

Willingham, M. C., Yamada, S. S., and Pastan, I., 1978, Ultrastructural antibody localization of alpha$_2$-macroglobulin in membrane-limited vesicles in cultured cells, *Proc. Natl. Acad. Sci. USA* **75**:4359–4363.

Willingham, M. C., Jay, G., and Pastan, I., 1979, Localization of the ASV *src* gene product to the plasma membrane of transformed cells by electron microscopic immunocytochemistry, *Cell* **18**:125–134.

Yamaizumi, M., Uchida, T., Okada, Y., and Furusawa, M., 1978, Neutralization of diphtheria toxin in living cells by microinjection of antifragment A contained within resealed erythrocyte ghosts, *Cell* **13**:222–232.

7

Molecular Bases of Neuronal Individuality

Lessons from Anatomical and Biochemical Studies with Monoclonal Antibodies

Lois Alterman Lampson

I. Introduction

Monoclonal antibody analysis has been particularly welcome for studies of the nervous system. The number of cell types, their delicate and often extensive processes, their dense interconnections, and the inability of mature cells to divide *in vitro* make it particularly difficult to obtain separated subpopulations for conventional immunization or antibody purification. Thus, the possibility of obtaining cell-type-specific antibodies by cloning the immune response to a mixed population is especially attractive.

A second consequence of the physical organization of neural tissue is that morphological criteria, rather than biochemical or physiological criteria, are frequently used to discriminate among different cell types. Because of this, microscopic assays have been especially important in characterizing antineuronal antibodies. Section IIA reviews experimental systems that have been particularly amenable to microscopic analysis, and discusses some generalizations that seem valid.

The necessary reliance on microscopic assays for immunological studies of the nervous system poses an important problem of interpretation. The microscopic assay is essentially a binding assay. When two cell types bind the same

---

Lois Alterman Lampson • Department of Anatomy, University of Pennsylvania School of Medicine, Philadelphia, Pennsylvania 19104.

antibody strongly, all that can be said is that they share a cross-reactive determinant, and, perhaps, that the determinant has the same subcellular localization in each case. This is no less a problem when one is dealing with monoclonal antibodies. The antibody combining site is small compared to the size of most proteins. Thus, molecules with very different structures, and possibly very different functions, can bind strongly to a monoclonal antibody if they share a single cross-reactive determinant. The difficulty of physically separating the different neuronal cell types that bind a single monoclonal antibody may prevent a definitive biochemical or functional comparison of the molecules expressed by each. Other aspects of this problem, and possible strategies for approaching it, are discussed in Sections IIB and IIC.

The particular interest of this laboratory is to use monoclonal antibodies to probe molecular bases of neuronal individuality: In what ways do neurons differ from other cell types, and from each other, in their biochemical composition, particularly at the cell membrane? Our experimental system for the study of human neuronal antigens is described in Section III. Our own studies of neuronal proteins are reviewed in Sections IV and V, and relevant studies from other laboratories in Sections VI and VII. This body of work is interpreted in terms of a model of cellular individuality in Section VIII.

As understanding of neuronal individuality increases, one practical development will be to apply that knowledge to the detection, classification, or treatment of neural tumors. Our approach to these clinical uses is described in Section IX.

II. Antibodies to Neural Antigens: A Review of Recent Work

A. Anatomical Studies: Lessons from Studies in Well-Characterized Systems

1. Antibodies of Predetermined Specificity

Monoclonal antibodies should be powerful tools for probing cellular individuality in the nervous system. They may be used to study one antigenic determinant at a time, and many techniques for localizing antibodies for analysis by light or electron microscopy are already well-established. Some of the most informative studies have come from experimental systems in which existing knowledge of the morphological and physiological properties of the different cells provides a framework for interpreting the antibody binding patterns. The nervous system of the leech is an example of such an experimental system in lower animals. The retina, where a few major cell types are formed into ordered layers, has served as one source of well-characterized tissue from vertebrates.

An early question that might be asked in such well-defined systems is this: To what extent is the anatomical distribution of single antigenic determinants, defined by monoclonal antibodies, consistent with principles of neuronal organization that have been established by morphological and functional criteria? Some examples of recent studies in which immunological work has supported previously established systems of neuronal classification, or given fresh evidence for widely held ideas about neuronal organization, are reviewed here.

Perhaps the broadest anatomical subdivision is that which distinguishes neurons of the central nervous system from those with their cell bodies in the periphery. Consistent with this traditional subdivision, monoclonal antibodies have been described with specificity for either central (Cohen and Selvendran, 1981) or peripheral neurons (Vulliamy et al., 1981).

The vertebrate retina provides an experimental system in which many finer neuronal subdivisions are easily recognized. Morphological and physiological criteria have been used to divide retinal neurons into five major classes (photoreceptors, horizontal cells, bipolars, amacrines, and ganglion cells), as well as many subclasses (Dowling, 1975; Kolb, 1979; Sterling, 1983). Barnstable has described a group of monoclonal antibodies to "new" antigens whose distributions fit cleanly within this scheme. The panel includes antibodies that recognize all photoreceptors or only rod photoreceptors, as well as antibodies that distinguish between neurons and glial cells (Barnstable, 1980). In a series of studies of well-defined molecules, Karten and colleagues have used both monoclonal and conventional antibodies to localize several different neuropeptides in the avian retina. They have also found distributions that fit well within the established anatomical scheme. Each of the peptides localizes to one of the major cell types, the amacrine cells, and, moreover, appears to define a characteristic subset of amacrine cells (Brecha et al., 1981; Karten and Brecha, 1980, 1981). As discussed by the authors, these findings agree in principle, and in some cases, in detail, with previous anatomical studies suggesting that the retina amacrine cells may contain as many as 20 different subclasses (reviewed in Sterling 1983).

Because of its well-ordered structure, the retina has frequently been used to explore the question of positional specificity. During development in lower vertebrates, cells from retina project onto corresponding positions of the optic tectum (reviewed in Fraser and Hunt, 1980). Although it has been difficult to define the mechanism by which this specificity is achieved, it is often suggested that molecular gradients may play a role. Trisler et al. (1981) have now described a monoclonal antibody that defines a topographic gradient in the chick retina. Besides providing fresh evidence for the existence of such gradients, the antibody should be an important probe for analyzing their biochemistry and mode of action.

In the nervous system of the leech, many neurons have been classified, not only by morphological criteria, but also according to function. The leech, therefore, provides a system in which it has been possible to ask whether functional subclasses of neurons do, as has been widely assumed, bear characteristic antigenic markers. This assumption has received striking support in the work of Zipser and McKay (1981). They have described monoclonal antibodies that are specific for small groups, or even pairs, of cells among the 400 neurons of the leech ganglion. The functions served by some of these groups or pairs had already been defined. In other cases, the particular groupings established by the antibodies have suggested additional functional relationships. The appeal of this experimental system is that the existing knowledge of the physiological connections and available techniques facilitate direct testing of the suggested functional relationships. Therefore, in the future, we may expect this system to tell us how frequently cross-reactions established by monoclonal antibodies actually have a functional basis.

An important feature of each of these examples is that knowledge of the target molecule or of the experimental system permitted a very directed screening of the antibodies. The monoclonal antibodies were originally chosen, sometimes among hundreds of others, because they were specific for a single neuropeptide, did define a gradient, or did define small subpopulations. The existing literature makes it clear that antibodies with these predetermined specificities can be found and that they can be of great help in refining our understanding of well-characterized neural tissue.

2. Newly Defined Antigens

Another application for monoclonal antibodies should be to help complete the characterization of parts of the nervous system that have not been as extensively studied by other methods. In these cases, one may not have the benefit of either predetermined target molecules (such as a specific neuropeptide) or extensive anatomical subdivisions to aid in choosing the most appropriate antibodies. This consideration led us to ask this question: Suppose one were to raise a series of antibodies to a well-defined tissue, and, without prior selection, examine their distribution. How frequently would the distribution of a single antibody map onto the existing morphological or functional classifications? In collaboration with Dr. Peter Sterling, we have used a panel of monoclonal antibodies to the cat retina to address this question.

Monoclonal antibodies were raised to a retina homogenate, and 19 that bound strongly to the retina in microscopic assays were studied. Monoclonal antibody A257 provides a striking example of the type of distribution we have seen. As illustrated in Figure 1, A257 fills cells, binding strongly in both the cytoplasm and nucleus. This makes it particularly easy to appreciate the binding pattern at the light level. Light and electron microscopic studies show that A257 cuts across the five major divisions of retinal neurons in an unanticipated way: The antibody stains ganglion cells; some, but not all, amacrine cells; and a few bipolar cells. The majority of the bipolar cells, the horizontal cells, and the photoreceptors are completely unstained, as are the Muller glial cells. The other antibodies we have analyzed, most of which are to cell membrane rather than internal antigens, display a similar kind of pattern. That is, they do discriminate between neurons and glial cells, and they also discriminate between subpopulations of neurons, but not in a way that would have been predicted from existing knowledge of the retina's organization. Existing knowledge of the cat retina can help us determine whether these reaction patterns can give new insight into functional relationships. The important point here is that the anatomical dis-

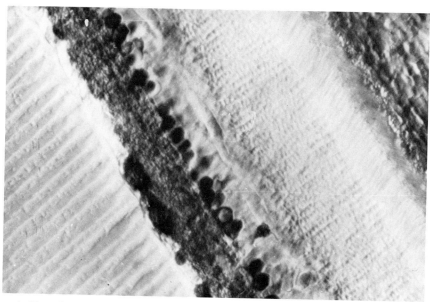

FIGURE 1. Monoclonal antibody A257 staining cat retina. The unlabeled antibody peroxidase–antiperoxidase (PAP) technique was used to stain a 50-μm section
of perfused cat retina. This antibody is able to stain
both cytoplasm and nuclei of some cell types, including
ganglion cells (examples are indicated by 1 in the drawing), amacrine cells (3), and occasional bipolar cells (4).
Staining is also seen within the processes of the inner
plexiform layer (2). At the same time, horizontal cells,
photoreceptors (5), and most bipolar cells are unstained. Electron microscopy confirms this pattern, and
shows that glial cell bodies and processes are also unstained (P. Sterling and L. Lampson, unpublished).

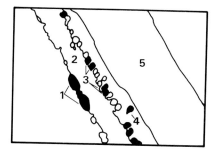

tribution of "new" antigens may frequently cut across the classifications that
would be established by more traditional criteria. Another example of this point
is seen among the anticerebellar antibodies recently described by Lagenauer *et
al.* (1980).

To summarize, recent work supports two conclusions about the use of
monoclonal antibodies in neural tissue. (1) When one has the advantage of
working with known molecules or a well-defined system, it is clearly possible to
select monoclonal antibodies that are specific for fine neuronal subpopulations
and to use these as immunological probes. (2) While monoclonal antibodies
should be important tools for clarifying less well-defined systems, great care
must be used in interpreting the binding patterns. If one does not have the
benefit of either a known molecule or a morphologically well-defined tissue to
aid in screening the antibodies, one cannot expect that the immunological classifications will necessarily coincide with independent morphological or functional
studies.

B. Biochemical Studies: Distinguishing between an Antigenic Determinant and the Molecule That Bears It

Two factors make it essential to complement anatomical studies with biochemical analysis. First, it is important to stress that a single antibody is specific for an antigenic determinant, rather than a whole molecule. Although the estimated size of an antigenic determinant may vary with the particular antigen–antibody combination and the assay, it is certainly small relative to the size of most proteins. Fewer than 10 amino acids, sugar residues, or nucleotides are sufficient to give maximal binding energy for most of the antibodies that have been studied (Kabat, 1966). This means that it is possible to obtain monoclonal antibodies to a variety of different determinants on a single molecule. Moreover, experience with molecules whose structures are well known demonstrates that different anatomical distributions may be obtained depending upon which antibody is used. The immunoglobulin molecule itself provides a very clear illustration of this point. Although immunoglobulins are the definitive marker for B lymphocytes, not every antiimmunoglobulin antibody will react with all B lymphocytes, or only B lymphocytes. An antibody to an immunoglobulin idiotype will react with at most a few clones of B lymphocytes. An antibody to the determinant on human immunoglobulin light chains that cross-reacts with β2-microglobulin (β2-m) (Gottlieb *et al.*, 1977) will react with all human cells that express β2-m, which includes most of the nucleated cells in the adult. Other examples are given in Table I. As these examples show, the anatomical distribution of a single molecule may be either broader or narrower than that observed with a particular monoclonal antibody. That is, the distribution of the immunoglobulin molecule is broader than would be seen with an antiidiotype antibody, and narrower than would be seen with an antibody to the β2-m cross-reactive determinant.

The second important point is that many molecules display tissue-specific differences in their structure. For example, Thy-1 and Ia are each expressed in the nervous system as well as in lymphoid and other tissues (Ting *et al.*, 1981; Williams and Gagnon, 1982). Each of these molecules displays tissue-specific variation in its carbohydrate composition (Barclay *et al.*, 1976; Cullen *et al.*, 1981). An antibody to the carbohydrate portion of these molecules might therefore display a narrower tissue distribution than would one to the common pro-

TABLE I

Anatomical Distributions That Would Be Observed with Different Antiimmunoglobulin Antibodies

Antibody specificity	Anatomical distribution
Immunoglobulin	All B lymphocytes
Light chains	All B lymphocytes
κ Light chains	Sixty percent B lymphocytes
λ Light chains	Forty percent of B lymphocytes
Idiotype	One or few clones of B lymphocytes
Ig/β2-m cross-reactive determinant	Most nucleated human cells

tein portion. Examples of families of molecules that express tissue-specific differences in the protein backbone itself include isozymes (Harris, 1979) and the intermediate filament subunits (discussed in Section VI.D).

Thus, when a monoclonal antibody to a previously uncharacterized molecule shows an apparently restricted anatomical distribution, one must ask whether the molecule that bears the antigenic determinant might belong to a family of functionally-related molecules with a broader distribution. Conversely, if a monoclonal antibody displays a broad or unexpected distribution, one must ask whether the molecules that bear the antigenic determinant are the same in the different cells or tissues. Possibilities in this case are that the molecules might be identical, they might have an obvious structural relationship (tissue-specific forms of Thy-1 or Ia), or they might have a more subtle structural or evolutionary relationship (Ig and β2-m). In addition, a monoclonal antibody may react with different molecules for which no functional, structural or evolutionary relationship is currently known. The reported cross-reaction between Thy-1 and intermediate filaments is an example (Dulbecco et al., 1981). In these cases, there is no a priori way of knowing whether the antibody has revealed an informative relationship as opposed to a "fortuitous" cross-reaction.

It is worth reiterating that the degree of homology between the members of a protein family may vary widely. At one end of the spectrum, we have the isozymes and the immunoglobulins. In these cases, members of a family may differ from each other by only a few amino acids. Approaching the other end of the spectrum, we have the intermediate filaments, which display gross differences in molecular weight and chain structure. Yet their physical properties, as well as recent amino acid sequence data, suggest a basis for the recently described immunological cross-reactivity, and strongly support thinking of the intermediate filaments as members of a family of functionally related proteins (Geisler et al., 1982; Lazarides, 1980; Pruss et al., 1981). Additional examples are discussed in Section VI. The point here is that the ability to recognize cross-reactions between nonidentical molecules should not be regarded as a weakness of monoclonal (or conventional) antibodies. Rather, these cross-reactions may often give very useful information about molecular relationships.

To summarize, in interpreting microscopic or other binding assays, it is essential to discriminate between the distribution of an antigenic determinant and the distribution of the molecule that bears the determinant. When a monoclonal antibody (or a conventional serum) does reveal cross-reactions between nonidentical molecules, this is not necessarily a "fortuitous" cross-reaction. Rather, the antibody may be revealing a family of functionally or evolutionarily related proteins. (This is discussed further in Section VI.)

C. Sources of Tissue for Biochemical Studies: The Potential of Cloned Cell Lines

One general impediment limits the biochemical studies: In order to compare the biochemical composition of molecules recognized by a single antibody in different cells, one must first separate the cells from each other. Although it is relatively simple to make this comparison at the level of whole tissues (brain versus peripheral nerve; brain versus retina; retina versus cortex; motor cortex versus visual cortex), it is much more difficult to achieve it for individual cell types (such as subpopulations of amacrine cells). Techniques that have been used or suggested include selective culture conditions to permit the growth of only some cell types; antibody-mediated killing of selected cells; and antibody-mediated separation of cells, such as by the fluorescence-activated cell sorter. In some cases, simple physical separations are also possible, such as isolation of large retinal ganglion cells by means of unit-gravity sedimentation (Kornguth et al., 1981). Clearly, as finer subpopulations are studied, these techniques become increasingly more difficult to use.

An alternative approach is to use cloned cell lines of known origin as antigenic models of different cell types. Previous experience in the lymphoid system, in which cell lines bearing markers associated with many different lymphocyte subpopulations and stages of differentiation are available, shows the potential value of this approach. At present, cloned neural cell lines are available from only relatively few cell types and species. The most commonly used include rodent lines derived from embryonic neural tissue, and human and rodent lines derived from neural tumors. Most of these lines have been categorized as corresponding to neurons, glia, or intermediate types (Stallcup et al., 1981), or to broad subdivisions within the first two categories [for example, granule cells or oligodendrocytes (Heitzmann et al., 1981)]. In generating and defining cells corresponding to finer subdivisions (such as subpopulations of amacrine cells), monoclonal antibodies should be of use both for isolating selected populations for expansion and for characterizing the resulting clones. The antibodies will be particularly important for classification, since the morphological criteria that form the basis of much in vivo discrimination between cell types will no longer be applicable to cell lines.

Perhaps the most important technical limitation in producing new cell lines is that, unlike mature lymphoid cells, differentiated neurons do not normally divide. Thus, it is not yet clear to what extent neuronal cell lines can be matched to adult neuronal cell types. Neuronal cell lines can express some properties of differentiated cells. For example, human neuroblastoma lines, which are derived from a tumor of the sympathetic neuroblast, can express properties associated with electrically excitable membranes, as well as neurotransmitters and enzymes of neurotransmitter biosynthesis (Biedler et al., 1973; Schlesinger et al., 1976; Tischler et al., 1977; West et al., 1977). In addition, we have found that neuroblastoma lines reflect the unusually weak expression of the major histocompatibility antigens that is seen in normal brain (Section IV).

The ability of neuronal cell lines to express differentiated properties may reflect that fact that these properties were already present in the immature cell of origin. Alternatively, expression of differentiated phenotypes may result from transformation or adaptation to tissue culture, or, when the cell line has been created by fusion, interaction between the two parental cells (Minna, 1978). Additional differentiated properties may also be revealed by in vitro differentiation of the cell lines (Imada and Sueoka, 1980; Littauer *et al.*, 1980). It is, of course, of great interest to know whether a particular differentiated phenotype is characteristic of the cell of origin or its progeny. In addition, the cell lines can serve as expedient, homogeneous sources of large quantities of cellular components (such as neuropeptides or their receptors), and this use is independent of whether the component is normally expressed by the cell of origin.

It seems likely that, as monoclonal antibodies are used to select cells for expansion and to characterize new and existing lines (Bechtol *et al.*, 1980; Heitzmann *et al.*, 1981; Kennett *et al.*, 1980; Seeger *et al.*, 1982; Stallcup *et al.*, 1981; Trisler *et al.*, 1979; Section IV), the lines will become increasingly useful for biochemical analysis of both developmental and adult phenotypes.

III. An Experimental System for Studying Neuronal Individuality in Human Tissue

A. Human Neuroblastoma-Derived Cell Lines for Biochemical Analysis

We have sought to establish an experimental system that would allow both anatomical and biochemical studies of mammalian neural antigens. In the human lymphoid system, normal tissue, tumors, and cloned cell lines have been used very successfully as sources of tissue, with the results obtained in one system frequently reinforcing those from the others. We have sought to establish a similar interplay in the nervous system. The heart of our system is a panel of human neuroblastoma-derived cell lines. Each cell line is derived from a different neuroblastoma tumor, which in turn represents a clonal expansion of a different sympathetic neuroblast.

Several types of studies support the idea of using neuroblastoma cell lines as a biochemical model for the original tumor. The cell lines and tumor also display many properties of normal neurons. Different neuroblastoma tumors and their derivative cell lines have been shown to express individual neurotransmitters or enzymes of neurotransmitter biosynthesis. Many of the cell lines express the action potential Na^+ ionophore, suggesting that they have excitable membranes. Other proteins that are specific for, or characteristic of, the nervous system, such as the neuron-specific enolase (NSE or 14-3-2) and Thy-1, are also synthesized by these cell lines (Biedler *et al.*, 1973; Herschman and Lerner, 1973; Schlesinger *et al.*, 1976; Seeger *et al.*, 1982; West *et al.*, 1977).

In studies with monoclonal antineuroblastoma antibodies, we have observed frequent cross-reactions between the cell lines and normal brain, and this agrees with studies using both monoclonal and conventional antibodies in other laboratories. However, the biochemical basis of most of these immunological cross-reactions has not been directly studied. Thus, in most cases, it is not possible to say whether a monoclonal (or conventional) antibody is recognizing the same molecule in the cell line as in normal neural tissue. Therefore, the studies with known molecules are the best current evidence that the cell lines (and tumors) can express individual phenotypes of normal neurons.

Our approach is to use these cloned lines as "antigen factories"—sources of freshly synthesized molecules produced by individual clones of cells—for biochemical analysis. The information we gain may help characterize the neuroblastoma tumor, which is a major solid tumor of early childhood (Evans, 1980). Information we gain from the study of the cell lines may also help us to understand normal neurons. The way in which this interplay has helped us to probe the neural expression of the molecules bearing the conventional major transplantation antigens (HLA-A,B,C molecules) is described in Section IV and in Lampson *et al.* (1983) and Lampson and Whelan (1983).

B. Complementary Microscopic Studies of Primary Tumors and Normal Tissue

An essential part of our approach is that results that are obtained with the cloned cell lines must be extended to primary tumors and normal nervous tissue. Because neither of these represent homogeneous, or easily separable, populations of cells, we must rely on microscopic analysis for much of this work. Many other laboratories have shown the feasibility of using frozen human material obtained at biopsy or autopsy for immunological studies. Because of the difficulty of obtaining such material at will, we have explored two additional approaches to anatomical analysis.

1. Paraffin Sections

One approach is to exploit the extensive collections of formalin-fixed, paraffin-embedded material, taken from both normal and malignant tissue, that are maintained in many hospitals. For appropriate antigen–antibody combinations, immunocytochemical techniques, such as the peroxidase–antiperoxidase (PAP) technique, can be used for studies of such material, at least when conventional antisera are used (Sternberger, 1979).

In asking whether this material is suitable for analysis with individual monoclonal antibodies, three independent factors must to be considered. (1) Some antigens might be destroyed by the fixation (4% formaldehyde) (many of our antibodies were initially screened against cells that had been "lightly" fixed in 0.1% glutaraldehyde). (2) Some molecules might be lost during the paraffin embedding and the attendant exposure to warm wax, acids, alcohol, and xylene. (3) Some determinants on a molecule might survive these procedures, whereas others would be destroyed. Thus, only some monoclonal antibodies to a given molecule might be usable. Our initial findings may be summarized as follows:

1. To test the effects of fixation, eight antineuroblastoma antibodies were chosen for their strong binding to neural tissue in radioimmunoassays using lightly fixed material. In two assays, binding to lightly fixed tissue was compared

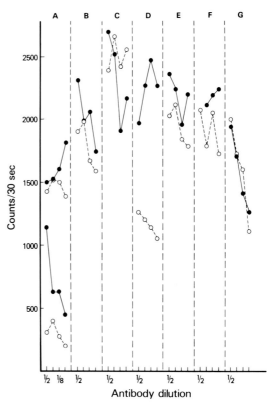

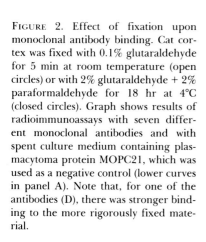

FIGURE 2. Effect of fixation upon monoclonal antibody binding. Cat cortex was fixed with 0.1% glutaraldehyde for 5 min at room temperature (open circles) or with 2% glutaraldehyde + 2% paraformaldehyde for 18 hr at 4°C (closed circles). Graph shows results of radioimmunoassays with seven different monoclonal antibodies and with spent culture medium containing plasmacytoma protein MOPC21, which was used as a negative control (lower curves in panel A). Note that, for one of the antibodies (D), there was stronger binding to the more rigorously fixed material.

to the binding to tissue that had been fixed in 4% aldehydes overnight. In seven of the cases, there was no difference in the extent of binding. In the eighth case, the binding was actually increased for the more rigorously fixed target tissue (Figure 2). Thus, for antibodies chosen at random from screenings against lightly fixed material, the more rigorous fixation did not usually destroy the antigenic determinants.

Of course, not every antigen will be unaffected or enhanced by fixation. For example, reactivity of L368, a monoclonal antibody to β2-microglobulin, was reduced when the concentration of fixative was increased from 0.1 to 4% aldehydes.

2. Four antibodies known to bind strongly to tissue that had been fixed in 4% aldehydes were tested in the PAP assay against paraffin-embedded tissue. We found that two of the antibodies bound strongly to the paraffin-embedded tissue, one bound weakly, and one did not show any detectable binding. Thus, while the paraffin embedding can cause loss of antigenic determinants over and above that resulting from the fixation procedure, many determinants can survive this treatment (J. Whelan and L. Lampson, unpublished; Sternberger *et al.*, 1982).

2. Species Cross-Reactions

A second approach to microscopic analysis, particularly for studies of normal tissue, is to exploit interspecies cross-reactions and perform microscopic studies in tissue obtained from perfused laboratory animals. We have found that many of the monoclonal antibodies we have raised to mammalian neural tissue do show cross-reactivity between humans, mice, rats, and cats. This is true whether the original immunogen was a human neuroblastoma-derived cell line or normal cat tissue (homogenized retina), and agrees with previous reports for both monoclonal and conventional antibodies.

As discussed above, we must confirm biochemically that the same molecules are being recognized in the different species. The antiretina antibody A257 provides a striking illustration of this point. In microscopic and radioimmunoassays, A257 binds strongly to the human neuroblastoma-derived cell line IMR-5 and displays the relatively uncommon intracellular distribution that had been seen in several neuronal cell types in the cat: The antibody stains the nucleus and cytoplasm, but not the outer membrane. However, when immunoblots were used to identify the polypeptide chains recognized in the different tissues, it was seen that A257 binds to human neuroblastoma and cat retina polypeptides of different apparent molecular weights (Figure 3). Presumably, closer correspondence between the sources of cat and human tissues would have increased the

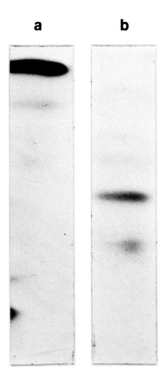

a   **b**

FIGURE 3. Analysis of A257 on immunoblots. Monoclonal antibody A257 (Figure 1) was allowed to bind to electrophoretically separated proteins from either (a) the neuroblastoma cell line IMR-5 or (b) normal adult cat retina. The procedure was as described in Fisher and Lampson, Appendix to this volume. Note that, although the antibody binds strongly to both tissues, in agreement with microscopic analysis, the predominant polypeptide chain that is recognized has a different apparent molecular weight in the two tissues.

likelihood of finding a similar molecule in the two species. The important point here is that even a strong cross-reaction and a similar subcellular distribution in microscopic assay do not ensure biochemical identity of the recognized molecules.

Thus, both clinical material preserved as paraffin sections, and perfused tissue of laboratory animals, may provide alternative sources of tissue for microscopic analysis with carefully selected antibodies. However, the effect of fixation and embedding and the possibility of cross-reactions between nonidentical molecules must be evaluated in each case.

3. Conclusions

As a system for study, the human nervous system offers the potential of immediate clinical applicability. Indeed, clinical interest has led to the establishment and characterization of many different cell lines from neuronal, glial, and other human cell types. By using monoclonal antibodies as probes for single molecules, the structure of individual molecules expressed by individual cells can be compared. The comparison can be made between different cell types (neurons versus glial or lymphoid cells) as well as between different cells of a single type (different neuronal cell lines). Microscopic assays can then be used to relate observations made on the cell lines to individual cells in primary tumors and in normal tissue. Existing collections of fixed material can provide one source of such tissue for appropriate antibodies. It may also be possible to exploit species cross-reactions, again for appropriate antibodies. Our laboratory is using this experimental approach to study the molecular bases of neuronal individuality, as described in Sections III.C, IV, and V.

C. Neurons versus Other Cell Types: Do Similarities or Differences Predominate?

Most mature mammalian neurons differ from other cell types in one or all of these ways: The neuron is incapable of division, it has an excitable membrane, it has a cell body in a specific place, it extends processes in specific directions, it makes specific synaptic contacts with other cells, and it recognizes and expresses characteristic neurotransmitters. One would expect that molecules serving each of these functions might serve as neuronal markers, particularly at the cell surface. At the same time, many other cellular components are very widespread or ubiquitous. In probing neuronal individuality, one might begin by asking which of these factors predominates. We have used monoclonal antibodies to ask this question at the level of the cell membrane: Are most of the molecules on the surface of a neuron widely distributed among other cell types, or do most of them serve more specific functions?

One might approach this problem by comparing neuronal membrane proteins *en masse* with membrane proteins of other cell types (reviewed in Moore,

1975). One problem with this approach is that, without knowing the function or finer structure of the proteins, it is not possible to be certain of the interpretation. For example, the Thy-1 molecule has the same protein backbone but a different carbohydrate structure in neurons and lymphocytes. If neuronal and lymphocyte membrane proteins were compared without realizing that one of the molecules was Thy-1, the different bands would be seen as different glycoproteins.

A second way of approaching this question is to examine individual major cell surface proteins one at a time. This approach has been used very successfully in the analysis of erythrocytes and lymphocytes (Branton *et al.*, 1981; Brown *et al.*, 1981), and monoclonal antibodies have now facilitated extending the approach to other cell types. Our studies of the neuronal expression of both known and newly defined molecules are described in Sections IV and V.

IV. Striking Paucity of HLA-A,B,C Molecules on Cells of Neuronal Origin

To begin our studies of the human neuronal surface, we chose the HLA-A,B,C molecules, which bear the conventional major transplantation antigens, for several reasons. The structure of the molecules has been intensively studied, their general tissue distribution is established, and well-characterized conventional and monoclonal antibodies, some of which we ourselves had raised, were already available. We expected that the study of these known molecules would help us to work out assay procedures to be used later for new molecules. In addition, two points lent this work a more theoretical interest. First, although the HLA-A,B,C molecules are generally thought to be present on most nucleated human cells, they are only poorly expressed by homogenates of whole brain. Since glial cell lines have been shown to express the molecules strongly, this suggested that neurons may express them only weakly. The second point is that the extensive structural studies of the HLA-A,B,C molecules have for the most part utilized material isolated from lymphoid cells. We were interested to know, therefore, whether there might be tissue-specific variations in the structure of the molecules.

A. HLA-A,B,C Function and Structure: Antibody Probes

The HLA-A,B,C molecules are important in several ways. As transplantation antigens, they form a principal barrier to successful organ transplantation. In addition, they are involved in cellular interactions in the immune response. A third important property is that a growing list of human diseases are associated with particular HLA phenotypes.

The clinical importance of these molecules has led to intensive study of their structure. The HLA-A,B,C molecules are a family of closely related proteins. In each case, the molecule is composed of two chains. The HLA chains, which are coded by the major histocompatibility complex on chromosome 6, are glycoproteins of 43,000 daltons apparent molecular weight. These chains are highly polymorphic. Approximately 20 alleles at the A locus, 40 at the B locus, and six at the C locus have been identified (Bodmer, 1981). For each of these molecules, the polymorphic HLA chain is linked to an invariant 12,000-dalton chain, β2-microglobulin.

Because of their clinical importance and the resulting knowledge of their structure, these molecules were among the first subjects for study with monoclonal antibodies (Barnstable *et al.*, 1978; Lampson *et al.*, 1978a; Parham and Bodmer, 1978). Of the many possible specificities, we have chosen two monoclonal antibodies that serve as very broad probes for these molecules. L368 recognizes β2-microglobulin, the invariant chain of all HLA-A,B,C molecules (Lampson and Levy, 1980). W6/32 recognizes a nonpolymorphic determinant on the native two-chain molecules (Barnstable *et al.*, 1978). A conventional rabbit antiserum to β2-microglobulin (Dako Immunoglobulins), which presumably contains antibodies to more than one determinant on that chain, was also used.

B. Striking Paucity of HLA-A,B,C on Neuroblastoma Cell Lines: Results from Four Kinds of Assays

In order to be able to compare the structure of the HLA-A,B,C molecules on neurons, glia, and lymphoid cells, we used a panel of human cell lines. In part because these experiments were intended as a model for later studies with new antibodies, we compared a number of different assays, as described below.

Among assays for cell surface determinants, the most convenient is the radioimmunoassay against glutaraldehyde-fixed target cells. We had previously established that the light fixation (0.1% glutaraldehyde for 5 min at room temperature) did not destroy the determinants recognized by L368 or W6/32 on lymphoid cells. Our standard assay employs cell pellets consisting of 250,000 fixed target cells. Under these conditions, we obtained strong binding of L368 and W6/32 to glial and lymphoid cells, but no consistent specific binding to four different neuroblastoma-derived cell lines (Figure 4). By increasing the number of neuroblastoma targets, we were able to reveal some binding with L368 and even weaker binding with W6/32 against some of the neuroblastoma lines (Lampson *et al.*, 1983).

Complement-mediated cytotoxicity is generally regarded as a potentially more sensitive assay for cell surface antigens. In collaboration with Dr. Roger Kennett, we used this assay to assess HLA-A,B,C expression on the different cell lines. In this case, the assay was not more sensitive than the binding assay. In three experiments, we detected no specific lysis of any of the neuroblastoma-derived lines, whereas the antibodies did lyse a B cell line, and a previously characterized antineuroblastoma antibody did lyse the neuroblastoma lines (Kennett *et al.*, 1982).

In order to be able to detect internal as well as cell surface determinants, we analyzed sections of fixed cells that had been embedded in agarose. This en-

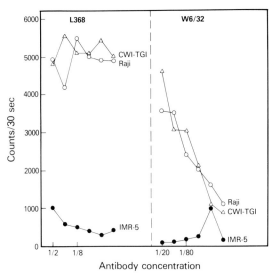

FIGURE 4. Binding of monoclonal antibodies to human cell lines. Monoclonal antibodies L368 and W6/32 were assayed against neuronal (IMR-5), glial (CW1-TG1), and lymphoid (Raji) cell lines in radioimmunoassay. Negative controls, described in Figure 2, were a few hundred counts/30 sec for the different cell lines (Lampson, 1981).

sured that cytoplasmic antigens would be directly exposed to antibody. The unlabeled antibody peroxidase–antiperoxidase (PAP) procedure was used to assess the binding of L368 and W6/32 to lymphoid, glial, and neuronal cell lines (Lampson and Whelan, 1983; Lampson *et al.*, 1983; and Lampson *et al.*, Appendix to this volume). The results of these assays are illustrated in Figure 5. Strong binding to lymphoid and glial cells was seen, with a dark rim of stain surrounding a less darkly stained cytoplasm. This characteristic pattern of stain agrees with the previously established subcellular localization of these antigens. However, even when 30-fold more concentrated antibodies were used, we detected no specific staining in the neuroblastoma lines.

The fourth assay in this series was a binding inhibition assay. In this case, detergent (Nonidet P-40) extracts of the cell lines were used to inhibit the binding of the monoclonal antibodies to a B-cell target (Lampson, Appendix to this volume). The advantages of this assay were that it had the potential to reveal both internal and cell surface antigens in unfixed tissue and that it allowed us to quantify the differences in HLA-A,B,C expression. In addition, this assay proved to be the most sensitive of the four assays in these experiments. As illustrated in Figure 6, we were able to obtain clear inhibition of both L368 and W6/32 with the neuroblastoma extracts. Yet, these extracts were clearly much less efficient inhibitors than were the glial or lymphoid extracts. In 10 experiments, the amount of B-cell extract needed to obtain 50% inhibition was compared to the amount of neuroblastoma or glial extract needed for 50% inhibition. We found that the neuroblastoma extracts were always less than 1% as efficient, per microgram of extract protein, than the B-cell extract, and the B-cell and glial cell extracts were about equally efficient (Lampson and Whelan, 1983).

Thus, in four different assays in which both internal and cell surface antigens of fixed or unfixed tissue might be revealed, neuroblastoma cell lines showed a striking paucity of HLA-A,B,C molecules as compared to glial or lymphoid lines. Indeed, our results suggest that the neuroblastoma cell lines are

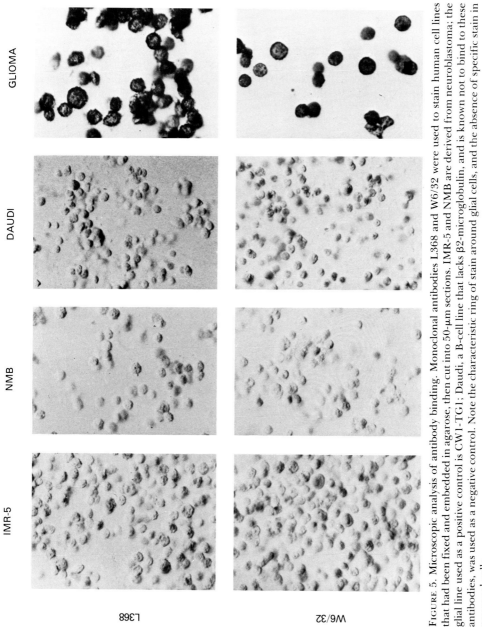

FIGURE 5. Microscopic analysis of antibody binding. Monoclonal antibodies L368 and W6/32 were used to stain human cell lines that had been fixed and embedded in agarose, then cut into 50-μm sections. IMR-5 and NMB are derived from neuroblastoma; the glial line used as a positive control is CW1-TG1; Daudi, a B-cell line that lacks β2-microglobulin, and is known not to bind to these antibodies, was used as a negative control. Note the characteristic ring of stain around glial cells, and the absence of specific stain in neuronal cells.

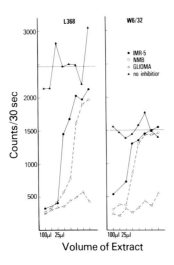

FIGURE 6. Binding inhibition assays. Diminishing volumes of cell extracts were used to inhibit the binding of a constant volume of monoclonal antibody (L368 or W6/32) to a human B-cell line. Extracts were prepared from the same starting cell concentration, and final protein concentrations varied by a factor of two or less. Solid line shows mean of values obtained with no inhibitor. Note that both neuronal (IMR-5 and NMB) and glial extracts do inhibit the antibodies, but the glial extract is much more efficient.

at the low end of the observed spectrum of HLA-A,B,C activity (Lampson *et al.*, 1983).

C. HLA-A,B,C Expression on Neuroblastoma Tumors and Normal Brain

As we continued to study HLA-A,B,C expression on neuroblastoma lines, it became of increasing interest to know whether the paucity of the molecules reflected a property of either the original tumor or normal neurons.

To study the tumor, we first used a microscopic assay to analyze metastatic neuroblastoma in bone marrow. Here, the tumor may appear as aggregates, which are readily identified by their morphology, as well as single cells. Normal bone marrow was used as a control. The results of this type of assay are illustrated in Figure 7. The majority ($\geq 96\%$) of the nucleated normal bone marrow cells were clearly stained with monoclonal antibody L368, in agreement with previous reports of HLA-A,B,C expression in this tissue (Brown *et al.*, 1979; Fitchen *et al.*, 1981). In contrast, many fewer of the single cells ($< 50\%$) in the neuroblastoma marrow were stained. More strikingly, all tumor aggregates appeared negative. The unstained aggregates were readily distinguished from clumps or groups of cells in the normal marrow, which were clearly stained (Lampson *et al.*, 1983).

These results confirm that the paucity of HLA-A,B,C is a characteristic of at least one form of neuroblastoma tumor rather than a culture artifact. They also suggest a possible use for the antibodies in helping to discriminate between tumor cells and HLA-A,B,C-rich normal tissue, as discussed in Section IX.

Previous studies had shown that normal human and mouse brain express at best weak HLA-A,B,C or H-2,K,D activity, respectively (Berah *et al.*, 1970; Schachner and Sidman, 1973; Williams *et al.*, 1980). We have confirmed this in our laboratory, using both radioimmunobinding assays and binding inhibition assays. We are now using the microscopic assay to directly compare the HLA-A,B,C expression on normal neurons and glial cells.

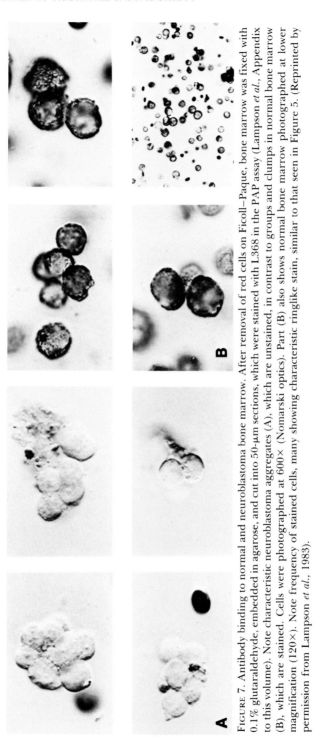

Figure 7. Antibody binding to normal and neuroblastoma bone marrow. After removal of red cells on Ficoll–Paque, bone marrow was fixed with 0.1% glutaraldehyde, embedded in agarose, and cut into 50-μm sections, which were stained with L368 in the PAP assay (Lampson et al., Appendix to this volume). Note characteristic neuroblastoma aggregates (A), which are unstained, in contrast to groups and clumps in normal bone marrow (B), which are stained. Cells were photographed at 600× (Nomarski optics). Part (B) also shows normal bone marrow photographed at lower magnification (120×). Note frequency of stained cells, many showing characteristic ringlike stain, similar to that seen in Figure 5. (Reprinted by permission from Lampson et al., 1983).

D. Possible Functional Significance of Weak HLA-A,B,C Expression on Neural Tissue and Tumors

In general, "foreign" antigens, such as viruses, must be associated with the host's own HLA-A,B,C molecules if they are to be the target of T-cell-mediated cytotoxicity (Dausset, 1981). This is relevant to our HLA results in three ways.

First, if normal neurons lack HLA-A,B,C molecules, they may be protected from T-cell-mediated cytotoxicity, even if they express viral or other inappropriate antigens. In theory, this may serve to protect postmitotic cells, such as neurons, which cannot be replaced. Second, if neurons lack HLA-A,B,C molecules, neurons in grafted neural tissue may be protected from T-cell-mediated killing, even if they come from donors expressing inappropriate HLA-A,B,C specificities, or they express other inappropriate antigens. Third, if tumor-specific antigens do not appear in conjunction with appropriate HLA-A,B,C molecules, then the tumor cells may also be protected from T-cell-mediated cytotoxicity. Thus, tumors or metastases with weak HLA-A,B,C expression may be relatively more successful in escaping host rejection (Bodmer, 1981). In this context, it is interesting to note that neuroblastoma can be a particularly aggressive tumor.

Of course, several other interpretations of weak neuronal HLA-A,B,C expression must also be considered. Low levels of HLA-A,B,C (compared to what is expressed on other cell types) may be sufficient to mediate T-cell restriction; HLA-A,B,C expression may increase under certain pathological conditions; or other molecules may serve as restriction elements in neural tissue. Direct microscopic analysis of normal and pathological neural tissue, and structural and functional studies of restriction in the T-cell-mediated killing of *neuronal* target cells are needed to test these possibilities.

E. Further Studies: Immunoprecipitation

In seeking the functional significance of the observed weak HLA-A,B,C expression on cells of neuronal origin, we have first sought to characterize the molecules that inhibit the monoclonal antibodies. First, we wish to know whether the binding inhibition assays reveal cross-reactive molecules rather than conventional HLA-A,B,C molecules. Immunoprecipitation studies have given us a partial answer to this question.

For immunoprecipitation, cell lines were labeled biosynthetically with [^{35}S]methionine or [^{3}H]-sugars, extracted with nonionic detergent (Nonidet P-40), and then incubated with antibody bound to *Staphylococcus aureus*, as described previously (Lampson, 1980). The precipitates were analyzed by SDS–polyacrylamide gel electrophoresis, on 10–20% gradient polyacrylamide slab gels, using the Laemmli buffer system. Monoclonal antibodies L368 and W6/32, as well as a conventional rabbit anti-β2-m serum, were used. The molecules precipitated from three neuroblastoma lines and one glial line were directly compared to the molecules precipitated from the B-cell line Raji.

These experiments have shown that all of the neural cell lines (neuronal and glial) do synthesize a polypeptide chain that comigrates with the β2-microglobulin precipitated from Raji (Lampson *et al.*, 1983). The experiments also

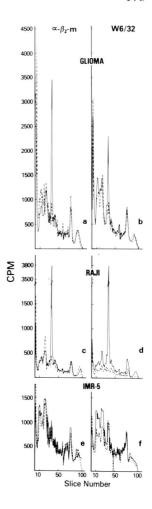

FIGURE 8. Immunoprecipitation from cell extracts. Cell lines were labeled biosynthetically with a mixture of [³H]-sugars, extracted with NP-40, and precipitated with anti-β2-m serum or with monoclonal antibody W6/32. The precipitates were analyzed by SDS–polyacrylamide gel electrophoresis on 10–20% polyacrylamide gradient slab gels. Precipitates from a glioma line (CW1-TG1) and Raji were electrophoresed on the same gel; precipitates from IMR-5 were also electrophoresed on the same gel with Raji precipitates. Individual lanes were cut into 1-μm slices and solublized in Econofluor + Protosol (New England Nuclear) for scintillation counting. Solid lines show precipitates with antibody; dashed lines show precipitates with appropriate controls (normal rabbit serum for the anti-β2-m, and normal mouse ascites for W6/32). Note that both antibodies precipitate a single specific glycopeptide from the glioma line, and this comigrates with the HLA chain from Raji. No specific HLA-like material is seen in the IMR-5 precipitates. (Reprinted by permission.)

show that the glial line synthesizes a glycoprotein that comigrates with the HLA chain from Raji (Figure 8). At the same time, we have been unable to visualize a specific HLA-like chain in the neuroblastoma extracts. This was true when either anti-β2-m serum or W6/32 was used, and whether the cells had been biosynthetically labeled with [³⁵S]methionine or [³H]-sugars. The results with extracts that had been labeled with [³H]-sugars are illustrated in Figure 8.

We are now using other strategies to characterize the molecule recognized by W6/32 on neuroblastoma cells. At present, we cannot say whether the conventional HLA chain is present in small quantities, present in an altered form, or absent. These questions are of interest in the functional context described above, and also because of the developing picture of qualitative and quantitative variations among HLA-A,B,C molecules and their analogs in other human cell types (Brown *et al.*, 1979; Cotner *et al.*, 1981; Law and Bodmer, 1978; Sunderland *et al.*, 1981; Trowsdale *et al.*, 1980; von Willebrand *et al.*, 1980; Ziegler and Milstein, 1979).

F. Summary and Conclusions

We have used well-characterized monoclonal antibodies in a variety of assays to study the expression of HLA-A,B,C molecules on a panel of human cell lines. These studies have revealed a striking paucity of HLA-A,B,C molecules on neuroblastoma-derived cell lines as compared to glial, lymphoid, and many other cell types.

An important aspect of these results is that they do not represent a culture artifact. Rather, the paucity of HLA-A,B,C is also a property of the tumor from which the neuroblastoma cell lines were derived, as well as a property of normal adult brain. Although it is, of course, necessary to test these correspondences directly in each case, these findings do support the general plan of using the neuronal cell lines to complement studies of more complex tissue.

The paucity of HLA-A,B,C in brain and neuroblastoma tumor has been discussed in terms of the role of HLA-A,B,C molecules in T-cell-mediated cytotoxicity. Further experiments are needed to test the several possible implications of our results.

V. Tissue Distribution of Newly Defined Molecules

We have also approached the question of neuronal individuality through analysis of antigens that are newly defined by monoclonal antibodies. We have worked with panels of monoclonal antibodies to two different kinds of mammalian neural tissue, human neuroblastoma-derived cell lines and normal adult cat retina. In each case, antibodies were selected for their ability to bind strongly to the immunizing neural tissue in radioimmuno- or microscopic assays. These assays were then used to ask how many of the antibodies were specific for the immunizing tissue.

The results of these initial assays were consistent with previous work from many other laboratories: Monoclonal antibodies that define a single tissue or cell type are infrequent. In these particular experiments, each of 200 antineuroblastoma antibodies also reacted with nonneuronal human cell lines or tissue, and 19/19 of the antiretina antibodies reacted with other cat tissues. In addition, we observed frequent interspecies cross-reactions between human, rodent, and cat tissue, and this is also in agreement with previous work.

As discussed in Section IIB, even a strong immunological cross-reaction and a similar subcellular distribution need not mean that a monoclonal antibody has identified the same molecule in different cells or tissues. In order to test this, a group of antibodies showing strong tissue cross-reactions were chosen for structural analysis of their antigens.

A. Analysis of Tissue Cross-Reactions by Immunoblots

For the structural analyses, we turned first to the immunoblot technique. Here, tissue extracts are first electrophoresed on SDS–polyacrylamide gels. The separated proteins are then electrophoretically transferred to nitrocellulose sheets. The nitrocellulose sheets are exposed first to monoclonal antibody, and

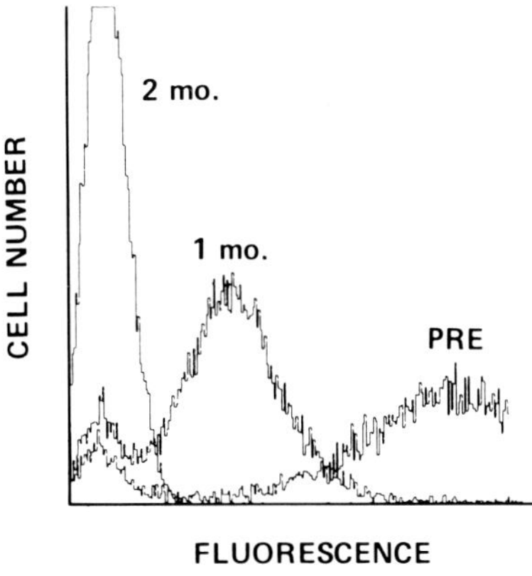

FIGURE 7. Blocking effect of human anti-mouse antibody. The binding of fluoresceinated anti-Leu-1 antibody to T leukemia cells *in vitro* was determined in the presence of serum taken from a patient at various times during his therapy. Fluorescence staining was measured on a fluorescence-activated cell sorter.

blocking activity of immune serum (Figure 7) is due to antiidiotype antibody, and cannot be removed by absorption of the serum on unrelated mouse Ig. It is clear, therefore, that the neutralizing effect of human anti-mouse antibody *in vivo* is due to a host immune response against both the constant region and the idiotype of the mouse monoclonal. These conclusions have important implications for the eventual use of human monoclonal antibodies for therapy. Such human antibodies may likewise evoke an antiidiotypic immune response.

C. Antigenic Modulation, Free Antigen Blockade, Immunoselection

The most dramatic example of antigenic modulation occurred in the study by Ritz and colleagues (1981), who used the anti-CALLA monoclonal antibody in patients with common ALL. The CALLA antigen was subsequently shown to disappear totally from the surface of leukemic cells within minutes after their exposure to the antibody *in vitro* (Pesando *et al.*, 1981). In the clinical trial, escape of leukemic cells from the effects of antibody *in vivo* was completely explained by antigenic modulation. Cell surface antigens vary in their propensity to undergo antibody-induced modulation. For instance, the Leu-1 antigen only partially modulates *in vitro*, and in the clinical trials with the anti-Leu-1 monoclonal antibody, some degree of modulation was observed but was overcome by intermittent dosing (Miller and Levy, 1981). Free antigen in the serum explained both the ineffectiveness of the antilymphoma monoclonal antibody in the study by Nadler and colleagues (1980) as well as the renal toxicity of high doses. One patient with adult T-cell leukemia treated with the anti-Leu-1 antibody was documented to release free antigen into the serum upon destruction of leukemic cells, whereupon a subsequent dose of antibody was rendered ineffective (Miller *et al.*, 1981). Low levels of free idiotype in the serum of a patient with B-cell lymphoma initially blocked the effect of antiidiotype monoclonal antibody, but this blockade was overcome with higher doses of antibody (Miller *et al.*, 1982). No clinical examples of immunoselection have been documented as yet since all relapses in antibody-treated patients have occurred with antigen-positive cells.

However, the true test of whether immunoselection will be an important problem will require larger numbers of patients achieving prolonged clinical remissions.

D. Therapeutic Effects

The primary purpose of all the initial clinical trials has been to define the toxicities and problems of monoclonal antibodies in man. However, in almost every case there was the opportunity to make some preliminary observations on therapeutic effects as well. In no instance has the maximum tolerated dose or the optimum schedule of monoclonal antibody administration been determined. Yet, some positive results have been described. Many of the studies have shown that leukemia cells can be cleared from the blood, at least temporarily (Ritz et al., 1981; Nadler et al., 1980; Miller and Levy, 1981; Dillman et al., 1982; Miller et al., 1981). In one case evidence has been presented to argue that cells were actually destroyed and not just redistributed (Miller et al., 1981). The first patient in whom a clinically significant response was achieved had a T-cell lymphoma with disease in skin, lymph nodes, and blood (Miller and Levy, 1981). He received 15 infusions of anti-Leu-1 antibody extending over a period of 10 weeks (Figure 8). Disease in all sites regressed after the first 2 weeks, but despite continued therapy, he never achieved a complete remission. Histological analysis of the regressing lesions disclosed fewer tumor cells but no evidence of infiltration by other reactive lymphoreticular cells. Small amounts of mouse antibody could be documented on the tumor cells in the skin. The disease eventually recurred, largely in

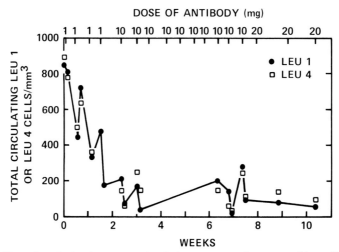

FIGURE 8. Effect of antibody therapy on circulating Leu-1- and Leu-4-positive cells. The relative number of Leu-1- and Leu-4-positive cells was determined by immunofluorescence staining and FACS analysis. Total circulating Leu-1- and Leu-4-positive cells were calculated from white blood cell counts.

new lymph node and skin sites, and the tumor cells that grew expressed the Leu-1 antigen. The most likely explanation for tumor cell resistance to therapy was a shortage of effector cells in the local tumor sites. This patient produced no anti-mouse antibody.

These observations on the anti-Leu-1 antibody have now been extended to another seven patients with cutaneous T-cell lymphoma. The therapeutic effects have been confirmed, with five of the seven patients achieving a partial response which was clinically meaningful. None of these patients achieved a complete response. Unlike the first patient, four of these subsequent patients made significant anti-mouse Ig antibody responses, and it is this response that led to the loss of clinical benefit.

Simultaneously, a series of eight patients with T-cell ALL, mostly children, were studied with anti-Leu-1 antibody infusions. In addition, many of these same patients received one or more other antibodies that were highly reactive with their leukemic cells. The other two antibodies studied, 12E7 (Levy et al., 1979) and 4H9, were of the IgG1 and IgG2a class, respectively, and, unlike anti-Leu-1, neither induced antigenic modulation. Some of these treatments included combinations of two or three antibodies. Many of these infusions resulted in transient reductions of circulating leukemic cells, but no lasting clinical benefit was achieved. In contrast to the patients with cutaneous T-cell lymphoma, these patients with refractory T-cell ALL had very rapidly progressive disease and were unstable clinically. For this reason, observations on the therapeutic effects were very limited and no conclusions can be drawn at this time about the relative effectiveness of the three different antibodies, the effects of multiple antibodies in comparison to single antibodies, or the therapeutic promise for monoclonal antibodies in general for this disease. For the time being, these studies in T-cell ALL have provided the phase I toxicity data to justify trials of antibody in patients with more limited tumor burdens.

E. Antiidiotype Antibody

The B-cell malignancies present a special opportunity to test the potential of antibody therapy. Each B-cell tumor expresses a unique cell surface Ig, which is common to all the members of the malignant clone and different from virtually all normal B cells of the host. The idiotype of the tumor cell surface Ig represents the closest approximation of a tumor-specific antigen available (Stevenson et al., 1977). It is the nonsecreting B-cell malignancies that are the prime candidates for antiidiotype therapy, since they are not associated with high serum levels of idiotype protein, which could block the effects of antibody. Diseases in this category include follicular lymphoma, Burkitt lymphoma, diffuse large-cell lymphoma, and chronic lymphocytic leukemia. One report has appeared on the treatment of a patient with CLL with antiidiotype antibodies (Hamlin et al., 1980). In that study, transient effects on circulating leukemia cells were noted, but there was considerable toxicity. The antibody preparation used in that case was a globulin fraction of an antiserum prepared in sheep. By contrast, a dramatic clinical result was achieved in one patient with follicular lymphoma with a monoclonal antiidiotype antibody (Miller *et al.*, 1982). This patient had failed other therapies and had growing disease in all lymph node sites, skin, liver, spleen, and bone marrow. He was treated with a monoclonal mouse IgG2b antibody in doses escalating from 1 to 150 mg. Low levels of serum idiotype initially blocked the antibody *in vivo*, but higher doses of antibody eventually reached tumor cells, whereupon the tumor began to regress (Figure 9). After eight doses of antibody over 4 weeks the therapy was discontinued. The patient entered a complete remission, which has continued now for over 1 year with no other therapy of any kind. There was no toxicity of therapy and the patient did not make an anti-mouse antibody response. The regressing lesions in this patient were shown to contain large numbers of macrophages and activated T cells. It is likely that such reactive cells were important in the antitumor effect of the antiidiotype antibody.

F. Use of Monoclonal Antibodies in Autologous Bone Marrow Transplantation

Bone marrow toxicity represents the limiting factor of most of the effective therapies for leukemia and lymphoma. Hematopoietic function can be restored to patients who have received otherwise lethal doses of chemotherapy or whole-body radiotherapy by transplantation. Appropriate clinical settings for this maneuver include malignant diseases that are not curable by conventional therapy, but in which it is suspected that higher doses of therapy would increase the

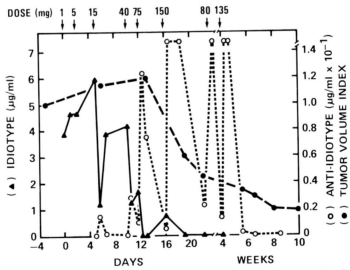

FIGURE 9. *In vivo* effects of antiidiotype. Levels of serum idiotype (triangles) and antiidiotype (open circles) are indicated over the course of therapy. The tumor response to antiidiotype therapy is represented by the plot of tumor-volume index (solid cirlces). Reprinted by permission of the *New England Journal of Medicine* **306**:517–522, 1983.

chances for cure. Bone marrow can be transplanted from donors who are histo-compatible; however, unless an identical twin is available, there is a risk of graft versus host disease when this is carried out. Alternatively, the patient's own bone marrow may be harvested prior to therapy, cryopreserved, and used to recon-stitute hematopoietic function after supralethal therapy. The disadvantage of this approach is that the transfused marrow may contain tumor cells. Antibodies can be used to eliminate contaminating tumor cells from such bone marrow specimens.

The use of antibodies to remove tumor cells from autologous bone marrow *in vitro* has many advantages over the use of antibodies for therapy *in vivo*. For instance, incubations can be performed under conditions that do not allow anti-genic modulation, such as reduced temperature. Circulating blocking factors can be removed. Heterologous complement can be added to lyse antibody-coated cells. Multiple treatments can be used to enhance elimination of tumor cells. The requirements for specificity of the antibody are far less; it must react with all tumor cells and spare hematopoietic stem cells, but it may react with other normal cells that are irrelevant for marrow engraftment.

Preliminary results are available from two ongoing clinical trials using monoclonal antibodies for autologous bone marrow transplantation in acute lymphocytic leukemia. Ritz *et al.* (1982) at the Sidney Farber Cancer Center have used the anti-CALLA monoclonal antibody for patients with common ALL; and Kaizer *et al.* (1982) at Johns Hopkins Medical School have used the anti-Leu-1 antibody for patients with T-cell ALL. The study designs are similar, in that patients who have relapsed at least once with the appropriate type of leukemia have been reinduced into remission with chemotherapy. At that point the bone marrow is harvested, treated with antibody and complement, and cryopre-served. The patients then receive supralethal radiotherapy and chemotherapy followed by infusion of the treated marrow. Both groups have established that marrow treated with antibody and complement *in vitro* and cryopreserved can successfully reconstitute hematopoietic function. At this point, it is too early to conclude whether or not the antibody treatment actually contributed to remis-sion maintenance, since leukemia cells are only presumed to have been present in the treated marrow.

G. Future Prospects

It is clear that monoclonal antibodies offer promise in the therapy of malig-nant disease. It is equally clear that their true role remains to be established and that they will certainly be used in conjunction with other effective modalities of treatment rather than as a substitute for them. Before that role can be found, their limitations, listed in Table VII, will have to be solved.

The most important limitation seems to be the effector cell system that eliminates antibody-coated cells *in vivo* and its finite capacity. Perhaps methods will be found to enhance or augment this system. Alternatively, it may be possi-ble to make the antibodies more toxic on their own, such as by arming them with radioactive or toxic substances. If antibodies were directly cytotoxic, the probem

TABLE VII
Limitations of Monoclonal Antibody Therapy in Man

Finite capacity to eliminate antibody-coated cells
   Antibody-dependent cellular cytotoxicity (ADCC)
   The reticuloendothelial system
Possible solutions
   Improve schedule of antibody administration
   Augment effector cells
   Treat minimal residual disease

Immunogenicity of mouse antibody
   Chronic therapy is ineffective
Possible solutions
   Induce tolerance to mouse Ig
   Use human antibodies
   Use antibody coupled to a cytotoxic agent

of their immunogenicity might disappear, since their toxicity would likely be expressed on the antibody-forming cell ("B-cell suicide") as well as on the tumor cell target.

Solid tumors may not be as susceptible to the therapeutic effects of antibodies as are the leukemias and lymphomas, which, as single cells, are exposed to the vascular and reticuloendothelial effector systems. Ultimately, whether they are used for leukemias or for solid tumors, it seems likely that antibodies will have maximum effect when the number of target cells is low. It is for this reason that clinical trials of antibody therapy will eventually need to be done as properly randomized, controlled studies in patients who are in remission but who are at high risk for eventual relapse. The studies being conducted at the present time are addressing the issues of toxicity and mechanism of antitumor effect. It is hoped that they will lay the foundation for the definitive studies of the future.

ACKNOWLEDGMENTS

The author's work was supported by grants CA-05838 and CA-21223 from the USPHS and IM 114 from the American Cancer Society. The assistance of Dr. David Asher and Herbert Amyx in the conduct of the chimpanzee experiments is gratefully acknowledged.

References

Badger, C. C., and Bernstein, I. D., 1983, Therapy of murine leukemia with monoclonal antibody against a normal differentiation antigen, *J. Exp. Med.* **157**:828–842.

Bernstein, I. D., Tam, M. R., and Nowinski, R. C., 1980a, Mouse leukemia: Therapy with monoclonal antibodies against a thymus differentiation antigen, *Science* **207**:68–71.

Bernstein, I. D., Nowinski, R. C., Tam, M. R., McMaster, B., Houston, L. L., and Clark, E. A., 1980b,

Monoclonal antibody therapy of mouse leukemia, in: *Monoclonal Antibodies. Hybridomas: A New Dimension in Biological Analyses* (R. H. Kennett, T. J. McKearn, and K. B. Bechtol, eds.), Plenum Press, New York, pp. 275–291.

Boyse, E. A., Stockert, E., and Old, L. J., 1967, Modification of the antigenic structure of the cell membrane by thymus-leukemia (TL) antibody, *Proc. Natl. Acad. Sci. USA* **58**:954–957.

Colvin, R. B., Cosimi, A. B., Burton, R. C., Kurnick, J. T., Struzziero, C., Goldstein, G., and Russell, P. S., 1982, Anti-idiotype antibodies in patients treated with murine monoclonal antibody, OKT3, *Fed. Proc.* **41**:363.

Dillman, R. O., Shawler, D. L., Sobol, R. E., Collins, H. A., Beauregard, J. C., Wormsley, S. B., and Royston, I., 1982, Murine monoclonal antibody therapy in two patients with chronic lymphocytic leukemia, *Blood* **59**:1036–1045.

Ehrlich, P., 1906, *Collected Studies on Immunity*, Wiley, New York, Volume 2, pp. 442–447.

Hamlin, T. J., Abdul-Ahad, A. K., Gordon, J., Stevenson, F. K., and Stevenson, G. T., 1980, Preliminary experience in treating lymphocytic leukemia with antibody to immunoglobulin idiotypes on the cell surface, *Br. J. Cancer* **42**:495–502.

Herlyn, D. M., Steplewski, Z., Herlyn, M. F., and Koprowski, H., 1980, Inhibition of growth of colorectal carcinoma in nude mice by monoclonal antibody, *Cancer Res.* **40**:717–721.

Johnson, R. J., Siliciano, R. F., and Shin, H. S., 1979, Suppression of antibody-sensitized cells by macrophages: Insufficient supply or activation of macrophages within large tumors, *J. Immunol.* **122**:379–382.

Kaizer, H., Levy, R., Brovall, C., Civin, C. I., Fuller, D. J., Hsu, S. H., Leventhal, B. G., Miller, R. A., Milvenan, E. S., Santos, G. W., and Wharam, M. D., 1982, Autologous bone marrow transplantation in T cell malignancies: A case report involving *in vitro* treatment of marrow with a pan-T cell monoclonal antibody, *J. Biol. Resp. Mod.* **1**:233–243.

Kirch, M. E., and Hammerling, U., 1981, Immunotherapy of murine leukemias by monoclonal antibody. I. Effect of passively administered antibody on growth of transplanted tumor cells, *J. Immunol.* **127**:805–810.

Kohler, G., and Milstein, C., 1975, Continuous cultures of fused cells secreting antibody of predefined specificity, *Nature* **256**:495–497.

Langlois, A. G., Matthews, T., Goloson, G. J., Thiel, H. J., Collins, J. J., and Bolognesi, D. P., 1981, Immunologic control of the ascites form of murine adenocarcinoma 755. V. Antibody directed macrophages mediate tumor cell destruction, *J. Immunol.* **126**:2337–2341.

Lanier, L. L., Babcock, G. F., Raybourne, R. B., Arnold, L. W., Warner, N. L., and Haughton, G., 1980, Mechanism of B cell lymphoma immunotherapy with passive xenogeneic anti-idiotype serum, *J. Immunol.* **125**:1730–1736.

Levy, R., Dilley, J., Fox, R. I., and Warnke, R., 1979, A human thymus-leukemia antigen defined by hybridoma monoclonal antibodies, *Proc. Natl. Acad. Sci. USA* **76**:6552–6556.

Miller, R. A., and Levy, R., 1981, Response of cutaneous T cell lymphoma to therapy with hybridoma monoclonal antibody, *Lancet* **2**:226–229.

Miller, R. A., Maloney, D. G., McKillop, J., and Levy, R., 1981, *In vivo* effects of murine hybridoma monoclonal antibody in a patient with T cell leukemia, *Blood* **58**:78–86.

Miller, R. A., Maloney, D. G., Warnke, R., and Levy, R., 1982, Treatment of B cell lymphoma with monoclonal anti-idiotype antibody, *New Engl. J. Med.* **306**:517–522.

Nadler, L. M., Stashenko, P., Hardy, R., Kaplan, W. D., Button, L. N., Kufe, D. W., Antman, K. H., and Schlossman, S. T., 1980, Serotherapy of a patient with a monoclonal antibody directed against a human lymphoma-associated antigen, *Cancer Res.* **40**:3147–3154.

Pesando, J. M., Ritz, J., Lazarus, H., Tomaselli, K. J., and Schlossman, S. F., 1981, Fate of a common acute lymphoblastic leukemia antigen during modulation by monoclonal antibody, *J. Immunol.* **126**:540–544.

Ritz, J., Pesando, J. M., Sallan, S. E., Clavell, L. A., Notis-McConarty, J., Rosenthal, P., and Schlossman, S. F., 1981, Serotherapy of acute lymphoblastic leukemia with monoclonal antibody, *Blood* **58**:141–152.

Ritz, J., Bast, R. C., Clavell, L. A., Herhcend, T., Sallan, S. E., Lipton, J. M., Feeney, M., Nathan, D. G., and Schlossman, S. F., 1982, Autologous bone marrow transplantation in CALLA-positive ALL following *in vitro* treatment with J5 monoclonal antibody and complement, *Lancet* **2**:60–63.

Sears, H. F., Mattis, J., Herlyn, D., Hayry, P., Atkinson, B., Ernst, C., Steplewski, Z., and Koprowski,

H., 1982, Phase-I clinical trial of monoclonal antibody in treatment of gastrointestinal tumors, *Lancet* **1:**762–765.

Shin, H. S., Hayden, M., Langley, S., Kaliss, N., and Smith, M. R., 1975, Antibody-mediated suppression of grafted lymphoma. III. Evaluation of the role of thymic function, non-thymus-derived lymphocytes, macrophages, platelets, and polymorphonuclear leukocytes in syngeneic and allogeneic hosts, *J. Immunol.* **114:**1255–1263.

Shin, H. S., Economou, J. S., Pasternack, G. P., Johnson, R. G., and Hayden, M. L., 1976, Antibody-mediated suppression of grafted lymphoma, IV. Influence of time of tumor residency *in vivo* and tumor size upon the effectiveness of suppression by syngeneic antibody, *J. Exp. Med.* **144:**1274– 1283.

Stackpole, C. W., and Jacobson, J. B., 1978, Antigenic modulation, in: *The Handbook of Cancer Immunology* (H. Waters, ed.), Garland STPM, New York, pp. 55–65.

Stevenson, G. T., Elliott, E. V., and Stevenson, F. K., 1977, Idiotypic determinants on the surface immunoglobulin of neoplastic lymphocytes: A therapeutic target, *Fed. Proc.* **36:**2268–2271.

Stratte, P. T., Miller, R. A., Amyx, H. L., Asher, D. M., and Levy, R., 1982, *In vivo* effects of murine monoclonal anti-human T cell antibodies in subhuman primates, *J. Biol. Resp. Mod.* **1:**137–148.

Wright, P. W., and Bernstein, I. D., 1980, Serotherapy of malignant disease, *Prog. Exp. Tumor Res.* **25:**140–162.

9

Monoclonal Antibodies to Human Neuroblastoma Cells and Other Solid Tumors

FRANK BERTHOLD

I. Introduction

My own interest in and work with monoclonal antibodies to human tumor cells originated from diagnostic and therapeutic experiences in children with solid tumors. Therefore, this chapter attempts primarily to review the present status of the ability of monoclonal antibodies to meet clinical needs, to point out problems and restrictions with the current available antibodies, and to show recent approaches to overcome them. A brief look at the general potential of monoclonal antibodies to tumor cells is followed by an overview concerning the actual available antitumor antibodies and the necessary requirements for diagnostic and therapeutic use in cancer patients. Special problems like specificity and heterogeneity, as well as recent advances in cytological detection of bone marrow metastasis, in radioimmunoimaging of bone metastasis, and in therapeutic efforts are discussed in detail for antineuroblastoma antibodies, the field of my own special interest in clinic and laboratory.

FRANK BERTHOLD • Department of Human Genetics, University of Pennsylvania School of Medicine, Philadelphia, Pennsylvania 19104, and Universitätskinderklinik, D 6300 Giessen, Federal Republic of Germany.

II. The Potential of Monoclonal Antibodies to Human Solid Tumor Cells

There are several reasons for the enthusiastic interest in the potential for monoclonal antibodies to be used as reagents for the analysis and clinical management of human malignancies.

1. Monoclonal antibodies can be used as probes for specific cell surface molecules. It is now well accepted that the different phenotypic characteristics of a given tumor, compared to their normal counterparts, often include abnormal growth, different morphological appearance, and altered antigenic pattern. Antigenic structures found on or in the malignant, but not the normal cell may provide an insight into the mechanisms of oncogenesis. Such antigens may result from new genetic information or from expression of normal genetic information at the wrong time and/or in altered quantities. These changes may result from either mutation or oncogenic viral infection. In addition, malignant cells frequently reveal an antigenic pattern that they share with their normal counterparts during certain stages of development (oncodevelopmental antigens). So far, a multitude of these normal developmental antigens has been demonstrated on leukemic cells (Reinherz et al., 1980; Reinherz and Schlossman, 1982; Griffin et al., 1981). The failure to demonstrate a truly tumor-specific antigen does not necessarily mean that it does not exist. With current techniques, it is possible to raise pure antibodies to unknown antigens. Unfortunately, the majority of antigens detected with monoclonal antibodies that have been reported to date seem not to be related directly to the specific oncogenic properties of the tumor cells. The combination of antibody production with transfection procedures should make it possible to eliminate the non-tumor-related immune responses and reveal whether or not tumor-specific information is expressed on the cell surface (see Kennett et al., Chapter 12, this volume). This should result in a better understanding of primary as well as secondary antigenic changes in malignancy.

2. Monoclonal antibodies may provide a tool for more accurate diagnosis of undifferentiated malignancies. Though the majority of malignancies can be confidently diagnosed from the clinical picture and the conventional histopathological analysis, there are heterogeneous groups of tumors that can be differentiated from each other only with difficulty (or not at all). For example, in the pediatric age group, one finds the so-called "small round cell neoplasm group" and the brain tumor group. Unfortunately, the choice of appropriate treatment depends on the correct classification of the tumor. Isolation and characterization of human precursor cells (Doering and Federoff, 1982) and an understanding of the processes involved in the initiation of differentiation (Lee et al., 1982a; Sidell, 1982) may help to identify monoclonal antibodies that can specify developmental stages and ultimately provide more appropriate, multidimensional classifications within the heterogeneous tumor group, thus supplementing the static picture of the conventional histology.

3. Monoclonal antibodies can provide a homogeneous reagent of defined specificity, constant affinity, and unlimited availability (Edwards, 1981). They

may therefore be considered a valuable aid in detecting minimal residual disease (Jonak *et al.*, 1982) and metastasis (Weinstein *et al.*, 1982), and in monitoring the blood level for the more or less specific products synthesized and released by some tumors (Ruddon, 1982).

4. Monoclonal antibodies to human tumor cells may overcome the major limitation of polyclonal serotherapy. These difficulties have included the difficulty of preparing antisera with desired specificity, the low antibody titer remaining after multiple absorption procedures, and the large quantities required for clinical use. Though reports about successful serotherapy with monoclonal antibodies are limited (Miller and Levy, 1981; Miller *et al.*, 1982; Levy *et al.*, Chapter 8, this volume), they seem to justify further efforts.

III. Monoclonal Antibodies to Human Tumor-Associated Antigens

Table I lists several reports of monoclonal antibodies made against tumor-associated antigens. Interestingly, many of these antibodies were raised against tumors with poor prognoses (e.g., melanoma, neuroblastoma), whereas there have been fewer reports describing antibodies raised against tumors with more favorable outlooks (e.g., Wilms tumor, leiomyosarcoma). This may be due to a variety of reasons, e.g., special need for more effective clinical procedures, availability of tumor lines, or antigenicity of the tumor.

Commonly, initial publications describing antitumor antibodies (Table I) do not contain enough information to allow one to classify them according to the requirements for diagnostic or therapeutic use listed in Table II. However, it should be pointed out that a successful application does not only depend on the characteristics of the antibody. There is increasing evidence from leukemia studies (Ritz and Schlossman, 1982; Levy *et al.*, Chapter 8, this volume) that while minimal residual disease has a chance to be treated successfully by monoclonal antibodies, their use for "bulky" disease may be an inappropriate goal at this time. Furthermore, success in clinical trials using monoclonal antibodies for clearing tumor cells from bone marrow *in vitro* depends on an effective therapeutic regimen (including drugs or total body irradiation) which is able to sufficiently kill the rest of the tumor in the patient's body. Another factor influencing the efficacy of treatment with antibodies is the unknown capacity of the effector cell system in the host to cope with tumor under the condition of treatment.

Recently, the use of monoclonal antibodies has helped to uncover previously unknown relationships between normal and tumor cells. Schwab *et al.* (1982) produced monoclonal antibodies against the Hodgkin cell line L428. The antigen detected by one hybridoma antibody (Ki-1) was found on Hodgkin and not on other tumor cells tested using immunoperoxidase staining techniques on frozen sections of biopsies. Subsequent studies (Stein *et al.*, 1982) on 24 frozen and 83 paraffin sections of Hodgkin tumors with a wide variety of markers and

TABLE I

Monoclonal Antibodies to Antigens Associated with Solid Tumors

Colon carcinoma	Herlyn *et al.* (1979), Koprowski *et al.* (1981)
Germ cell tumors and terato-carcinomas	Solter and Knowles (1978), Kapadia *et al.* (1981), McIlhinney *et al.* (1981), Moshakis *et al.* (1981)
Glioblastoma	Wikstrand *et al.* (1981), Schnegg *et al.* (1981), Carrel *et al.* (1982)
Hodgkin disease	Schwab *et al.* (1982)
Leiomyosarcoma	Deng *et al.* (1981)
Lung cancer	Cuttitta *et al.* (1981), Sikora and Wright (1981), Mazauric *et al.* (1982)
Mammary carcinoma	Solter and Knowles (1978), Kapadia *et al.* (1981), McIlhinney *et al.* (1981), Moshakis *et al.* (1981), Andrews *et al.* (1982)
Melanoma	Koprowski *et al.* (1978), Yeh *et al.* (1979), Herlyn *et al.* (1980), Mitchell *et al.* (1980), Galloway *et al.* (1981), Imai *et al.* (1981), Carrel *et al.* (1982), Liao *et al.* (1981)
Neuroblastoma	See Tables III–VI
Osteosarcoma	Hosoi *et al.* (1982), Price *et al.* (1982)
Ovarian carcinoma	Bast *et al.* (1981)
Prostatic cancer	Frankel *et al.* (1982)
Tumor markers:	
CEA	Mitchell *et al.* (1980), Accolla *et al.* (1980), Kupchik *et al.* (1981)
α-Fetoprotein	Uotila *et al.* (1980)
Acid phosphatase	Naritoku and Taylor (1982)

monoclonal antibodies confirmed this result. They demonstrated also for Hodgkin and Sternberg cells a lack of markers found on null, B and T lymphocytes, monocytes, macrophages, and erythropoietic and thrombopoietic cells. In contrast, granulocyte-related antigens were demonstrable (TU5, TU6, TU9, 3C4). Immunostaining on frozen sections of normal lymph nodes and tonsils consistently detected a few Ki-1-positive cells around, between or at the inner rim of the follicular mantles. These otherwise unidentified cells might be the normal counterparts of Hodgkin and Sternberg–Reed cells.

Monoclonal antibodies against teratocarcinomas and germ cell tumors (Table I) were used to detect stage-specific cell-surface changes in the development of human germ cell tumor lines (Neville *et al.*, 1982) analogous to the development of hematopoietic cells. Treatment with the phorbol ester TPA revealed both morphological alterations (enlargement, flattening of cells, cytoskeletal rearrangements) and changes in the surface marker expression (loss of LICR LON-10.2 receptor, loss of peanut agglutination, expression of the SSEA-1 antigen), suggesting differentiation of the tumor cells toward an extraembryonic cell type.

Trojanowski *et al.* (1982) were able to demonstrate the probable neuronal origin of esthesioneuroblastoma (previously classified as APUDomas, *a*mine-*p*recursor *u*ptake and *d*ecarboxylation). They found that these tumor cells contained both types of intermediate filaments and were immunoreactive for neurofilament proteins, but not for vimentin and glial filaments. These are characteristics of cells of neural origin.

TABLE II

Required Characteristics of Monoclonal Antibodies in Terms of Diagnostic or Therapeutic Uses for Cancer Patients

Application	Requirements
Histological or cytological diagnosis	Tissue specificity to tumor cells on a single-cell level Knowledge of incidence of inter- and intratumor heterogeneity
Serum tests	Antigen specificity Antigen shed into the blood by the tumor High avidity to the shed antigen
In vivo radioimmunodetection	Stable antibody–isotope complex High tumor/tissue binding ratio and failure to destroy essential cells (e.g., bone marrow stem cells or nervous tissue) High avidity of the antibody–isotope complex to the tumor cells No or minimal antigen modulation by the tumor
In vitro treatment of metastatic tumor cells in bone marrow	Tissue specificity Cytotoxic antibody or stable complex with, e.g., toxins, cytostatic drugs, magnetic microspheres, radiosensitizers, or mononuclear cells No or minimal antigen modulation by the tumor
Serotherapy	Tumor specificity (at least "operationally"; see text) Cytotoxic antibody or stable complex with, e.g., toxins, cytostatics, radiosensitizers, or mononuclear cells No antigen modulation No antigen-negative tumor cells Knowledge of *in vivo* turnover rate and the immune response of the host against the antibody

IV. Monoclonal Antibodies to Human Neuroblastoma Cells

The major characteristics of monoclonal antibodies reportedly binding to human neuroblastoma cells are listed in Tables III–V. They vary considerably in terms of specificity, recognized antigen (if known), and usefulness in detecting neuroblastoma cells. Only four of the antibodies were raised by immunization with neuroblastoma cells (Table III). The majority of "antineuroblastoma antibodies" available at present result from immunizations with other neural crest-related antigenic material (glioblastoma cells, melanoma cells, fetal brain homogenate) (Table IV) or from immunizations with cells with no evident oncodevelopmental relationship (thymocytes, lymphatic leukemia cells, lung cancer cells) (Table V). Some of these results seem to suggest some relationship in embryological development between neural crest descendants, leukopoietic cells, and lung tissue. Binding of monoclonal antibodies to neuroblastoma and lung cancer are also reported by Minna (1981) and Hollinshead (1982), and to neuroblastoma and hematopoietic cells by Susimoto et al. (1982), supporting earlier results obtained with heterologous antisera (Reif and Allen, 1964; Seeger et al., 1979). The biological importance of their implied relationships depends, of course, on the function of the molecules for the cell.

A. Specificity

There is no truly neuroblastoma-specific monoclonal antibody reported. Some antibodies in Table IV might be viewed as tumor-specific, i.e., binding to tumor cells (of different origins) but not to normal ones. However, in most instances there are very few data presented supporting the lack of reactivity, especially on the faster growing tissues (bone marrow, gastrointestinal and urogenital epithelium, skin). Tissue specificity for bone marrow can be considered for some antibodies, e.g., HSAN1.2 (Table III), A2B5, 1H8cl2, 1H8cl3, 390, UJ127, UJ13A, 44, 11-1, 25-6 (Table IV). It is of interest that one of the antibodies (A2B5) with the highest degree of specificity, having virtually no cross-reactions to bone marrow and leukemic cells, resulted from immunization against chicken embryonic retinal cells, i.e., from an extraordinarily different system. In contrast, three of four antibodies raised against neuroblastoma cells show various degrees of binding to normal and malignant hematopoietic cells. It should be stressed that conclusions about tissue specificity based on the lack of binding to homogenates must be viewed as inadequate. That is also true for FACS analyses when estimating only the distribution pattern on the screen. Both methods are unable to detect the binding of an antibody to a quantitatively minor cell population (e.g., stem cells, megakaryocytes in bone marrow). In all instances, immunocytological or immunohistological analyses have to be done to screen the binding reactions on a single-cell level. The most sensitive technique currently being considered is the immunoperoxidase method (Sternberger, 1979; Becker et al., 1981; Hancock et al., 1982; see also Appendix, this volume). However, since in bone marrow the hematopoietic stem cells have not yet been identified, it remains problematical, if not impossible, to claim true nonreactivity on a qualitative basis (presence versus absence of binding) and moreover at a quantitative level (minimal or low versus no binding). This difficulty is circumvented by the term *"operationally tumor-specific"* for practical purposes, which means reactivity to tumor cells in a given tissue without cross-reactions to a majority of cells and without toxicity to essential cells. As in the use of drugs, "side effects" in a certain, well-defined range are tolerated, leaving open the question, what kind of cell is ultimately responsible for the side effects and to what degree?

Neville *et al.* (1982) pointed out that the lack of tissue or cell specificity for a certain monoclonal antibody may be disappointing in one respect but potentially interesting in another. Such cross-reactivity may result from the occurrence of the same molecule (or epitope) on the cell surface of different cell types, which is not surprising since the cell membranes have a similar structure and share many functions. This would be even less surprising if the carbohydrate portion of glycoproteins (Momoi *et al.,* 1980) or glycolipids turned out as the major antigenic determinant, since similar terminal carbohydrate sequences are common in different cell types (Rauvala and Finne, 1979).

One aspect of monoclonal antibody production that has not been developed to its full potential is the use of a monoclonal antibody for purification of tumor-associated antigens as a step in producing antibodies against other determinants on the same molecules. Such an immunization protocol has the potential for producing antibodies with either a more restricted or less restricted specificity compared to the original antibody. Indeed, *in vitro* immunization (this volume, Appendix) using the isolated antigen defined by antibody PI153/3 (Momoi *et al.,* 1980) resulted in production of 31 antineuroblastoma antibodies with quite different specificity in comparison to antibody PI153/3. Most of them revealed a broader reactivity pattern; however, two (11-1, 25-6, Table IV) did not show any cross-reactions with bone marrow cells, as PI153/3 did. Interestingly, the strong cell-membrane (processes and soma) related binding pattern of PI153/3 to neuroblastoma cells was contrasted with the whole cell staining with antibodies 11-1 and 25-6 (immunoperoxidase method, unpublished observation).

B. Heterogeneity

Whereas some antibodies bind to all neuroblastoma cells tested so far (PI153/3, HSAN 1.2, Table III) the majority show various degrees of "false-negative" results in terms of diagnostic reliability. Kemshead *et al.* (1981c) reported that the monoclonal antibody A2B5 reacted with cells in only 70% of bone marrow aspirates, all of which were heavily infiltrated with neuroblastoma cells. A second antibody from this group, M1/N1 (Kemshead *et al.,* 1981a), shows quantitative binding differences when tested on various cell lines, e.g., binding to the neuroblastoma cell line CHP-100 is about four times greater than to CHP-126. Again, by means of antibody M1/N1, metastatic cells in bone marrow were identified in only five of eight cases. Using quantitative absorption techniques,

TABLE III

Characteristics of Monoclonal Antibodies to Human Neuroblastoma Raised by Immunization with Neuroblastoma Lines

Monoclonal antibody	Immunogen	Antigen identified	Specificity	Reference
PI153/3	Human neuroblastoma line (IMR-6) coated with anti-human mouse serum	Glycoprotein 20 kdaltons	Neuroblastoma, some glioblastomas, some retinoblastomas, melanomas, B-ALL, most non-B, non-T ALL, hairy cell leukemia, NHL, CLL, pre-B and mature B lymphocytes No binding to: AML, CML (11/12), erythroleukemia, medulloblastoma, monocytes, myelo- and erythropoietic cells, T cells, plasma cells	Kennett and Gilbert (1979), Momoi *et al.* (1980), Greaves *et al.* (1980), Kemshead *et al.* (1982a), Jonak *et al.* (1982)
C10.115	Human neuroblastoma line (LA-N1)	No	Neuroblastoma (6/8), T-ALL (3/4), AML (3/4) No binding to: non-B, non-T ALL, T-CML, teratoma, medulloblastoma, glioma, sarcoma, carcinoma (colon, blad-	Seeger *et al.* (1980), Danon *et al.* (1981)

der, lung), peripheral blood cells

| M1/N1 | Human neuroblastoma line (CHP-100) | No | Neuroblastoma, CML, blasts, single T-ALL lines; myelopoietic cells (promyelocytes—neutrophils), eosinophils, fetal and adult brain. No binding to: non-B, non-T ALL, AML blasts, erythropoietic and red blood cells, lymphocytes | Kemshead et al. (1981a) |
| HSAN 1.2 | Human neuroblastoma line (SMS-SAN) | No | Neuroblastoma, ganglioneuroma (1/2), Wilm tumor, Ewing sarcoma (1/2), fetal and adult brain, newborn kidney. No binding to: ALL, NHL, CLL, AML, Hodgkin cells, rhabdomyosarcoma, oat cell carcinoma, melanoma, glioma, bone marrow cells, fibroblasts, sympathetic ganglia, adrenal, kidney, liver, lung, thyroid, ovary | Reynolds and Smith (1981, 1982) |

TABLE IV

Characteristics of Monoclonal Antibodies to Human Neuroblastoma Raised by Immunization with Neural Crest Antigens except Neuroblastoma

Monoclonal antibody	Immunogen	Antigen identified	Specificity	Reference
CG-12	Glioblastoma line (LN-18)	No	Neuroblastoma (1/1), glioblastoma (17/37), melanoma, medulloblastoma, fetal and adult brain. No reaction to: B-, T-, non-B, non-T ALL lines, myeloid cell line (K-562), carcinoma (endometrial, cervical, mammary, colon), rhabdomyosarcoma, meningeoma	Schnegg et al. (1981)
Anti-glioma MCA	Glioblastoma line D54	No	Neuroblastoma, glioblastoma, fibroblasts. No reaction to: carcinoma (cervical, ovarian, bladder, colon, prostata), sarcoma (osteosarcoma, leitomyosarcoma, fibrosarcoma), melanoma, peripheral blood cells, brain, liver, spleen, kidney, muscle, lung	Wikstrand et al. (1982a)
G13-C6	Glioblastoma line (LN-18)	No	Neuroblastoma (1/3), glioblastoma (9/13), melanoma, fetal brain. No reaction to: carcinoma (colon, endometrial, lung), meningeoma, fibroblasts, peripheral blood cells	Carrel et al. (1982)
7.51, 7.60	Melanoma line (CaCL 78-1)	No	Neuroblastoma, melanoma, retinoblastoma, glioblastoma, fetal brain. No reaction to: carcinoma (colon, cervical, lung, oral), fibroblasts, amniotic epithelium	Liao et al. (1981)
376	Melanoma line (UCLA-SO-M14)	No	Neuroblastoma, glioma, melanoma (2/4), sarcoma, lung, fetal tissues except brain. No reaction to: carcinoma (colon, bladder, lung), teratoma, fibroblasts, lymphocytes, erythrocytes, fetal and adult brain	Seeger et al. (1981)

	Immunogen	Antigen	Reactivity	Reference
Me 1,2,3,4,5	Melanoma line (Me 43, IGR3) (membrane-enriched fractions)	No	Neuroblastoma, melanoma, glioblastoma No reaction to: carcinoma (colon, cervical, mammary), fibroblasts, peripheral blood cells, fetal brain	Carrel et al. (1982)
705F6	Melanoma line	95 kdaltons	Neuroblastoma, melanoma, glioblastoma, carcinoma, sarcoma, leukemia lines (3/7), fetal cell lines No reaction to: B lymphoid cell lines	Saxton et al. (1982a,b)
A2B5	Chicken embryo retinal cells	Ganglioside GQ	Neuroblastoma, retinoblastoma, some leukemias (ALL, AML); adult brain No reaction to: nearly all acute leukemias (ALL, AML), B-NHL, erythroleukemia, bone marrow cells	Eisenbarth et al. (1979), Kemshead et al. (1981c)
7H10cl4	Fetal brain (months 4–6)	No	Neuroblastoma (1/1), glioblastoma, medulloblastoma, Hodgkin cells, fetal tissues (brain, liver, spleen, thymus), adult spleen No reaction to: carcinoma, sarcoma, CML, T-ALL, B-ALL, peripheral blood cells, fetal lung, fibronectin	Wikstrand et al. (1981, 1982b)
4D2cl6	Fetal brain (months 4–6)	No	Neuroblastoma (1/1), glioblastoma, fetal tissues (brain, spleen, liver), adult spleen No reaction to: carcinoma, sarcoma, ALL, AML, brain, skin, peripheral blood cells, fetal lung, fibronectin	Wikstrand and Bigner (1982)
1H8cl2	Fetal brain (months 4–6)	No	Neuroblastoma (2/3), glioblastoma (9/14), melanoma (2/3), medulloblastoma, fetal tissues (brain, liver, spleen), adult spleen No reaction to: brain, thymus (adult), lymph node, liver, lung, kidney, skin, pancreas	Wikstrand et al. (1982b)
1H8cl3	Fetal brain (months 4–6)	No	Neuroblastoma (2/3), glioblastoma (7/14), medulloblastoma, fetal fibroblasts (2/3) No reaction to: brain, thymus (adult), lymph node, liver, lung, kidney, skin, pancreas	Wikstrand et al. (1982b)

(continued)

TABLE IV (Continued)

Monoclonal antibody	Immunogen	Antigen identified	Specificity	Reference
390	Fetal brain (week 12)	Thy-1, 25 kdaltons	Neuroblastoma (9/10), glioblastoma (2/3), rhabdomyosarcoma, leiomyosarcoma, osteosarcoma (1/2), teratoma, fibroblasts, brain (adult fetal), kidney No reaction to: medulloblastoma, melanoma, carcinoma (bladder, colon, lung), hematopoietic cells, thymocytes, adult adrenal gland	Seeger (1982a), Seeger et al. (1982)
UJ308	Fetal brain	180–200 kdaltons	Neuroblastoma, normal neural tissue, promyelocytic leukemia (HL60) No reaction to: fetal tissues (spleen, liver, kidney, muscle)	Kemshead et al. (1982a)
UJ127, UJ13A	Fetal brain	220–240 kdaltons (UJ127)	Neuroblastoma, normal neural tissue No reaction to: bone marrow cells, fetal tissues (spleen, liver, kidney, muscle)	Kemshead et al. (1982a)
44	Fetal brain	No	Neuroblastoma, adult brain, non-B, non-T ALL No reaction to: B-ALL, T-ALL, fibrosarcoma, neurofibromatosis, bone marrow cells	Kim, Berthold, and Kennett[a]
11-1, 25-6	Isolated antigen of antibody PI153/3	No	Neuroblastoma, non-B, non-T ALL, fibroblasts No reaction to: bone marrow cells	Berthold and Kennett[a]

[a]Unpublished observation.

Seeger (1982b) found considerable variation in antigen expression (1000-fold range) for tumors from patients with neuroblastoma stages II, III, and IV. This also applies to the binding of the same antibody (390) to astrocytic cells. Wikstrand and associates have demonstrated that some apparent differences in binding may be diminished by using more sensitive techniques (Wikstrand et al., 1981; Wikstrand and Bigner, 1982). They showed the binding of the monoclonal antibodies 4D2 cl6 and 7H10 cl4 to only 5/14 and 13/14, respectively, of glioblastoma cell lines using the radioimmunoassay (1/3 and 1/3, respectively, of neuroblastoma lines). With the peroxidase–antiperoxidase technique, however, binding of either antibody could be detected on every cell line (13/13 of glioblastoma cell lines, 1/1 of neuroblastoma). Thus, the sensitivity was enhanced from 36 to 100% for 4D2 cl6 on glioblastoma lines. Another point to consider is a possible change in antigen expression with time, particularly in vivo under selective chemotherapy or in vitro following cultivation of tumor cells. Kemshead et al. (1981b) reported that the neuroblastoma cells of a patient changed their antigen profile over a 5-month period of chemotherapy.

In general, it remains to be ascertained whether the heterogeneity is due to different cell types predominating under different physiological conditions or to progressive clonal variation of the tumor cell population.

C. Detection of Bone Marrow Metastasis

Using polyclonal antisera to an epithelial membrane antigen, Dearnaley et al. (1981) detected breast cancer cells in bone marrow samples in a significant number of patients otherwise regarded as being free of metastatic disease. By means of immunohistological analysis, they found 21 out of 74 positive samples, in contrast to 11 out of 74 recognized by employing other methods, including light microscopy. The need to detect micrometastasis applies in particular to the clinical management of neuroblastoma. There is a striking discrepancy between the 97% response rate (partial and complete remissions) to chemotherapy and the 13% disease-free survival after 30 months (Berthold et al., 1982) (Figure 1). It is thought to result from the difficulty in verifying a complete remission by conventional methods. Data from Green et al. (1981) and our group (Berthold et al., 1982) support this interpretation. The results show that the achievement of complete versus partial remission as currently determined influences only the median survival time (14.4 and 13 months for partial remission patients, 22 and 17 months for complete remission patients). It does not influence the survival rate. Apparently the 90% nonsurviving patients never really gain complete remission. In other childhood malignancies, a correlation exists between response rate and final outcome. Monoclonal antibodies against neuroblastoma are beginning to prove as useful in detecting bone marrow metastasis as the polyclonal antisera mentioned above, according to Jonak et al. (1982). Using a double-labeling technique with PI153/3 (an antineuroblastoma antibody that binds to all neuroblastoma cells tested so far) in combination with anti-B-lymphocyte antibody P3B1-C3 (to identify cross-reacting normal lymphoid and leukemic cells),

TABLE V
Characteristics of Monoclonal Antibodies to Human Neuroblastoma Raised by Immunization with Hematopoietic and Lung Cancer Cells

Monoclonal antibody	Immunogen	Antigen identified	Specificity	Reference
NA1-34	Thymocytes	45–49 kdaltons + 12 kdaltons (B$_2$-like)	Neuroblastoma (CHP-100), cortical thymic lympho-cytes, T-ALL blasts. No binding to: melanoma, astrocytoma, medulloblastoma, retinoblastoma, B-ALL line, bone marrow cells, platelets, spleen, liver, brain	McMichael et al. (1979), Kemshead et al. (1982a)
OKT 6	Thymocytes	45–49 kdaltons + 12 kdaltons (B$_2$-like)	Neuroblastoma (CHP-100) (2/2), T-ALL blasts (2/3), cortical thymic lymphocytes (70%), Langerhans cells (skin). No binding to: bone marrow cells	Reinherz et al. (1980), Kemshead et al. (1982a)
OKT 9	Thymocytes	180 kdaltons	Neuroblastoma (CHP-100, -212), T-ALL blasts, cortical thymic lymphocytes (10%), immature thymocytes. No binding to: bone marrow cells	Reinherz et al. (1980), Kemshead et al. (1982a)
BA-1	Pre-B-ALL line (Nalm6-M1)	No	Neuroblastoma, pre-B-ALL, most non-B non-T ALL, most NHL, CLL, erythroleukemia (K562), melanoma, astrocytoma, granulocytes. No binding to: medulloblastoma, retinoblastoma, AML blasts, red blood cells, platelets, T lymphocytes	Abramson et al. (1981), Kemshead et al. (1982a)
BA-2	Pre-B-cell line (Nalm6-M1)	24 kdaltons	Neuroblastoma, non-B, non-T ALL (77%), T-ALL (18%), B-CLL (50%), melanoma, retinoblastoma, some mononuclear bone marrow cells (3%). No binding to: astrocytoma, medulloblastoma, red blood cells, granulocytes, peripheral mononuclear cells, most bone marrow mononuclear cells (97%)	Kersey et al. (1981), Kem-shead et al. (1982a)
ALB 7, 8, 9	ALL cells	No	Neuroblastoma, B lymphocytes, myelopoietic cells (promyelocyte–granulocyte)	Boucheix et al. (1982)
525 A5, 534, T8 538, T12	Small cell lung cancer line (NCI-H69)	No	Neuroblastoma (3/3), small cell lung cancer, breast cancer (2/3), normal kidney (only antibodies 534T8 and 538T12). No binding to: bronchoalveolar carcinoma, large cell lung cancer, leukemias, myeloma, lymphoma, osteosarcoma, mesothelioma, hypernephroma, melanoma, fetal and normal lung cells, spleen, liver, skeletal muscle, kidney (only antibody 525A5), fibroblasts, erythrocytes, B lymphoblastoid lines	Cuttitta et al. (1981)

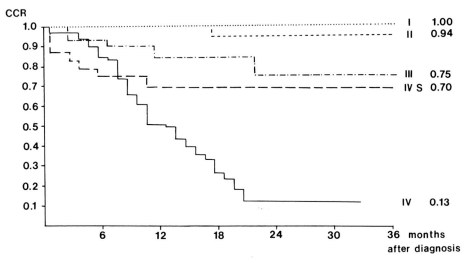

FIGURE 1. Survival rate in complete continuous remission (CCR) of children with neuroblastoma according to stage. German Pediatric Oncology Group Trial NBL 79. Stage I (n = 16) (···); stage II (n = 18) (–––); stage III (n = 41) (–·–); infants, stage IV-S (n = 24) (— —); children over 1 year, stage IV (n = 74) (——).

they were able to detect single tumor cells. Table VI lists other determinants, usually not present on human neuroblastoma cells, which may be helpful in such double-labeling techniques.

The fact that certain monoclonal antibodies do not react with all tumors of a given type, as discussed in the previous section on heterogeneity, also poses a problem that must be overcome when using the antibodies to detect metastases. It has been found that the use of a panel of monoclonal antibodies can also be used to effectively circumvent this technical problem (Hellström *et al.*, 1982; Kemshead *et al.*, 1983).

TABLE VI

Antigenic Structures or Receptors Usually Not Present (or in
Very Low Density) on Human Neuroblastoma Cells

Missing macromolecule	Reference
Ia-Like antigen (HLA)	Howe *et al.* (1980, 1981), Lampson and Fisher (1982)
Neurofilament	Lee *et al.* (1982a,b), Osborn *et al.* (1982)
Microtubule-associated protein MAP 2	Izant and McIntosh (1980)

D. Radioimmunodetection

Monoclonal antibodies offer the possibility of more specific radioimaging of primary tumor and metastasis than do conventional techniques (Young and L'Heureux, 1978). The fact that conventional 99m technetium bone scans and skeletal X rays produce incongruous results concerning bone metastasis in neuroblastoma (Kaufman *et al.*, 1978; Howman-Files *et al.*, 1979; Sty *et al.* 1979) indicates the need for more sensitive methods. A mouse model system has been investigated by Goldman *et al.* (1982). They gave mice bearing human neuroblastoma cells intravenous injections of three I^{125}-labeled antineuroblastoma monoclonal antibodies. Measuring the level of radioactivity in the tumor and a range of mouse organs as well as scanning by means of a gamma camera showed the selective uptake by the tumor. A second group (Ghose *et al.*, 1981) used only the Fab_2 part of the antibody for radiolabeling, resulting in a clearer localization of the intracerebral C1300 transplant (mouse neuroblastoma). Successful tumor imaging in sarcoma patients was recently reported (Brown *et al.*, 1983) using a ^{125}I-labeled mouse monoclonal antibody reacting with a variety of human sarcomas, but giving minimal reaction with normal tissues. The monitor detected known tumor in all seven patients as early as 15 min after antibody administration. Analysis of tissue specimens obtained 48 hr later showed increased radioactivity in the tumor tissue from all patients, ranging from 3.4 to 49.3 times the highest amounts found in normal tissue. However, the increased uptake of radioactivity by liver and spleen reveals some unspecific radioimmunoimaging, probably due to the phagocytosis by reticuloendothelial cells. The variability in uptake by six separate lung metastases in one patient (labeling index ranging from 0.9 to 16.9, normal lung = 1) also indicates the problems due to heterogeneity in antigen expression or to other factors that may affect the localization of the labeled antibody in a given tumor mass (vascularization, tumor cell necrosis).

E. Differential Diagnosis

The diagnosis of neuroblastoma is usually not difficult based on histological investigation or elevated urinary catecholamines and presence of typical tumor clumps in the bone marrow. On the other hand, cases without elevated urinary catecholamines (15%) or with a histological picture of anaplasia (15%) are very difficult to differentiate from other small cell tumors (lymphoma, Ewing sarcoma, rhabdomyosarcoma) even by means of electron microscopy, biochemistry, and cell culture studies (Berthold *et al.*, 1982). Pritchard and co-workers (1982) used a panel of 26 monoclonal antibodies to establish an antibody profile for each type of tumor. Distinct patterns of reactivity have emerged and allowed confident discrimination between non-Hodgkin lymphoma and neuroblastoma. In two cases, antibody studies led to the correction of the initial diagnosis (Kemshead *et al.*, 1983).

F. Therapeutic Possibilities

The difficult therapeutic situation in children over 1 year of age with disseminated neuroblastoma (Finklestein *et al.*, 1979; Nitschke *et al.*, 1980; Ninane *et al.*, 1981; Berthold *et al.*, 1982) contrasts markedly with the relatively good prognosis in infants (stage IV-S) and with the generally "manageable" disease in localized stages I–III (Figure 1). The availability of monoclonal antibodies has therefore renewed the interest in immunotherapy. There are three areas in which attempts to use monoclonal antibodies in therapeutic efforts are likely to be productive:

1. *In vitro* clearing of micrometastatic neuroblastoma from bone marrow. Marrow could be removed and the tumor cells killed *in vitro* by exposing to specific interacting antibodies (Table II). Meanwhile, the patient could be treated by total body irradiation and a high-dose drug regimen toxic to tumor and bone marrow to eradicate the residual disease, in particular the bone metastases. The *in vitro*-treated marrow could then be infused to reconstitute the hematopoietic system. Kemshead and co-workers (Kemshead *et al.*, 1982b,c) used polystyrene microspheres containing 27% magnetite to remove neuroblastoma cells from bone marrow. After binding a cocktail of monoclonal antibodies to the tumor cells, microspheres coated with anti-mouse immunoglobulin were added in excess and the sample placed in a magnetic field. Ninety-seven to ninety-nine percent of neuroblastoma cells could be removed with this procedure.

2. Induction of differentiation. The unique capability of neuroblastoma in infants to regress and mature spontaneously (Evans *et al.*, 1976; Nossal, 1976) suggests it may be fruitful to search for a way to initiate this process in tumors in older children. There is also increasing data on *in vitro* differentiation of mouse neuroblastoma C1300 (Prasad, 1975; Tank and Weiner, 1982; Revoltella *et al.*, 1982). Similar recent results on human neuroblastoma (Sidell, 1982) and occasional reports of *in vivo* induction of differentiation using papaverine (Helson, 1975; Imashuku *et al.*, 1977) further support this approach. Kennett *et al.*, (1982) found three out of 80 monoclonal antibodies to inhibit the proliferation of the leukemia cell line Reh. They concluded that these antibodies may react with membrane receptors involved in normal growth control processes. It is not unlikely that one could find similar antineuroblastoma monoclonal antibodies.

3. Serotherapy of minimal residual disease with neuroblastoma-specific monoclonal antibodies. None of the antibodies listed in Tables III–V appear to fulfill the proposed criteria for *in vivo* application (Table II), and therefore the lack of reports of this kind of therapy is not surprising. Cross-reaction with closely related normal neuroectodermal antigens (brain, some endocrine glands) and with blood precursor cells may, in fact, prevent the classification of these antibodies as "operationally tumor-specific" in the context of intravenous administration. On the other hand, with regard to *in vitro* serotherapy, Hurwitz and Danon (1982) were able to demonstrate a specific delivery of adriamycin to *in vitro* neuroblastoma cells by a cocktail of monoclonal antibodies.

V. Summary and Conclusions

The past few years have seen the beginning of many enthusiastic attempts to apply monoclonal antibody technology to the analysis and therapy of human tumors. As these applications have developed, there have been both encouraging results and, at the same time, a greater awareness of the technical problems that must be overcome before these new reagents can be applied in systematic and routine ways. We are at the stage now where a good deal of work is still necessary to reach the potential that clearly exists.

As stated by Neville (1982), "The pathological and clinical potential of monoclonal antibodies can only be surmised at this time. The euphoric phase may be almost over; now the hard work will begin—to derive reagents with specificity for particular purposes. Nevertheless, the scientific and medical rewards will well justify such future effort."

ACKNOWLEDGMENTS

This work was supported by a grant from Deutsche Krebshilfe (Mildred-Scheel-Stipendium 300/402/528/2). I thank Dr. Roger H. Kennett for his continuing support and encouragement of this chapter.

References

Abramson, C. S., Kersey, J. H., and LeBien, T. W., 1981, A monoclonal antibody (BA-1) reactive with cells of human B lymphocyte lineage, *J. Immunol.* **126**:83–88.

Accolla, R. S., Carrel, S., and Mach, J. P., 1980, Monoclonal antibodies specific for carcinoembryonic antigen and produced by two hybrid cell lines, *Proc. Natl. Acad. Sci. USA* **77**:563.

Andrews, P. W., Goodfellow, P. N., Shevinsky, L. H., Bronson, D. L., and Knowles, B. B., 1982, Cell-surface antigens of a clonal human embryonal carcinoma cell line: Morphological and antigenic differentiation in culture, *Int. J. Cancer* **29**:523–531.

Bast, R. C., Feeney, M., Lazarus, H., Nadler, L. M., Colvin, R. B., and Knapp, R. C., 1981, Reactivity of a monoclonal antibody with human ovarian carcinoma, *J. Clin. Invest.* **68**:1331.

Becker, G. J., Hancock, W. W., Kraft, N., Lanyon, H. C., and Atkins, R. C., 1981, Monoclonal antibodies to human macrophage and leucocyte common antigens, *Pathology* **13**:669.

Berthold, F., Kracht, J., Lampert, F., Millar, T. J., Müller, T. H., Reither, M., and Unsicker, K., 1982, Ultrastructural, biochemical and cell-culture studies of a presumed extraskeletal Ewing's sarcoma with special reference to differential diagnosis from neuroblastoma, *J. Cancer Res. Clin. Oncol.* **103**:293–304.

Berthold, F., Treuner, J., Brandeis, W. E., Evers, G. Haas, R. J., Harms, D., Jürgens, H., Kaatsch, P., Michaelis, J., Niethammer, D., Prindull, G., Riehm, H., Winkler, K., and Lampert, F., 1982, Neuroblastomstudie NBL 79 der Gesellschaft für Pädiatrische Oukologie—Zwischenbericht nach 2 Jahren, *Klin. Paediatr.* **194**:262–263.

Boucheix, C., Perrot, J. Y., Mirshani, M., Fournier, N., Billard, M., Bernadou, A., and Rosenfeld, C., 1982, Monoclonal antibodies against acute lymphoblastic leukemia differentiation antigens (meeting abstract), in: *First International Workshop on Human Leukocyte Differentiation Antigens*, Hospital Saint-Louis, Paris, France, p. AP-4.

Brown, J. M., Graeger, J. A., and Das Gupta, T. K., 1983, Tumor localization studies in sarcoma patients using a radiolabeled monoclonal antibody (meeting abstract), *Hybridoma* **2**:136.

Carrel, S., De Tribolet, N., and Mach, J.-P., 1982, Expression of neuroectodermal antigens common to melanomas, gliomas, and neuroblastomas. I. Identification by monoclonal anti-melanoma and anti-glioma antibodies, *Acta Neuropathol. (Berl.)* **57**:158–164.

Cuttitta, F., Rosen, S., Gazdar, A. F., and Minna, J. D., 1981, Monoclonal antibodies that demonstrate specificity for several types of human lung cancer, *Proc. Natl. Acad. Sci. USA* **78**:4591–4595.

Danon, Y. L., Rayner, S. A., Kaminsky, E., and Seeger, R. C., 1981, *Human neuroblastoma and acute leukemia cells common antigen defined with monoclonal antibody* (meeting abstract), *Isr. J. Med. Sci.* **17**:1096.

Dearnaley, D. P., Sloane, J. P., Ormerod, M. G., Steele, K., Coombes, R. C., Clink, H. M., Powles, T. J., Ford, H. T., Gazet, J. T., and Neville, A. M., 1981, Increased detection of mammary carcinoma cells in marrow smears using antisera to epithelial membrane antigen, *Br. J. Cancer* **44**:85.

Deng, C., El-Awar, N., Cicciarelli, J., Terasaki, P. I., Billing, R., and Lagasse, L., 1981, Cytotoxic monoclonal antibody to a human leiomyosarcoma, *Lancet* **1**:403–405.

Doering, L. C., and Federoff, S., 1982, Isolation and identification of neuroblast precursor cells from mouse neopallium, *Dev. Brain Res.* **5**:229–233.

Edwards, P. A. W., 1981, Some properties and applications of monoclonal antibodies, *Biochem. J.* **200**:1.

Eisenbarth, G. S., Walsh, F. S., and Nirenberg, M., 1979, Monoclonal antibody to a plasma membrane antigen of neurons, *Proc. Natl. Acad. Sci. USA* **76**:4913–4917.

Evans, A. E., Gerson, J., and Schnaufer, L., 1976, Spontaneous regression of neuroblastoma, *Natl. Cancer Inst. Monogr.* **44**:49.

Finklestein, J. Z., Klemperer, M. R., Evans, A., Bernstein, I., Leikin, S., McCreadie, S., Grosfeld, J., Hittle, R., Weiner, J., Sather, H., and Hammond, D., 1979, Multiagent chemotherapy for children with metastatic neuroblastoma: A report from children's cancer study group, *Med. Pediatr. Oncol.* **6**:179–188.

Frankel, A. E., Rouse, R. V., and Herzenberg, L. A., 1982, Human prostate-specific and shared differentiation antigens defined by monoclonal antibodies, *Proc. Natl. Acad. Sci. USA* **79**:903.

Galloway, D. R., Imai, K., Ferrone, S., and Reisfeld, R. A., 1981, Molecular profiles of human melanoma-associated antigens, *Fed. Proc.* **40**:231.

Ghose, T., Ramakrishnan, S., Kulkarni, P., Blair, A. H., Vaughan, K., Nolido, H., Norvell, S. T., Belitsky, P., and Bonavida, B., 1981, Use of antibodies against tumor-associated antigens for cancer diagnosis and treatment, *Transplant. Proc.* **13**:1970–1972.

Goldman, A., Pritchard, J., and Kemshead, J. T., 1982, Selective localization of radiolabeled monoclonal antibodies to human neuroblastoma xenografts in a nude mouse model (meeting abstract), in: *Fourteenth Annual Meeting of the International Society of Pediatric Oncology,* Berne, Switzerland, pp. A12.

Greaves, M. F., Verbi, W., Kemshead, J., and Kennett, R. H., 1980, A monoclonal antibody identifying a cell surface antigen shared by common acute lymphoblastic leukemias and B lineage cells, *Blood* **56**:1141–1144.

Green, A. A., Hayes, F. A., and Huster, H. O., 1981, Sequential cyclophosphamide and doxorubicine for induction of complete remission in children with disseminated neuroblastoma, *Cancer* **48**:2310.

Griffin, J. D., Ritz, J., Nadler, L. M., and Schlossman, S. F., 1981, Expression of myeloid differentiation antigens on normal and malignant myeloid cells, *J. Clin. Invest.* **68**:932.

Hancock, W. W., Becker, G. J., and Atkins, R. C., 1982, A comparison of fixatives and immunohistochemical techniques for use with monoclonal antibodies to cell surface antigens, *Am. J. Clin. Pathol.* **78**:825–831.

Hellström, K. E., Hellström, I., and Brown, J. P., 1982, Human tumor-associated antigens identified by monoclonal antibodies, *Springer Semin. Immunopathol.* **5**:127–146.

Helson, L., 1975, Management of disseminated neuroblastoma, *Cancer* **25**:264–267.

Herlyn, M., Steplewski, Z., Herlyn, D., and Koprowski, H., 1979, Colorectal carcinoma-specific antigen: Detection by means of monoclonal antibodies, *Proc. Natl. Acad. Sci. USA* **76**:1438.

Herlyn, M., Clark, W. H., Mastangelo, M. J., Guerry, D. J. V., Elder, D. E., LaRosse, D., Hamilton, R., Bondi, E., Tuthill, R., and Steplewski, Z., 1980, Specific immunoreactivity of monoclonal anti-melanoma antibodies, *Cancer Res.* **40**:3602.

Hollinshead, A. C., 1982, Human lung tumor markers—Biological basis and clinical studies, *Cancer Detect. Prev.* **5**:255.

Hosoi, S., Nakamura, T., Higashi, S., Yamamuro, T., Toyama, S., Shinomiya, K., and Mikawa, H., 1982, Detection of human osteosarcoma-associated antigen(s) by monoclonal antibodies, *Cancer Res.* **42**:654.

Howe, A. J., Seeger, R. C., Molinaro, G. A., and Ferrone, S., 1980, HLA-DR (Ia-like) antigens on human tumor cells, *Clin. Res.* **28**:104A.

Howe, A. J., Seeger, R. C., Molinaro, G. A., and Ferrone, S., 1981, Analysis of human tumor cells for Ia-like antigens with monoclonal antibodies, *J. Natl. Cancer Inst.* **66**:827–829.

Howman-Giles, R. B., Gilday, G. L., and Ash, J. M., 1979, Radionuclide skeletal survey in neuroblastoma, *Radiology* **131**:497.

Hurwitz, E., and Danon, Y. L., 1982, A conjugate of adriamycin-anti-neuroblastoma monoclonal antibodies inhibits neuroblastoma cell *in vitro* (meeting abstract), in: *Tenth Annual Meeting of the International Society for Oncodevelopmental Biology and Medicine*, Sapporo, Japan, p. A68.

Imai, K., Ny, A. K., and Ferrone, S., 1981, Characterization of monoclonal antibodies to human melanoma-associated antigens, *J. Natl. Cancer Inst.* **66**:489.

Imashuku, S., Todo, S., Amano, T., Mizukawa, K., Sukimoto, T., and Kusunoki, T., 1977, Cyclic AMP in neuroblastoma, ganglioneuroma and sympathic ganglia, *Experientia* **33**:1507.

Izant, J. G., and McIntosh, J. R., 1980, Microtubule-associated proteins: A monoclonal antibody to MAP2 binds to differentiated neurons, *Proc. Natl. Acad. Sci. USA* **77**:4741–4745.

Jonak, Z. L., Kennett, R. H., and Bechtol, K. B., 1982, Detection of neuroblastoma cells in human bone marrow using a combination of monoclonal antibodies, *Hybridoma* **1**:349–368.

Kapadia, A., Feizi, T., and Evans, M. J., 1981, Changes in the expression and polarization of blood group I and i antigens in post-implanatation embryos and teratocarcinomas of mouse associated with cell differentiation, *Exp. Cell Res.* **131**:185–195.

Kaufman, R. A., Thrall, J. H., Keyes, J. W., Jr., Brown, M. L., and Zakem, J. F., 1978, False negative bone scans in neuroblastoma metastatic to the ends of long bones, *Am. J. Radiol.* **130**:131.

Kemshead, J. T., Bicknell, D., and Greaves, M. F., 1981a, A monoclonal antibody detecting an antigen shared by neural and granulocytic cells, *Pediatr. Res.* **15**:1282–1286.

Kemshead, J. T., Greaves, M. F., Walsh, F., Cahyen, A., and Parkhouse, M., 1981b, Monoclonal antibodies to human neuroblastoma reveal a heterogeneity in antigenic expression within the tumor (meeting abstract), *Proc. Am. Assoc. Cancer Res.* **22**:399.

Kemshead, J. T., Walsh, F., Pritchard, J., and Greaves, M., 1981c, Monoclonal antibody to ganglioside GQ discriminates between haemopoietic cells and infiltrating neuroblastoma tumor cells in bone marrow, *Int. J. Cancer* **27**:447–452.

Kemshead, J. T., Fritschy, J., Asser, U., Sutherland, R., and Greaves, M. F., 1982a, Monoclonal antibodies defining markers with apparent selectivity for particular haemopoietic cell types may also detect antigens on cells of neural crest origin, *Hybridoma* **1**:109–123.

Kemshead, J. T., Rembaum, A., Ugelstad, J., and Malpas, J. S., 1982b, The potential use of monoclonal antibodies and microspheres containing magnetic compounds to remove neuroblastoma cells from bone marrow, *Proc. Am. Soc. Clin. Oncol.* **1**:C-143.

Kemshead, J. T., Ugelstad, J., Rembaum, A., and Gibson, F., 1982c, Monoclonal antibodies attached to microspheres containing magnetic compounds, used to remove neuroblastoma cells from bone marrow taken for autologous transplantation (meeting abstract), in: *Fourteenth Annual Meeting of the International Society of Pediatric Oncology*, Berne, Switzerland, p. A21.

Kemshead, J. T., Fritschy, J., Goldman, A., Malpas, J. S., and Pritchard, J., 1983, Use of panels of monoclonal antibodies in the differential diagnosis of neuroblastoma and lymphoblastic disorders, *Lancet* **1**:12–15.

Kennett, R. H., and Gilbert, F., 1979, Hybrid myelomas producing antibodies against a human neuroblastoma antigen present on fetal brain, *Science* **203**:1120–1121.

Kennett, R. H., Jonak, Z. L., Momoi, M., Glick, M. C., and Lampson, L. A., 1982, Analysis of cell surface molecules on human neuroblastoma cells and leukemia cells, in: *Proceedings of the First*

John Jacob Abel Symposium on Drug Development (J. T. August, ed.), The Johns Hopkins University School of Medicine, Baltimore, Maryland, pp. 91–107.

Kersey, J. H., LeBien, T. W., Abramson, C. S., Newman, R., Sutherland, R., and Greaves, M., 1981, p24: A human leukemia-associated and lymphohemopoietic progenitor cell surface structure identified with monoclonal antibody, *J. Exp. Med.* **153:**726–731.

Koprowski, H., Steplewski, Z., Herlyn, D., and Herlyn, M., 1978, Study of antibodies against human melanoma produced by somatic cell hybrids, *Proc. Natl. Acad. Sci. USA* **75:**3405.

Koprowski, H., Herlyn, M., Steplewski, Z., and Sears, H. F., 1981, Specific antigen in serum of patients with colon carcinoma, *Science* **212:**53.

Kupchik, H. Z., Zurawski, V. R., Hurrel, J. G., Zamcheck, N., and Black, P. H., 1981, Monoclonal antibodies to carcinoembryonic antigen produced by somatic cell fusion, *Cancer Res.* **41:**3306.

Lampson, L. A., and Fisher, C. A., 1982, Monoclonal antibody analysis of human neural tumors (meeting abstract), *Fed. Proc.* **41:**411.

Lee, V., Trojanowski, J. Q., and Schlaepfer, W. W., 1982a, Induction of neurofilament triplet proteins in PC12 cells by nerve growth factor, *Brain Res.* **238:**169–180.

Lee, V., Wu, H. L., and Schlaepfer, W. W., 1982b, Monoclonal antibodies recognize individual neurofilament triplet proteins, *Proc. Natl. Acad. Sci. USA* **79:**6089–6092.

Liao, S.-K., Clarke, B. J., Kwong, P. C., Brickenden, A., Gallie, B. L., and Dent, P. B., 1981, Common neuroectodermal antigens on human melanoma, neuroblastoma, retinoblastoma, glioblastoma and fetal brain revealed by hybridoma antibodies raised against melanoma cells, *Eur. J. Immunol.* **11:**450–454.

Mazauric, T., Mitchell, K. F., Letchworth, G. J., Koprowski, H., and Steplewski, Z., 1982, Monoclonal antibody-defined human lung cell surface protein antigens, *Cancer Res.* **42:**150.

McIlhinney, R. A. J., Dinsdale, E., and Neville, A. M., 1981, A monoclonal antibody to the murine teratoma F9: An immunocytochemical demonstration of tissue specificity, *Diagn. Histopathol.* **4:**129.

McMichael, A. J., Pilch, J. R., Galfré, G., Manson, D. Y., Fabre, J. W., and Milstein, C., 1979, A human thymocyte antigen defined by a hybrid myeloma monoclonal antibody, *Eur. J. Immunol.* **9:**205–210.

Miller, R. A., and Levy, R., 1981, Response of cutaneous T cell lymphoma to therapy with hybridoma monoclonal antibody, *Lancet* **2:**226.

Miller, R. A., Maloney, D. G., Warnke, R., and Levy, R., 1982, Treatment of B-cell lymphoma with monoclonal anti-idiotype antibody, *N. Engl. J. Med.* **306:**517.

Minna, J., 1981, Preparation and potential clinical applications of monoclonal antibodies against human tumors (meeting abstract), in: *Monoclonal Antibodies and Breast Cancer*, July 29, 1981, NCI—Veterans Administration Medical Oncology Branch, Bethesda, Maryland.

Mitchell, K. F., 1980, A carcinoembryonic antigen (CEA) specific monoclonal hybridoma antibody that reacts only with high molecular weight CEA, *Cancer Immunol.* **10:**1.

Mitchell, K. F., Fuhrer, J. P., Steplewski, Z., and Koprowski, H., 1980, Biochemical characterization of human melanoma cell surfaces: Dissection with monoclonal antibodies, *Proc. Natl. Acad. Sci. USA* **77:**7287.

Momoi, M., Kennett, R. H., and Glick, M. C., 1980, A membrane glycoprotein from human neuro-blastoma cells isolated with the use of a monoclonal antibody, *J. Biol. Chem.* **255:** 11914–11921.

Moshakis, V., McIlhinney, R. A. J., Raghaven, D., and Neville, A. M., 1981, Monoclonal antibodies to detect human tumors: An experimental approach, *J. Clin. Pathol.* **34:**314.

Naritoku, W. Y., and Taylor, C. R., 1982, A comparative study of the use of monoclonal antibodies using three different immunohistochemical methods: An evaluation of monoclonal and polyclo-nal antibodies against human prostatic acid phosphatase, *J. Histochem. Cytochem.* **30:**253.

Neville, A. M., Foster, C. S., Moshakis, V., and Gore, M., 1982, Monoclonal antibodies and human tumor pathology, *Hum. Pathol.* **13:**1067–1081.

Ninane, J., Pritchard, J., and Malpas, J. S., 1981, Chemotherapy of advanced neuroblastoma: Does adriamycin contribute?, *Arch. Dis. Child.* **56:**544.

Nitschke, R., Cangir, A., Crist, W., and Berry, D. H., 1980, Intensive chemotherapy for metastatic neuroblastoma: A southwest oncology group study, *Med. Pediatr. Oncol.* **8:**281.

Nossal, G. J., 1976, Spontaneous regression of cancer: Summary and profile for the future, *Natl. Cancer Inst. Monogr.* **44:**145.

Osborn, M., Altmannsberger, M., Shaw, G., Schauer, A., and Weber, K., 1982, Various sympathetic derived human tumors differ in neurofilament expression, *Virchows Arch.* **40:**141–156.

Prasad, K. N., 1975, Differentiation of neuroblastoma cells in culture, *Biol. Rev.* **50:**129.

Price, M. R., Pimm, M. V., and Baldwin, R. W., 1982, Complement dependent cytotoxicity of anti-human osteogenic sarcoma monoclonal antibodies, *Brit. J. Cancer* **46:**601.

Pritchard, J., Malpas, J. S., and Kemshead, J. T., 1982, Monoclonal antibodies help in the differential diagnosis of "small round cell" childhood tumors (meeting abstract), in: *Fourteenth Annual Meeting of the International Society of Pediatric Oncology*, Berne, Switzerland, p. A10.

Rauvala, H., and Finne, J., 1979, Structural similarity of the terminal carbohydrate sequences of glycoproteins and glycolipids, *FEBS Lett.* **97:**1.

Reif, A. E., and Allen, J. M. V., 1964, The AKR thymic antigen and its distribution in leukemias and nervous tissue, *J. Exp. Med.* **120:**413.

Reinherz, E. L., and Schlossman, S. F., 1982, The characterization and function of human immunoregulatory T lymphocyte subsets, *Pharmacol. Rev.* **34:**17–22.

Reinherz, E. L., Kung, P. C., Goldstein, G., Levey, R. H., and Schlossman, S. F., 1980, Discrete stages of human intrathymic differentiation: Analysis of normal thymocytes and leukemic lymphoblasts of T-cell lineage, *Proc. Natl. Acad. Sci. USA* **77:**1588–1592.

Revoltella, R. P., Businaro, R., Lauro, G., and Toesca, A., 1982, Tumor-associated neural differentiation antigens detected on C1300 neuroblastoma cells by hybridoma monoclonal autoantibodies, *Cell. Immunol.* **68:**75–92.

Reynolds, C. P., and Smith, R. G., 1981, Monoclonal antibody to human neuroblastoma-associated antigen (meeting abstract), *Proc. Am. Assoc. Cancer Res.* **22:**402.

Reynolds, C. P., and Smith, R. G., 1982, A sensitive immunoassay for human neuroblastoma cells, in: *Hybridomas in Cancer Diagnosis and Treatment* (M. S. Mitchell and H. F. Oettgen, eds.), Raven Press, New York, pp. 235–240.

Ritz, J., and Schlossman, S. F., 1982, Utilization of monoclonal antibodies in the treatment of leukemia and lymphoma, *Blood* **59:**1–11.

Ruddon, R. W., 1982, Tumor markers in the recognition and management of poorly differentiated neoplasms and cancers of unknown primary, *Semin. Oncol.* **9:**416–426.

Saxton, R. E., Mann, B. D., Irie, R. F., Morton, D. L., and Burk, M. W., 1982a, Monoclonal antibodies to human melanoma: Identification of two unique proteins on the tumor cell membrane (meeting abstract), *Proc. Am. Assoc. Cancer Res.* **23:**1040.

Saxton, R. E., Mann, B. D., Morton, D. L., and Burk, M. W., 1982b, Monoclonal antibodies to 125 kd and 95 kd proteins on human melanoma cells: Comparison with other monoclonal-defined melanoma antigens, *Hybridoma* **1:**433.

Schnegg, J. F., Diserens, A. C., Carrel, S., Accolla, R. S., and de Tribolet, N., 1981, Human glioma-associated antigens detected by monoclonal antibodies, *Cancer Res.* **41:**1209–1213.

Schwab, U., Stein, H., Gerdes, J., Lemke, H., Kirchner, H., Schaadt, M., and Diehl, V., 1982, Production of a monoclonal antibody specific for Hodgkin and Sternberg–Reed cells of Hodgkin's disease and a subset of normal lymphoid cells, *Nature* **299:**65–67.

Seeger, R. C., 1982a, Expression of human Thy-1 by neuroblastoma, glioma, sarcoma, and teratoma cells, in: *Hybridomas in Cancer Diagnosis and Treatment* (M. S. Mitchell and H. F. Oettger, eds.), Raven Press, New York, pp. 231–234.

Seeger, R. C., 1982b, Neuroblastoma: Clinical perspectives, monoclonal antibodies, and retinoic acid, *Ann. Intern. Med.* **97:**873–884.

Seeger, R. C., Zeltzer, P. M., and Rayner, S. A., 1979, Onco-neural antigen: A new neural differentiation antigen expressed by neuroblastoma, oat cell carcinoma, Wilm's tumor, and sarcoma cells, *J. Immunol.* **122:**1548–1555.

Seeger, R. C., Danon, Y. L., Zeltzer, P. M., Maidman, J. E., and Rayner, S. A., 1980, Expression of fetal antigens by human neuroblastoma cells, *Prog. Cancer Res. Ther.* **12:**344.

Seeger, R. C., Rosenblatt, H. M., Imai, K., and Ferrone, S., 1981, Common antigenic determinants on human melanoma, glioma, neuroblastoma, and sarcoma cells defined with monoclonal antibodies, *Cancer Res.* **41:**2714–2717.

Seeger, R. C., Danon, Y. L., Rayner, S. A., and Hoover, F., 1982, Definition of a Thy-1 determinant on human neuroblastoma, glioma, sarcoma, and teratoma cells with a monoclonal antibody, *J. Immunol.* **128**:983–989.

Sidell, N., 1982, Retinoic acid-induced growth inhibition and morphologic differentiation of human neuroblastoma cells *in vitro*, *J. Natl. Cancer Inst.* **68**:589.

Sikora, K., and Wright, R., 1981, Human monoclonal antibodies to lung-cancer antigens, *Br. J. Cancer* **43**:696.

Solter, D., and Knowles, B. B., 1978, Monoclonal antibody defining a stage-specific mouse embryonic antigen (SSEA-1), *Proc. Natl. Acad. Sci. USA* **75**:5565–5569.

Stein, H., Gerdes, J., Schwab, U., Lemke, H., Mason, D. Y., Ziegler, A., Schienle, W., and Diehl, V., 1982, Identification of Hodgkin and Sternberg–Reed cells as a unique cell type derived from a newly-detected small-cell population, *Int. J. Cancer* **30**:445–459.

Sternberger, L. A., 1979, *Immunocytochemistry*, Wiley, New York, pp. 104–169.

Sty, J. R., Babbitt, D. P., Casper, J. T., and Boedecker, R. A., 1979, 99 mTc-methylene diphosphonate imaging in neural crest tumors, *Clin. Nucl. Med.* **4**:12.

Susimoto, T., Sawada, T., Kusunoki, T., and Minowda, J., 1982, Presence of neuroblastoma surface membrane antigens cross-reacting with monoclonal antibody primarily developed against hematopoietic cells (meeting abstract), in: *Proceedings of the Japanese Cancer Association 41st Annual Meeting*, Osaka, Japan, p. 425.

Tank, A. W., and Weiner, N., 1982, Induction of tyrosine hydroxylase by glucocorticoids in mouse neuroblastoma cells: Enhancement of the induction by cyclic AMP, *Mol. Pharmacol.* **22**:421–430.

Trojanowski, J. Q., Lee, V., Pillsbury, N., and Lee, S., 1982, Neuronal origin of human esthesioneuroblastoma demonstrated with anti-neurofilament monoclonal antibodies, *N. Engl. J. Med.* **307**:159–161.

Uotila, M., Engvall, E., and Rouslahti, E., 1980, Monoclonal antibodies to human alphafetoprotein, *Mol. Immunol.* **17**:791.

Weinstein, J. N., Parker, R. J., Keenan, A. M., Dower, S. K., Morse III, H. C., and Sieber, S. M., 1982, Monoclonal antibodies in the lymphatics: Toward the diagnosis and therapy of tumor metastases, *Science* **218**:1334–1337.

Wikstrand, C. J., and Bigner, D. D., 1982, Expression of human fetal brain antigens by human tumors of neuroectodermal origin as defined by monoclonal antibodies, *Cancer Res.* **42**:267–275.

Wikstrand, C. J., Pegram, C. N., and Bourdon, M. A., 1982, Expression of human fetal brain antigens (FBA) by human glioblastoma (HGL) cells as defined by monoclonal antibodies (MCA) (meeting abstract), *Proc. Am. Assoc. Cancer Res.* **22**:304.

Wikstrand, C. J., Bigner, S. P., and Bigner, D. D., 1982a, Antigenic heterogeneity of an established human glioma cell line (HGCL) and eight single cell derived clones as defined by specific anti-glioma monoclonal antibodies (MCA) (meeting abstract), *Proc. Am. Assoc. Cancer Res.* **23**:1070.

Wikstrand, C. J., Bourdon, M. A., Pegram, C. N., and Bigner, D. D., 1982b, Human fetal brain antigen expression common of tumors of neuroectodermal tissue origin, *J. Neuroimmunol.* **3**:43–62.

Yeh, M., Hellström, J., Brown, J. P., Warner, G. A., and Hranson, J. A., 1979, Surface antigens of human melanoma identified by monoclonal antibody, *Proc. Natl. Acad. Sci. USA* **76**:2927.

Young, G., and L'Heureux, P. L., 1978, Extraosseous tumor uptake of 99m technetium phosphate compounds in children with abdominal neuroblastoma, *Pediatr. Radiol.* **7**:159.

10
Monoclonal Antibodies and Immunoparasitology

S. Michael Phillips and Deni M. Zodda

I. Introduction

The newly emerging discipline of immunoparasitology has extensively borrowed from and contributed to the more general field of immunology. Initially immunoparasitology benefited from technology developed by the more advanced discipline of immunology. More recently immunoparasitology has developed to the point that it clearly is capable of making significant and unique contributions to our understanding of immune response mechanisms. For example, vital information has been provided on the role of the eosinophil, mechanisms of genesis and modulation of granulomatous hypersensitivity, and genetic control of both host and parasite responses during infection. Clearly the approaches in immunoparasitology have become increasingly concordant to those of general immunology. Hence, it comes as no surprise that monoclonal antibody technology has been embraced by immunoparasitology and extensively utilized in the study of parasitic diseases. Areas of emphasis have included the preparation of purified reagents and the selective identification of antigenic determinants involved in antiparasite reactions. In addition to these general areas, there are also areas of emphasis unique to the field of immunoparasitology. These include:

1. Seroepedemiological studies to assess the incidence, prevalence, and morbidity of parasitic diseases.

S. Michael Phillips • Allergy and Immunology Section, University of Pennsylvania School of Medicine, Philadelphia, Pennsylvania 19104.   Deni M. Zodda • SmithKline Diagnostics, Sunnyvale, California 90486.

2. The preparation of reagents for use in vaccines for either immunoprophylaxis or the control of morbidity.
3. The elucidation of mechanisms of resistance and morbidity in both experimental and clinical infections.

The difficulties of preparing purified, biologically relevant antigens has limited the development of sophisticated immunoparasitological studies. Thus, monoclonal antibodies have been especially useful as reagents for the identification and purification of specific epitopes. It is the goal of this chapter to review some of the more salient advances in immunoparasitology that have been facilitated by the use of monoclonal antibodies. The discussion will be limited to parasites important to human disease.

II. The Use of Monoclonal Antibodies in Specific Parasitic Diseases

A. Malaria

The analysis of immune mechanisms and antigenicity in malaria is difficult, as more than 100 species of plasmodia are known. Most of these have relatively restricted host ranges and life cycles, characterized by a number of discrete stages (Figure 1). Each stage is unique in terms of physiology, morphology, and antigenic composition. Infection of the vertebrate host occurs when an infective mosquito injects malaria sporozoites while ingesting blood. The sporozoites are carried to the liver, where they invade parenchymal cells and divide asexually to form merozoites. The merozoites burst out of their host cell and infect new parenchymal cells. This hepatic or exoerythrocytic cycle can be repeated a number of times. Eventually, the merozoites enter the bloodstream. They infect erythrocytes and begin a cycle of asexual intraerythrocytic development. There are three sequential, morphologically distinct, intraerythrocytic stages known as ring forms, trophozoites, and schizonts. A small portion of the merozoites that invade erythrocytes differentiate into sexual forms, male (micro-) and female (macro-) gametocytes. When a mosquito ingests blood containing gametocytes, sexual reproduction occurs in the gut of the mosquito. Sporozoites are the progeny of this reproduction. They migrate to the salivary gland and are subsequently injected into the blood of the mosquito's next victim.

Numerous studies have suggested that there are multiple, immunologically unique markers and reactions for each parasite species and stage. Monoclonal antibodies have been extensively used to dissect a portion of this diversity (Cox, 1981; Taylor et al., 1981; Boyle et al., 1982; Nardin et al., 1982; R. S. Nussenzweig, 1982). Attempts have been made to identify antigens as potential sources of defined vaccines, improve the specificity and sensitivity of serodiagnosis, and identify potential mechanisms of resistance and morbidity.

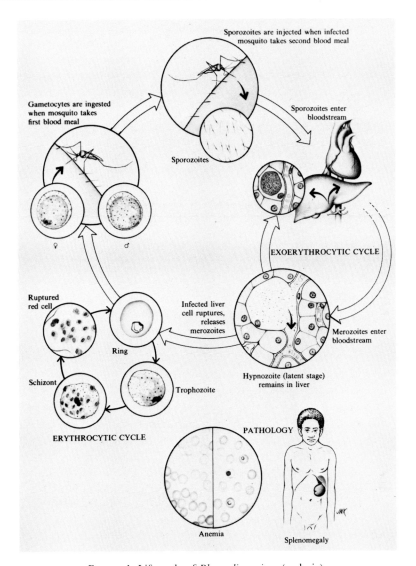

FIGURE 1. Life cycle of *Plasmodium vivax* (malaria).

1. Identification and Characterization of Merozoite Antigens

Protective monoclonal antibodies have been produced against merozoites of *Plasmodium yoelii, P. knowlesi,* and *P. falciparum.* Initial studies by Freedman *et al.* (1980) reported the recognition of a number of classes of antigens, using criteria of surface membrane distribution and polyacrylamide gel electrophoresis patterns. In addition, two of the antibodies were biologically active *in vivo.* They reduced the level of infection (i.e., parasitemia) in *P. yoelii*-infected mice. When two monoclonal antibodies were injected into the same recipient mouse, the infection was controlled more effectively than when the antibodies were injected into different mice. These data suggest that at least two antigens are involved in the induction of resistance. Furthermore, the injection of the monoclonal antibody attenuated the infection by confining it to reticulocytes. The ability to passively protect appeared to be related to the providing of sufficient time for the host to develop a protective immune response.

Holder and Freeman (1981) have produced two monoclonal antibodies used in immunoadsorption chromatography to isolate two antigens from *P. yoelii* intraerythrocytic forms. They isolated a high-molecular-weight (HMW) antigen (230,000 daltons), which is apparently a native polypeptide that fragments during development. Each fragment contains the relevant epitope. The HMW antigen is located on the parasite's surface. The second antigen, a 235,000-dalton protein, can be isolated from intracellular organelles. Both of these antibodies were able to protect mice against infection with *P. yoelii*. Indirect immunofluorescence (IIF) studies indicated that the antigens recognized by the protecting monoclonal antibodies were not expressed externally on infected erythrocytes. The authors concluded that the antibody-mediated protection against malaria may act at the level of free merozoites in inhibiting invasion of the host erythrocytes.

Epstein *et al.* (1981) reported that protection *in vitro* against merozoite-induced *P. knowlesi* infections was provided by monoclonal antibodies directed against specific surface determinants. The exact nature of the *in vivo* mechanisms of action of the monoclonal antibodies directed against merozoites is not clear. Epstein *et al.* (1981) have demonstrated that monoclonal antibodies possess the ability to block merozoite reinvasion of erythrocytes by agglutinating the parasites *in vitro*. The activity of the antibody appeared to be related to its binding of a membrane protein weighing approximately 250,000 daltons. This protein is precipitable by monoclonal antibodies and infected monkey serum. It has been demonstrated on two geographically isolated *P. knowlesi* strains.

Perrin *et al.* (1980,1981) described a series of monoclonal antibodies produced by injection of *P. falciparum* into mice. These monoclonal antibodies were capable of inhibiting parasite reinvasion and intraerythrocytic development *in vitro*. They also obtained a monoclonal antibody from *P. berghei*-infected mice that also inhibited *P. falciparum* growth *in vitro*. This is presumptive evidence for a "common protective" antigen on murine and human malarias. The "protective antibodies" recognized antigens of different molecular weight. One recognized a 41,000-dalton polypeptide; the second recognized polypeptides of 82,000 and 41,000 daltons; the third recognized a 140,000-dalton polypeptide (Perrin and Dayal, 1982). Myler *et al.* (1982) have produced monoclonal antibodies that inhibit the invasion of erythrocytes by *P. falciparum* merozoites.

Perrin and Dayal (1982) have reviewed the identification of specific *P. falciparum* antigens, associated with different asexual erythrocytic stages, and the analysis of *P. falciparum* polypeptides released *in vitro* and recognized by human immune serum. They have been studying the relationship between the previously identified "knob" antigens of *P. falciparum* and those molecules detected by monoclonal antibodies. They have also purified antigens recognized by inhibitory monoclonal antibodies, studied the synthesis and derivation of antigens from higher molecular weight polypeptides, begun the utilization of monoclonal antibodies as probes in recombinant DNA experiments, and evaluated antibodies for their seroimmunodiagnostic potential (Perrin, personal communication).

In other epidemiological studies, McBride *et al.* (1982) have demonstrated that monoclonal antibodies against blood forms of *P. falciparum* detect considerable antigenic diversity. Species isolates were characterized *vis-à-vis* the ability of certain monoclonal antibodies to react specifically with merozoites or trophozoites or both in an attempt to analyze the antigenic relationships between strains of different geographic origins. Typing with the monoclonal antibodies enabled the identification of different strains of the malarial parasite and suggested a degree of heterogeneity not previously suspected. The importance of these geographically constrained antigens has recently been emphasized by *in vitro* binding studies using monoclonal antibodies and long-term *P. falciparum* cultures by Schofield *et al.* (1982), although the biological significance of these antigens is not yet established.

2. Identification and Characterization of Sporozoite Antigens

Monoclonal antibodies against the sporozoite stage of *P. berghei* (NK65) were first reported by Yoshida *et al.* (1980). In this study, a monoclonal antibody was found to bind diffusely over the surface of the parasite, leading to a circumsporozoite precipitation (CSP) reaction. This monoclonal antibody immunoprecipitated a protein with a molecular weight of approximately 44,000 daltons (Pb44). The antigen appeared on only 50% of immature sporozoites, persisted in early exoerythrocytic stages, and was absent from the blood forms of *P. berghei* (Aikawa *et al.*, 1981b). The biological importance of the antigen was established when incubation of sporozoites *in vitro* with the antibody against Pb44 abolished the infectivity of these sporozoites (Yoshida *et al.*, 1980). Recent *in vitro* studies by Hollingdale (1982) have suggested that the monoclonal antibodies or their Fab fragments prevent sporozoite entry into target cells. Additional studies by Potocnjak *et al.* (1980) demonstrated that as little as 10 μg of monoclonal antibody directed against Pb44 was effective in mediating protection *in vivo*. Metabolic labeling studies of *P. berghei* sporozoites using [³⁵S]methionine demonstrated the existence of several intracellular polypeptide precursors of Pb44 (Yoshida *et al.*, 1981).

Subsequently, monoclonal antibodies against *P. berghei*, recognizing both specific and common determinants of sporozoites and erythrocytic forms, have been reported by Groot *et al.* (1982). Van Meirvenne (personal communication) has reported that an antigen of slightly higher molecular weight (53,000 daltons) can be isolated from the closely related *P. berghei* anka strain. This antigen reacts strongly with the monoclonal antibody directed against Pb44 from the NK65 strain. He has also observed that immunity between the two *P. berghei* strains can be cross-induced with the two antigens. A similar experience was reported by Ramsey and Charoenvit (1982, and personal communication).

Monoclonal antibodies have been used to identify protective antigens on sporozoites of *P. knowlesi* (a primate malaria) by Cochrane *et al.* (1982) and *P. falciparum* and *P. vivax* (both human malarias) by Nardin *et al.* (1982). Additional studies have suggested that these antigens are intimately related to those responsible for the circumsporozoite precipitation reaction (Santoro *et al.*, 1982). However, the specificity of the different detecting monoclonal antibodies varies. Some demonstrate exquisite stage and species specificity, while others show more diverse cross-reactivity (V. Nussenweig, 1982). Preliminary studies on peptide maps by Santoro *et al.* (1982) using monoclonal antibodies have shown 30–80% structural homology among a number of murine and primate malarial species. It is suggested that this homology may facilitate attempts at cloning relevant genes for the large-scale production of antigens for use as vaccines.

R. S. Nussenzweig (1982) reported the production of a monoclonal antibody that recognizes an antigen on *P. falciparum* sporozoites similar to one precipitated by immune human sera. This antibody was able to produce significant but not complete reduction of sporozoite infectivity following inoculation of parasites into splenectomized chimpanzees.

3. Identification and Characterization of Gamete Antigens

Studies by R. S. Nussenzweig (1982) demonstrated that male and female gametes of the avian parasite *P. gallinaceum* share certain surface determinants, since single monoclonal antibody reacted with gametes of both sexes. Agglutination of male gametes *in vitro* by Rener *et al.* (1980) was accomplished by using two monoclonal antibodies. This phenomenon demonstrated synergism *in vitro* and correlated with *in vivo* studies showing synergistic inhibition of oocyst development if the mosquitoes ingested monoclonal antibodies with blood containing gametocytes. Similar events were observed if vertebrate hosts were immunized with gametocytes prior to infection, as demonstrated with *P. yoelii* in rodents (Mendis and Targett, 1979) and *P. knowlesi* in primates (Gwadz and Greene, 1978). Subsequent studies by Aikawa *et al.* (1981a) have demonstrated that the pattern of agglutination of male gametes varied, depending on the monoclonal antibody used. One monoclonal antibody might cause agglutination in loose clusters, while others produced long, ropelike bundles of agglutinated parasites. The difference in the agglutination patterns appeared to be related to the distribution of antigens on the surfaces of the gametocytes. These studies further suggested that the effective blockade of fertilization was dependent on antibodies that coated the entire surface of the gamete rather than on those that produced a specific focal interaction.

4. Summary

Through the use of monoclonal antibodies, a large number of species and stage-specific antigens have been identified and isolated. In addition, many of the monoclonal antibodies have demonstrated their biological relevance by their ability to adoptively transfer resistance. Many can be used to purify antigens that can actively immunize against subsequent challenge by viable parasites. These studies, as summarized by Cox (1981, 1982), have produced a number of potential protective antigens and might enable a "quantum jump from the use of crude homogenates as vaccines to cocktails of characterized polypeptides, much more likely to be acceptable in human medicine than anything in experimental use at the present time."

B. Schistosomiasis

Schistosomiasis is a disease caused by several distinct species of the genus *Schistosoma*. The three major species *S. mansoni*, *S. japonicum*, and *S. hematobium* produce similar, although not identical, disease in man. Infection is initiated by the penetration of free-swimming cercariae. The cercariae enter the blood stream and, after several passages through the circulation, are trapped in the lungs. Schistosomulae then migrate to the liver, to undergo growth and development. Male and female worms mate and migrate as one to the mesenteric and pudendal veins of the host. Here, egg deposition occurs. The eggs are passed in the urine or feces of the host and hatch into free-swimming miracidia, which infects the appropriate snail vector. Following additional growth and development, asexual reproduction occurs and cercariae are liberated to complete the life cycle.

Although knowledge of the parasite and the host responses to infection are limited, there is much evidence to suggest that immunological mechanisms are intimately related to resistance and morbidity (Phillips and Colley, 1978). Considerable recent emphasis has centered on a definition of the nature and biological relevance of parasite antigens to resistance and morbidity. Thus, it comes as no surprise that monoclonal antibodies are increasingly used in the study of schistosomiasis.

1. Schistosoma mansoni

Verwaerde *et al.* (1979) were the first to describe monoclonal antibodies from rat–rat hybrids that participated in antibody-dependent, cell-mediated *in vitro* cytotoxic reactions against *S. mansoni* schistosomulae. Subsequently, this research group at Lille has described a number of monoclonal antibodies of various classes with a variety of *in vivo* and *in vitro* activities. A certain IgG2a monoclonal antibody (IPL Sm1) injected prior to challenge resulted in significant protection of syngeneic rats against challenge with *S. mansoni* cercariae (Grzych *et al.*, 1982). This antibody also possessed the ability to mediate eosinophil-dependent cytotoxicity *in vitro*. More recently, this monoclonal antibody has been used to isolate specific surface antigens (Dissous and Capron, 1982a,b; Dissous *et al.*, 1982). The protecting IgG2a antibody precipitated a 38,000-dalton antigen extracted from the surface of schistosomes. Surface antigens of similar

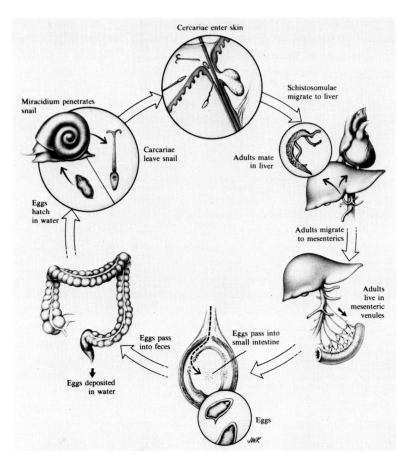

FIGURE 2. Life cycle of *Schistosoma mansoni* (schistosomiasis).

molecular weight had been previously shown to react with sera from infected mice, monkeys, and humans (Dissous *et al.*, 1981; Dissous and Capron, 1982a). This surface antigen was present on cercariae, newly transformed schistosomules, and schistosomules incubated *in vitro* for 24 hr. The antigen could not be isolated from detergent extracts of surface-labeled lung stage schistosomules. Additional studies suggested that the 38,000-dalton antigen was probably derived from a relatively recently synthesized, higher molecular weight moiety.

Taylor and Butterworth (1982) have described the production of mouse monoclonal antibodies against surface antigens of *S. mansoni* schistosomules. These antibodies were detected by radioimmunoassay and immunofluorescence. Although the antibodies initially described did not have demonstrable antibody-dependent cell-mediated cytotoxicity (ADCC) or complement-dependent cytotoxic activity *in vitro*, they were capable of precipitating specific membrane antigens. Subsequently, D. W. Taylor and A. E. Butterworth (personal communication) have described an IgG monoclonal antibody recognizing a 24,000-dalton pI 6.5 antigen. When mixed with schistosomules prior to their injection, the antibody reduces the subsequent adult worm burden. Work in that laboratory is currently emphasizing the use of the monoclonal antibodies to identify antigenic products, previously recognized by serum obtained from infected immune patients, and to confirm biological activity in rodents (A. E. Butterworth, P. Dalton, R. F. Sturrock, J. Ouma, and K. Siongo, personal communication). In other studies, the same group (J. Cordingley, D. W. Taylor, and A. E. Butterworth, personal communication) has found that mRNA can be produced from cercariae or adult worms and translated *in vitro*. The various products can be detected on sodium dodecyl sulfate (SDS) polyacrylamide gel electrophoresis (PAGE).

Smith *et al.* (1982) similarly reported the production of a biologically active IgM monoclonal antibody against *Schistosoma mansoni*. This antibody possessed the ability to passively immunize mice against *S. mansoni* infection and mediated complement-dependent cytotoxicity *in vitro* against schistosomules. It is of interest that the surface determinant appeared to be present on schistosomules, adult worms, and miracidia but was not detected on cercariae or lung schistosomules. Unlike polyspecific immune antiserum having considerable cross-reactivity with various species of flukes, these studies strongly suggested that the monoclonal antibodies described by Smith *et al.* (1982) may be preferable as immunological reagents because they recognized only *S. mansoni* antigens. This contention has been recently substantiated by the work of Catty *et al.* (1983). They measured circulating immune complexes, containing parasite-specific antigen and antibodies, in the circulation of infected humans, utilizing monoclonal antibodies and indirect inhibition ELISA techniques.

D. Harn (personal communication) has described a large series of monoclonal antibodies with *in vitro* cytotoxic ability. They are being used for antigen purification and as DNA transcriptional probes. He has identified five monoclonal antibodies which protect mice in passive transfer studies; the most active is an IgG2a affording a 51% reduction of lung schistosomule and adult worm recovery. The target antigen is apparently present for up to 72 hr on the surface of newly formed schistosomules. This antigen is labile under conditions of reduction and alkylation and treatment with SDS.

Our laboratory (Hafez *et al.*, 1983, 1984; Phillips, 1982; Zodda and Phillips, 1982; Zodda *et al.*, 1983) has been using monoclonals to study *S. mansoni* antigens, mechanisms of resistance, and morbidity. Over 100 monoclonal antibodies against *S. mansoni* antigens have been produced by fusion of splenocytes from *S. mansoni*-infected mice with SP2/0 myeloma cells. Antibody activity was assessed by a number of criteria, including: ELISA and RIA binding; an inhibition ELISA using 4 M KC extracts of cercariae and adult worms, soluble egg antigen (SEA), and purified antigenic preparations; indirect immunofluorescence, antibody-dependent cell-mediated cytotoxicity (ADCC), and complement-dependent cytotoxicity using living schistosomules; circumoval precipitation (COP) and cercarienhullen activity; effects on transmembrane potentials; and immunoprecipitation or adsorption of antigens.

These studies established the feasibility of producing large numbers of monoclonal antibodies and using them in antigen identification. Under appropriate conditions, monoclonal antibodies could detect less than 0.01 μg/ml of schistosome antigen (Hafez *et al.*, 1983, 1984). The monoclonal antibodies recognized a wide spectrum of antigenic determinants. The specificity of the monoclonal antibodies ranged from high cross-reactivity to extreme restriction. The distribution of the determinants within genus, species, and stages for a variety of antigenic preparations could be reliably analyzed with monoclonal antibodies where polyspecific antisera gave confusing data. Facilitated by the support of the Edna McConnell Clark Foundation, these monoclonal antibodies are available to any interested investigators upon request.

Following the generation of these monoclonal antibodies and a preliminary description of the antigens recognized by them, our attention has focused on the phenomenon of biological activity as determined by protection against infection (Zodda and Phillips, 1982). Furthermore, monoclonal antibodies have been used to pursue antigens related to protection and basic mechanisms of resistance. First, we identified a monoclonal antibody 3AF12-D6 (D6) possessing the ability to passively transfer resistance to syngeneic mouse recipients at a level similar to that demonstrable with immune mouse serum (Zodda and Phillips, 1982). A dose−response curve comparing the volume of monoclonal antibody transferred and the resultant protection is illustrated in Figure 3. This experiment demon-

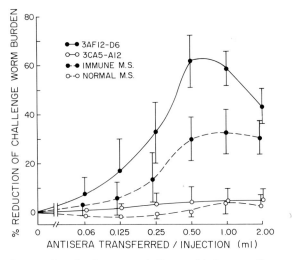

FIGURE 3. The adoptive transfer of resistance to challenge with *S. mansoni* by monoclonal antibody. Increasing amounts of ascites fluid containing specific monoclonal antibodies, control ascitic fluid, immune mouse serum, or normal mouse serum were injected into male CB6F$_1$/J mice. Injections were performed on two occasions, 12 hr before and 12 hr after challenge with *S. mansoni* cercariae. Significant resistance was noted when monoclonal antibody S80-3AF12-D6 was used, with maximum resistance observed utilizing 0.5–1.0 ml injection. Larger quantities of monoclonal antibody actually resulted in a reduction of this resistance. Immune mouse serum (M.S.) was similarly capable of producing a significant reduction of challenge worm burden in transfer experiments. However, the level of protection was somewhat less than that observed with the D6 hybridoma ascitic fluid. Normal mouse serum (M.S.) and another ascitic fluid (3CA5-A12) produced no significant protection.

TABLE I

Activity of Selected Anti-Schistosoma mansoni Monoclonal Antibodies against Schistosome Life Cycle Stages[a]

Monoclonal antibody	Schistosome antigen[b]			
	SCI	SEA	SWI	Sch
3AF12-D3	0.2[c]	0.8	0.1	2+[d]
3AE5-D1	0.3	0.5	0.5	NEG
3AF12-D6	0.5	1.0	0.2	4+
CH12-H1	1.8	2.0	0.2	4+
2CC7-D3	1.5	0.2	0.2	NEG
IMS[e]	>2.0	2.0	>1.5	4+

[a]See Appendix of this volume for experimental details, which are adapted from Zodda *et al.* (1983).
[b]SCI: soluble cercarial immunogen, ELISA. SEA: soluble egg antigen, ELISA. SWI: soluble worm immunogen, ELISA. Sch: living schistosomules, IIF.
[c]OD at 492 nm in ELISA using undiluted culture supernatant.
[d]Intensity of fluorescence in indirect immunofluorescence using undiluted culture supernatant.
[e]Immune mouse serum (1 : 500).

strates that the antibody has a potent protective ability. Of interest is the fact that larger amounts of the D6 antibody, rather than resulting in increased resistance, actually produced a decreased resistance. These findings are compatible with results in other parasite models, which showed that there may be an optimal molecular ratio of antibody and relevant immunogen. Excess antibody does not always result in maximum resistance to parasites. For example, Cochrane *et al.* (1981, and personal communication) have indicated that excessive amounts of monoclonal antibody may result in decreased resistance to challenge by *P. berghei* sporozoites.

The D6 monoclonal antibody was evaluated using the ELISA and IIF techniques. The direct binding and inhibition of binding by soluble antigen were studied. These studies clearly indicated that D6 antibody was capable of recognizing antigens present in various stages of the schistosome (Table I). The antibody titers of D6 against soluble cercarial immunogen, soluble worm immunogen (4 M KCl surface extracts), and soluble egg antigen were significant using ELISA criteria. However, strong cercarial binding *per se* was not an adequate explanation for protection. For example, 2CH12-H1 and 2CC7-D3 bound SCI strongly, but did not protect in adoptive transfer experiments. In addition, the ELISA titers against SCI and the IFF titers against living schistosomules are not necessarily correlated. Therefore, the ability to protect apparently lay in the ability of the D6 antibody to recognize a determinant of unique biological activity.

When D6 was compared to other monoclonal antibodies using IIF and ELISA binding assays, several phenomena became evident (Figure 4). The absolute titer of D6 was not the highest observed in either detection system; however, D6 antibody had a relatively higher titer directed against the surface of the living schistosomules by the IIF criteria, while its ELISA titer directed against 4 M KCl cercarial extract was more modest. The relative strength of IIF reaction implied

Figure 4. Comparison of hybrid-oma ascitic fluid activity utilizing criteria of surface indirect immunofluorescence and ELISA. Indirect immunofluorescence was performed utilizing intact living *S. mansoni* schistosomules previously produced by rat skin penetration. Anticercarial ELISA titers were calculated utilizing soluble cercarial immunogen produced by 4 M KCl extraction of *S. mansoni* cercariae. The results indicate that a wide range of antibody binding characteristics are expressed by the various ascitic fluids. Some express high titers in both assays, and others express high titers in only one of the two assays. The 3AF12-D6 antibody demonstrates a significant titer in both assays; however, the IIF titer is relatively greater than that demonstrated in ELISA in spite of the greater sensitivity of the latter test.

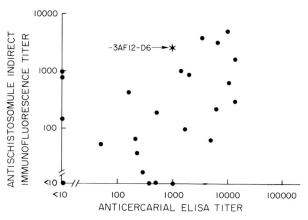

specificity for a surface determinant. Therefore, in comparison to other monoclonal antibodies, D6 is relatively more specific for an antigen present on the surface of the intact form. This contention is supported by the titers of antibody and the ease with which binding can be inhibited (Table II). Both binding titers and inhibition criteria confirm this conclusion.

These studies also demonstrate that there exist clear differences in the performance of these monoclonal antibodies with respect to the mode of assay. This may be because a given antibody may be highly selective in its binding of intact versus extracted membranes. These findings suggest that certain antigens, in a functional sense, may be created or destroyed by the method of extraction. A given antigen may be expressed on a fractionated membrane in a manner that makes it either more or less salient than its expression on the intact membrane. Thus, these studies would indicate that membrane fractionation, while necessary, represents a "double-edged" sword in that the mode of fractionation may influence the array of expressed antigens.

The data suggest that both quantitative and qualitative aspects of antigen recognition are important. The intact membrane should represent a closer analogy to the structure encountered by the infected host than does the fractionated antigen. This finding suggests that continual monitoring of purification, using techniques such as the inhibition of binding to the intact schistosomules and/or biological effects in terms of resistance, are required during antigen fractionation.

The quantitative binding studies suggested that the D6 does not have extremely high or low functional avidity when compared to other, nonprotecting monoclonal antibodies. Figure 5 illustrates that the binding affinity (functional avidity) of the monoclonal antibodies, as judged by the slope of the binding

TABLE II

Comparison of Monoclonal Antibody Recognition of Cercarial Antigens Using Criteria of Direct Binding and Antigen Inhibition

Monoclonal antibody	Ab binding titer[a]		Ratio IIF/ELISA	Antigen inhibition[c] (μg/ml)		Ratio[b] IIF/ELISA
	IIF	ELISA		IIF	ELISA	
N34-25	850	2000	0.42	3.8	5.3	0.71
N158-1	100	1600	0.06	1.4	2.0	0.70
N122-9	2300	5200	0.44	7.6	14.5	0.52
3AF12-D6	2800	1000	2.80	6.4	3.8	1.68
3CA5-A12	[d]	1080	—	[d]	6.4	—
7BO3-C8	160	[d]	—	2.9	[d]	—

[a] Extrapolated reciprocal of highest dilution demonstrating a positive reaction using the criteria of IIF or ELISA.
[b] Ratio of IIF titer/ELISA titer.
[c] Concentration of soluble cercaria immunogen that results in a 50% inhibition binding using IIF or ELISA criteria.
[d] Titer is not significant. Ratio cannot be calculated.

curves, varies over a wide range, as do the titers, as judged by intercepts. The slope and intercepts of the D6 myeloma binding curve were greater than, less than, or equivalent to those shown by other monoclonal antibodies that do not show protection.

It is unlikely that the class or subclass of a given monoclonal antibody determines its protective capability. The work of Grzych *et al.* (1982) suggest that IgG2a may be important in the rat for the induction of protection; however, protecting mouse-derived monoclonal antibodies of the IgM, IgG1, and IgG2 classes and subclasses have been observed. Conversely, the majority of monoclonal antibodies fail to protect, regardless of their class or subclass.

It is also clear that there are a number of antigenic determinants on the surface of the schistosomule, which can be recognized but are not necessarily related to resistance. It is suggested that the D6 monoclonal antibody preferentially recognizes an antigen on the surface of the schistosomule. For reasons that are not obvious, this antigen is uniquely related to protection.

Obviously, the monoclonal antibodies chosen to illustrate these points are somewhat arbitrary, as other monoclonals may have profiles that are more similar to D6; however, these do not share the ability to protect in adoptive transfer. There are no obvious relationships between absolute and relative titers, functional avidity, ease of inhibition of binding, and the ability to protect against infection.

The antigens of radiolabeled crude membranes produced by 4 M KCl extraction have been precipitated using D6 or other hybridomas and protein A beads. The immune precipitates have subsequently been reduced with mercap-

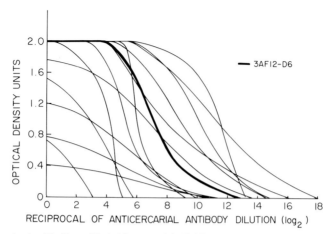

FIGURE 5. Quantitative binding of hybridoma ascitic fluids to SCI utilizing ELISA criteria. Increasing amounts of monoclonal antibody were incubated with SCI complexed to plates as previously described. The results indicate that a rather broad range in the absolute titers for the antibodies (judged by intercept analysis) and a very broad range of functional avidity (judged by the slope of the binding curves) are presented by these ascitic fluids. There was no obvious relationship between titer and functional affinity. In addition, the 3AF12-D6 antibody (heavy line) showed a titer and functional avidity that lay well within the extremes of these characteristics as demonstrated by other (nonprotecting) hybridoma ascitic fluids.

toethanol and run on slab SDS PAGE. The banding patterns were detected using overlay autoradiography (Figure 6). The D6, as well as other monoclonal antibodies, precipitated discrete structures. The major antigen appeared to have a molecular weight of approximately 130,000 daltons. Detergent extraction of membrane has produced a number of lower molecular weight antigens. It is of interest that other monoclonal antibodies, selectively chosen for illustrative purposes, can produce an apparently similar banding pattern. However, these other monoclonal antibodies do not protect, and therefore it is postulated that there may be multiple antigenic determinants that are recognized. Clearly, competitive inhibition studies, utilizing other radiolabeled purified monoclonal antibodies, will be necessary to resolve this question. The recent discovery of several other "protecting" monoclonal antibodies ought to facilitate this analysis (Phillips and Fox, unpublished observations). Ultimately, the monoclonal antibodies must serve as sophisticated "lectinlike" probes to establish the three-dimensional structure of the antigen in question.

In addition, this antigen represents approximately 0.3% of the total membrane antigenic mass of the parasite, judged by quantitative immunoaffinity chromatography. The antigen can be detected both *in vitro* by a variety of immunoprecipitation, inhibition, and transfer techniques and *in vivo* by the ability of monoclonal antibody to specifically effect increased rates of clearance of that antigen.

Studies relating to mechanisms of immunopathology utilizing monoclonal antibodies have also commenced. It has been possible to utilize monoclonal antibodies as specific markers for unique determinants of the egg, parenthetically the source of pathology. The first monoclonal antibody directed against a specific schistosome egg antigen (MSA$_1$) was reported by Hillyer and Pelley (1980). This antibody (F5) possessed the ability to produce a COP reaction. However, the determinant recognized is not stage-specific (Zodda *et al.*, 1983). Dresden *et al.* (1983) have reported a monoclonal antibody specific for proteinases found in *S. mansoni* eggs. This antibody is capable of effectively inhibiting these enzymes obtained from eggs, but only partially inhibiting the proteinases obtained from adult worms. The authors feel there is a relatively close steric relationship between the relevant egg and adult worm determinants, but that these determinants may not be identical. In addition, some of the monoclonal antibodies produced in our laboratory lead to a significant augmentation of the size of the granulomas about the egg when transferred to infected recipient animals. In addition, these antibodies can cause a COP reaction, which is known to result from an antigen–antibody reaction (Doughty and Phillips, unpublished observations). These latter results may imply that a critical informational bridge is supplied by the antibody.

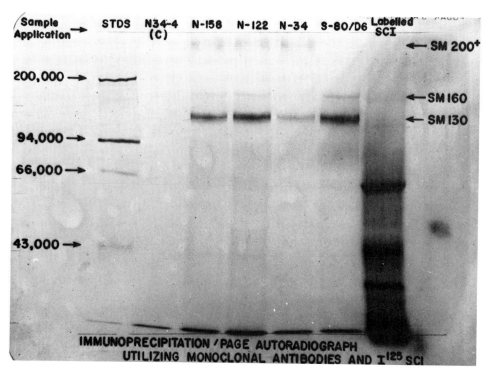

FIGURE 6. SDS PAGE autoradiograph of ^{125}I-cercarial antigen (SCI) precipitated by 3AF12-D6. Track 1, standards. Track 2, antigen precipitated by control AF not recognizing *S. mansoni*. Tracks 3–5, antigen precipitated by nonprotecting monoclonal antibody AF. Track 6, antigen precipitated by AF-containing monoclonal antibody 3AF-D6. Track 7, unprecipitated antigen.

2. Schistosoma japonicum

Monoclonal antibodies against *S. japonicum* have been utilized extensively by Mitchell *et al.* (1981) and Cruise *et al.* (1981a) as an immunodiagnostic tool for the detection of *Schistosoma japonicum* antigen using a competitive radioimmunoassay. Virtually no cross-reactivity was observed with other flukes, such as *Fasciola hepatica*, *Paragonimus westermani*, *Clonorchis sinensis*, and *S. mansoni* as well as several other helminths or protozoans.

One particular monoclonal antibody (I.134) is directed against a 23,000-dalton surface protein of adult *S. japonicum* worms. This antibody has been extremely useful as a reagent for the immunodiagnosis of *S. japonicum* in the Philippines. The data show that the antibody has excellent specificity (0% false positives to date) and adequate sensitivity (less than 10% false negatives to date) (G. F. Mitchell, personal communication). In addition, there appeared to be a gross correlation between the presence of high fecal egg counts and the ability of host serum to inhibit the binding of monoclonal antibodies.

These monoclonal antibodies have been demonstrated to be effective in mediating a COP reaction (Cruise *et al.*, 1981b). This simple, inexpensive immunodiagnostic test is based on a visible immunoprecipitation reaction around *S. japonicum* eggs *in vitro*. The data suggest the feasibility of using a monoclonal antibody under field conditions to overcome previously described difficulties in standardization using antisera (Garcia *et al.*, 1981).

C. Trypanosomatidiases

The family trypanosomatidae contains the causative agents for a broad spectrum of diseases, including leishmaniasis, Chagas disease, and African sleeping sickness. The parasites causing each disease have unique life cycles. Although they are too diverse to describe here in detail, we will give examples of life cycles in each case. In general, attempts at seroepidemiology have been frustrated by a lack of antigen definition. Hence, the initial use of monoclonal antibodies has been for the better definition of cell surface, family, species, and subspecies antigens of the trypanosomatidae.

1. Leishmaniasis

The many species of *Leishmania* cause a broad spectrum of diseases, ranging from cutaneous (*L. tropica*, *L. mexicana*) to mucocutaneous (*L. braziliensis*) to visceral (*L. donovani*) leishmaniasis (Figure 7). However, these species are morphologically identical and have immunological cross-reactivity. These characteristics have frustrated previous attempts to establish the precise seroepidemiological criteria required to assess the prevalence and impact of each species. The ability to distinguish species and subspecies from primary patient isolates is a prerequisite for the establishment of rational control and treatment programs. A variety of techniques, such as buoyant density of nuclear and kinetoplast DNA,

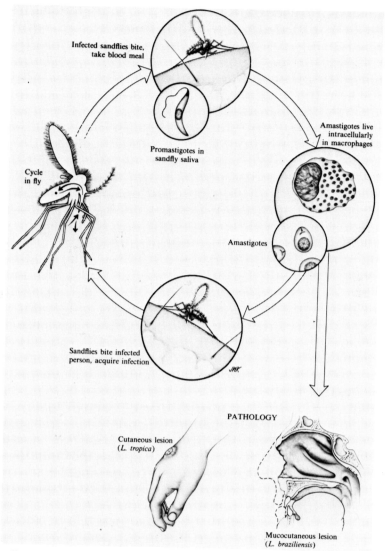

FIGURE 7. Life cycle of *Leishmania tropica* and *L. braziliensis* (leishmaniasis).

electrophoretic mobility of isozymes, serotyping, analysis of growth patterns, and electron microscopic criteria, have been used to differentiate *Leishmania* species. However, as reviewed by McMahon-Pratt and David (1982), these techniques are cumbersome and there is still a need for a convenient serodiagnostic tests for leishmaniasis. Monoclonal antibodies have proven useful in identifying antigens important for serodiagnosis and the understanding of immunity.

Monoclonal antibodies capable of distinguishing between the new world species of *Leishmania* (*L. braziliensis* and *L. mexicana*) were first described by Pratt and David (1981). Clear differentiation between these two species could be accomplished utilizing a panel of monoclonal antibodies in an RIA against membrane antigens. Unlike antisera obtained from infected humans, almost all of the monoclonals did not cross-react with *T. cruzi* epimastigotes, but could recognize a third species, *L. hertigi*. The monoclonal antibodies were shown to be reactive with glutaraldehyde-fixed promastigotes, suggesting field applicability. Recently, Pratt and David (1982) demonstrated the ability of a panel of antibodies to differentiate between subspecies of *L. braziliensis*. They differentiated between *L. braziliensis panamensis*, *L. b. braziliensis*, and *L. b. guyanensis*. The antibodies used in both studies were derived using cells from mice specifically immunized with membrane antigens.

Studies by Handman and Hocking (1982) described monoclonal antibodies derived from cells of *L. tropica*-infected mice, which demonstrated both stage-specific and cross-reactive antigens. One monoclonal antibody recognized the promastigote exclusively, while others recognized antigens shared between the promastigote and amastigotes. Common antigens shared between *L. tropica*, *L. mexicana*, and *L. donovani*, and even an antigen that appears to be ubiquitous on *Leishmania* species and *Crithidia fasiculata* (an insect parasite), were identified. Several of these monoclonal antibodies detected parasite antigens on the surface of *L. tropica*-infected macrophages and possessed the ability to inhibit parasite growth in macrophages *in vitro*. De Ibarra *et al.* (1982) have produced a number of monoclonal antibodies that recognize a variety of *L. tropica* antigens and were species- and stage-specific. However, a number of their antibodies recognized a matrix of antigens that were associated with organelles and were not species-specific.

In confirmation of these studies, Constantine and Anthony (1983) have described 29 monoclonal antibodies directed against *L. braziliensis* and 23 against *T. cruzi*. These reagents showed significant quantitative and qualitative differences with respect to cytoplasmic and/or flagellar antigen recognition patterns as determined by immunofluorescence. The labeling of *L. braziliensis* was either granular or intensely homogeneous, whereas with *T. cruzi* labeling was discretely paranuclear. Species specificity was limited to antibodies exhibiting reactivity to granular components in the cytoplasm and to an organelle thought to be the kinetoplast. Monoclonal antibodies against nongranular components of promastigotes and amastigotes of *L. braziliensis* cross-reacted with similar components in *T. cruzi* epimastigote. It was of interest that the species-specific monoclonal antibodies were IgM and the cross-reacting antibodies IgG (primarily IgG1). Subsequent studies by this group have demonstrated that the majority of the flagellar mass of the trypanosomatidae, which is the most highly cross-reactive component, has been identified as actin and tubulin, which are indistinguishable from those from mammalian cells (Anthony, personal communication).

These studies suggested that following the attainment of a wide repertoire of monoclonal antibodies, it will be possible to discriminate among species and subspecies of *Leishmania*. They also suggest that unique antigenic structures of *Leishmania* and other trypanosomatidae might be detected.

2. New World Trypanosomiasis: Chagas Disease

Chagas disease (Figure 8) is a chronic debilitating disease caused by *Trypanosoma cruzi*, affecting an estimated 12 million people in South and Central America. Initial studies using monoclonal antibodies have attempted to differentiate between *T. cruzi* and other trypanosomatidae, such as *Leishmania*, and to identify stage-specific antigens, as discussed in the section on leishmaniasis.

Two classes of glycoproteins from *T. cruzi* have been defined, one isolated by phenol extraction (Colli, 1979) and the other by detergent extraction. This latter class has been shown to be composed of two major subsurface glycoproteins. One glycoprotein had a molecular weight of 90,000 daltons and is present on all stages of the parasite (Snary and Hudson, 1979). This glycoprotein was initially purified by PAGE chromatography and shown to protect mice against lethal *T. cruzi* infection. The second glycoprotein had a molecular weight of 72,000 daltons and was found in epimastigotes and metacyclic amastigotes.

Snary *et al.* (1981) have used monoclonal antibodies obtained from mice immunized with *T. cruzi* epimastigotes to study these antigens. One monoclonal antibody was epimastigote specific. It bound to Y, Peru, and Tulahuén strain epimastigotes, but did not bind to Y strain amastigotes or trypomastigotes. The corresponding antigen had a molecular weight of 72,000 daltons (representing 0.04% of the total cell protein) and a carbohydrate content of 52%. Immunization with the purified glycoprotein, however, did not protect mice against a lethal infection with blood trypomastigotes. The 72,000-dalton glycoprotein, found only on the insect-derived stages of *T. cruzi*, protected only against metacyclic trypomastigote challenge. More recently, Snary (1982) has isolated the 90,000-mol. wt. glycoprotein, which immunized animals against blood stream challenge. Antibodies against both of the glycoproteins were present in human Chagasic serum.

Recent work by Araujo *et al.* (1982) has produced 17 monoclonal antibodies against *T. cruzi* and characterized their immunoglobulin classes, subclasses, and specificites for various stages of the parasite. Some recognized amastigotes, others epimastigotes, and others recognized antigens present in both stages. Immunofluorescence localization studies showed that the antibodies recognizing amastigotes and promastigotes bound to the extremities of the amastigotes and the region of the flagellar pouch of the epimastigotes. The monoclonal antibodies were capable of detecting *T. cruzi* antigens in the serum of infected mice and supernatants from infected cell cultures. These data indicate that monoclonal antibodies may become useful for antigen isolation and diagnostics.

Work by Hoff and Pratt (R. Hoff, D. M. Pratt, and J. R. David, personal communication) has provided additional clarification of the strain-specific antigens of *Trypanosoma cruzi*. Six monoclonal antibodies, all IgG, were specific for the epimastigote stage of the Y strain and other recently isolated stocks from Brazil. The antibodies did not react with Y-strain blood from trypomastigotes, with epimastigotes of *T. rangeli*, or promastigotes of *L. donovani chagasi*. Thus, the monoclonal antibodies appeared to recognize strain-, species-, and stage-

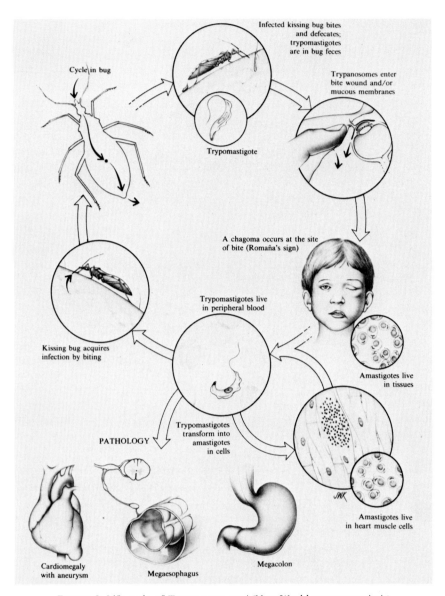

Figure 8. Life cycle of *Trypanosoma cruzi* (New World trypanosomiasis).

specific antigens. Interestingly, the antibodies failed to react with laboratory strains of *T. cruzi*. Studies by Anthony *et al.* (1981) have shown that monoclonal antibodies can differentiate between two closely related species of trypanosomes, *T. cruzi* and *T. rangeli*. These antibodies appeared to be reactive with different antigens based on their immunofluorescence staining patterns of cytoplasm, plasma membrane, and flagellum of epimastigotes.

Recent studies by Wood *et al.* (1982) have provided insights into the possible pathogenesis of Chagas disease. These investigators have described a monoclonal antibody raised against rat dorsal root ganglia. This antibody labeled *T. cruzi* amastigotes and epimastigotes and recognized an antigenic determinant on mammalian neurons. The authors suggested that common neuronal and trypanosomal antigens recognized by the antibody may be important in the pathogenesis of the disease.

3. African Trypanosomiasis

Old World trypanosomiasis, or African sleeping sickness, is caused by two major subspecies of hemoflagellates: *Trypanosoma brucei gambiense* and *T. b. rhodesiense*. Analysis is complicated due to the existence of multiple developmental stages (Figure 9), including: the infective metatrypomastigote (injected intradermally by the tsetse fly); the blood form trypomastigote; the procyclic trypomastigotes; and the epimastigote (which develops within the vector). In addition, antigenic variation exhibited by the trypanosome within its host represents an interesting, although complicating phenomenon. The course of disease is marked by a succession of parasitemic peaks, each represented by a restricted family of antigenic variants, defined by unique variant-specific surface glycoproteins (VSSG) (Cross, 1975). Each variant apparently multiplies and stimulates an appropriate protective immune response, which results in variant-specific destruction. In turn, new variant forms appear. Initial studies using monoclonal antibodies have attempted to define these VSSGs in an effort to understand various aspects of the genetic control of their expression. The identification and characterization of both unique and common antigens for use in serodiagnostic studies, for vaccination, and to aid in the understanding of resistance mechanisms has also been facilitated by the use of monoclonal antibodies.

Pearson and Anderson (1980) produced monoclonal antibodies against purified VSSGs and used a series of microimmunoadsorption columns and two-dimensional gel electrophoreses to determine certain biological and biophysical characteristics of the VSSG antigens. Lyon *et al.* (1981) have analyzed VSSGs of the Wellcome strains of *T. rhodesiense*. In both studies, exquisite specificity for a given variant within the antigenic serodeme was observed.

Additional studies have been performed by Campbell *et al.* (1981) and Mansfield (1981, and personal communication). These monoclonal antibodies produced from spleen cell donors exposed to infection, whole trypanosomes, or less pure VSSGs reacted against both variant-specific and nonspecific antigens. Some monoclonal antibodies reacted with all variants rather than just the homologous one, as found with immunization techniques using more purified antigens. Numerous patterns were seen in indirect immunofluorescence studies, with frequent labeling of subcellular organelles, such as mitochondria, kinetoplasts, nucleus, or flagella. These studies are currently being extended to study the nature of immune regulation by an analysis of idiotypic–antiidiotypic diversity and to better define parameters of parasite infection.

Studies by Esser *et al.* (1981, 1982) have provided special insight into the relationship between vector and host stages. These investigators have suggested

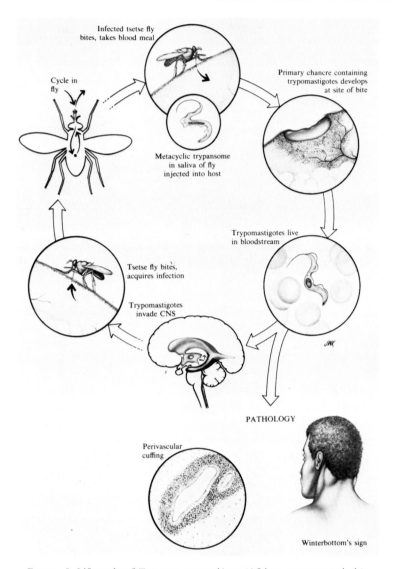

Figure 9. Life cycle of *Trypanosoma gambiense* (African trypanosomiasis).

that metacyclic trypanosomes are heterogeneous with respect to their variant antigen types and that the antigenic types expressed within the metacyclic forms are independent of the variant strain used to infect the tsetse fly. In addition, various trypanosome isolates from the same endemic area have been used to produce identical VSSGs. This suggests some restriction on the ultimate number of possible VSSGs. The first wave of parasitemia of blood-form-infected and metacyclic-innoculated mice express metacyclic VSSGs by day 5 of infection. In addition, the metacyclic VSSGs represent immunologically relevant antigens in that four of six variant-specific monoclonal antibodies abolished infectivity by homologous metacyclic trypanosomes. Additional studies from the same laboratory (K. Esser, personal communication) have included studies of *T. rhodesiensi* blood-form VSSGs. Monoclonal antibodies, which neutralized specific variant infectivity, identified three different antigenic epitopes for one specific VSSG.

Monoclonal antibodies are also being utilized in DNA cloning experiments for the preparation of large quantities of VSSGs. These glycoproteins may be used in discrete vaccine programs and for analysis of genetic control mechanisms (Pearson *et al.*, 1981; Lyon *et al.*, 1981).

D. Filariasis

Filariasis is a diverse group of diseases characterized by highly specialized tissue-dwelling nematodes (Figure 10). Female worms are ovoviviparous, releasing microfilariae, which subsequently survive for prolonged periods in the host's blood or skin. Transmission is accomplished by ingestion of microfilariae by arthropod vectors, in which the parasites develop into infective third-stage larvae. Because of the close relationship between various species and strains of filariae, antigen fractionation and serodiagnosis, especially during the long and critical prepatent period, have been difficult. The wide variety of organisms causing clinical disease and their recognized antigenic cross-reactivity have necessitated the development of more precise antigenic definition.

The advent of hybridoma technology has facilitated efforts to develop sensitive and specific immunodiagnostic tests for filarial infections. The monoclonal antibodies could enable the development of techniques that are more sensitive and capable of detecting earlier infections, and therefore facilitate more accurate serodiagnosis and rational assessment of therapy (Haque *et al.*, 1982). Des Moutis *et al.* (1983) have produced monoclonal antibodies from B cells obtained from "LOU" rats immunized with *Onchocerca volvulus* somatic extracts and rat myeloma cells (IR98F). The resultant monoclonal antibodies were assayed in an RIPEGA assay developed by Santoro *et al.* (1978). These monoclonal antibodies were able to detect circulating antigen in the serum of individuals infected with *O. volvulus*. There were also small but detectable levels of antigen in sera of individuals infected with other filariids (*Brugia malayi, Loa loa*) and even helminths (*S. mansoni*). This degree of cross-reactivity, however, was much lower than that shown by immune sera. The detected polysaccharide antigen appeared to be from the microfilarial cuticle and had a molecular weight of approximately 50,000 daltons. Unfortunately, the level of circulating antigen did not correlate with intensity of infection, judged by "skin snip" assay. It was concluded that it may be necessary to use a battery of several monoclonal antibodies, each reacting with different epitopes possibly on different molecules, to fully define the spectrum of human infection. In addition, it would be necessary to measure both antibody and antigen.

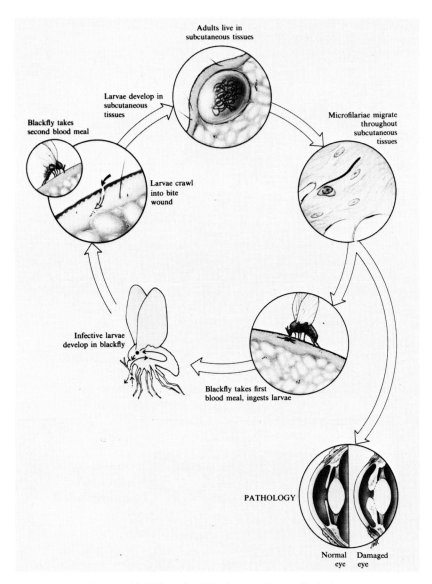

FIGURE 10. Life cycle of *Onchocera volvulus* (filariasis).

The ability to measure responses to infective larvae and microfilaria is also critical with respect to the determination of protective and transmission inhibitory immunity. In this context, studies by M. M. Canlas and W. F. Piessens (personal communication) have indicated that monoclonal antibodies can be developed against microfilaria, L3 infective larvae, and adult stages of *B. malayi*. Monoclonal antibodies capable of reacting specifically with extracts from microfilariae, but not with adult or L3 larvae, were produced. Other monoclonal antibodies could react with infective L3 stages or with adult worms. Most of the monoclonal antibodies were cross-reactive with other stages and recognized multiple bands in PAGE; however, some recognized only a single band, suggesting exploitable limits on heterogeneity.

E. Toxoplasma gondii

A number of laboratories have reported the production of murine hybridomas producing anti-*Toxoplasma* monoclonal antibodies. These have become useful tools in identifying and isolating individual antigens of *T. gondii* and have permitted an initial elucidation of the antigenic nature, topology, and function of these epitopes. Initial studies by Araujo *et al.* (1980) used an ELISA technique to detect antigens of the parasite in culture lysates, the peritoneal fluids of infected mice, and the sera of humans acutely infected with *T. gondii*. Subsequently, this group described initial studies on the characterization of membrane antigens of *Toxoplasma* (Handman *et al.*, 1980). Using two-dimensional PAGE analysis of radioiodinated surface proteins, four major structures of molecular weights 43,000, 35,000, 27,000, and 14,000 daltons were detected. Different precipitation patterns were obtained with different monoclonal antibodies and sera obtained from humans infected with *Toxoplasma*. Handman and Remington (1980) developed additional monoclonal antibodies capable of recognizing membrane and cytoplasmic antigens of *T. gondii* tachyzoites (Figure 11). Discrete localization, beaded irregular staining, and smooth rim fluorescence patterns were obtained. In contrast, polyspecific antiserum produced solid rim patterns. No obvious correlation between the pattern of fluorescence and the nature of the precipitated antigenic fragments was found. Subsequently, the utility of ELISA techniques to detect monoclonal antibodies against *T. gondii* was confirmed by Naot and Remington (1981). Sethi *et al.* (1980) presented data on eight functional hybridomas directed against *T. gondii* monitored by indirect immunofluorescence and radioimmunoassay. Further studies on the antigenic fractionation of monoclonal antibodies and a summary of the current state of the art with regard to the precise molecular weights and PAGE characteristics of identified structures are provided by Sethi (1982), who also reviews the variety of molecular separation techniques used in a number of laboratories. A summary of previous studies indicated that of the 35 previously described monoclonal antibodies, six reacted exclusively against cytoplasmic, 25 against membrane, and four against both components. A suggestion was made that a comparison of various strains of *T. gondii* with monoclonal antibodies might provide evidence for additional antigenic disparities.

Studies using monoclonal antibodies have also provided valuable information relative to potential models of phagocytosis and intracellular killing. Monoclonal antibodies that expressed cytotoxicity against *T. gondii* and were produced using spleen cells exposed to *T. gondii in vitro* have been described (Sethi and Brandis, 1981). Hauser and Remington (1981) demonstrated that monoclonal antibodies to *Toxoplasma* facilitated phagocytosis of this organism and prepared

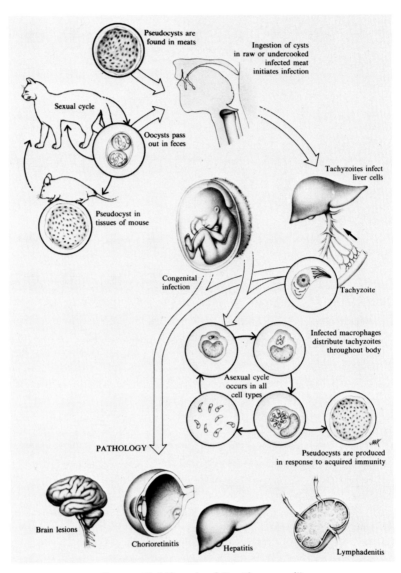

FIGURE 11. Life cycle of *Toxoplasma gondii.*

the organisms for intracellular destruction. This destruction could be demonstrated in normal peritoneal phagocytic monocytes. Similarly, Sethi *et al.* (1981) demonstrated that the monoclonal antibodies were probably of biological relevance since *T. gondii* trophozoites precoated with specific monoclonal antibody could not survive within normal murine macrophages. The investigators suggested that macrophage-derived complement components did not account for the killing of antibody-coated trophozoites within the normal peritoneal macrophage. This killing was solely an intracellular event. They postulated that the antibody-coated trophozoites may induce the fusion of lysosomes with the pha-gocytic vacuole containing the *Toxoplasma*, a process leading to parasite killing.

III. Future Applications of Monoclonal Antibodies in Immunoparasitology

Section II has amply demonstrated that monoclonal antibodies are ex-tremely useful in a number of venues. This is especially important for the defini-tion of those antigens and immune mechanisms that are relevant to protective or pathological immune responses. However, a number of additional applications appear promising, and this section summarizes a few of these.

A. Analysis of Idiotypic Networks

A number of recent observations using monoclonal antibodies have impli-cated idiotypic regulatory networks in a number of parasitic conditions. Studies by Potocnjak *et al.* (1982) have described an immunoradiometric assay of general applicability. This assay uses the principle of inhibition of interactions between monoclonal antibodies and antiidiotypic antibody by parasite antigen. The assay was specific for an epitope that was uniquely restricted to a given strain of malaria and had the additional advantage that it did not require the use of purified antigen. The ability to detect antigens that might not be readily detect-able using adherence techniques due to size or charge characteristics was an additional strength. Finally, the procedure could pick out minor components from a complex mixture of molecules and confirmed the "mirror hypothesis" by demonstrating the inhibition of an antiidiotypic response by antigen.

Somewhat analogous studies have been performed by Mitchell *et al.* (1983). These investigators have clearly demonstrated the ability of a monoclonal anti-body previously shown to react with antigens obtained from *S. japonicum* para-sites to react in an idiotypic–antiidiotypic (id/anti-id) matrix. Using a competitive radioimmunoassay, these investigators demonstrated inhibition of the binding of ^{125}I-labeled monoclonal antibody to *S. japonicum* adult worm antigen by monoclonal antiidiotype antibodies bound to plates and *vice versa*. Solid phase immunoadsorption studies demonstrated that the id/anti-id reactants could be removed specifically and appropriately by using adsorption columns that recog-nized either whole immunoglobulin, idiotypes, or the antigen. A 23,000-mol. wt. surface protein reactive with sera from infected individuals appeared to be the target of the specific monoclonal antibody (I-134). The anti-id antibodies would not substitute for an antigen in the competitive RIAs if one crossed species barriers, and there was significant evidence to suggest that the id/anti-id reac-tions were extremely complex. They involved the recognition not only of cir-culating antigen, but also of circulating antiidiotype antibody (Cruise *et al.*, 1981a).

Attempts to modulate lung granuloma hypersensitivity using monoclonal antibodies and idiotype immunization (Mitchell *et al.*, 1982) have resulted in partial inhibition of lung granuloma formation in experiments with IgM monoclonal antibodies. However, the effectiveness of this procedure was contingent on a number of parameters, including the genetically determined response of the strain of mouse studied and the source of the COP-positive IgM monoclonal antibody.

Direct evidence for the modulation of resistance or morbidity in *S. mansoni* by idiotypic networks has not yet been obtained. Indirect evidence, however, supports this contention. For example, the IgG2a monoclonal antibody, possessing the ability to mediate ADCC reactions directed against schistosomules *in vitro* and produce protection *in vivo*, can be effectively blocked by the use of another IgG3 monoclonal antibody (A. Capron, personal communication). Similar observations have been made by Butterworth (personal communication) on the ability of one monoclonal antibody to block the ADCC activity of another. Observations in our laboratory are concordant with these observations. Immunoaffinity-purified antigen can be shown to be cleared in an accelerated manner in normal animals injected with protecting monoclonal antibody. However, this accelerated clearance and *in vivo* protection are not observed when infected animals are used. These data suggest that certain factors in the infected animal preclude the effective recognition of the relevant epitope by a protective monoclonal antibody.

Finally, the work of Sacks *et al.* (1982) appeared to conclusively implicate the importance of idiotypic–antiidiotypic reactions in mediating resistance in parasitic disease. These investigators specifically immunized animals against a variety of monoclonal antibodies that were directed against specific clones of trypanosomes. Following immunization, the recipient animals demonstrated decreased levels of parasitemia and an increased frequency to switch to other variants. The studies were interpreted as indicating that antiidiotypic sensitization can lead to an immune response that is capable of recognizing the original "antigen." This is compatible with antiidiotypic regulation of the immune response.

B. Engineering of Cloned Variants

Since many parasites represent proliferating systems, the use of monoclonal antibodies for specific selection is possible. Of particular interest in this regard is the recent work of Kaspar *et al.* (1983). Using the technique of chemical mutagenesis in the presence of a selecting cytotoxic monoclonal antibody, these investigators have succeeded in producing a *Toxoplasma gondii* mutant that specifically lacks a defined membrane antigen of approximately 22,000 daltons. This technology appears especially promising, not only for use in toxoplasmosis, but also with any other proliferating protozoan. In addition, the use of monoclonal antibodies for negative selection might be possible. For example, the utilization of antibodies directed against cell populations capable of responding to a given antigen or with unique metabolic requirements may be feasible.

C. Extended Seroepidemiology

Besides extending the sensitivity and specificity of conventional seroepidemiological approaches, monoclonal antibodies promise to allow the definition of responses to unique restricted antigens. These responses or antigens might be better correlated with proximity to exposure, level of parasite burden, resistance, or propensity toward morbidity. In addition, the selective removal of cross-reacting antigens might improve specificity dramatically (Craig et al., 1981). Better definition of the totality of disease transmission may be possible with the extension of techniques to study not only host but also vector epidemiology. For example the technique described by Potocnyjak et al. (1982) permits the qualitative measurement of parasite infection in single mosquitoes.

D. Targeted Chemotherapy

The covalent linkage of cytotoxic agents to monoclonal antibodies to improve selectivity of attack would appear especially promising in parasitic therapeutics. Such an approach, as summarized by Edwards and Thorpe (1981), has already been shown to be feasible in tumor systems (Krolick et al., 1980).

E. Molecular Probing of Genomes

As already mentioned, monoclonal antibodies have been used in a number of laboratories as molecular probes for products of DNA transcription and to begin the elucidation of basic aspects of the genetic basis of variant expression. In addition, such analysis may be useful in the exclusion mode as well. For example, Simpson et al. (1982) have recently used monoclonal antibodies directed against histocompatibility antigens to identify nuclear probes. Their analysis demonstrated that host histocompatibility antigens observed on the surface of S. mansoni worms cannot be of parasite origin since the parasite lacked the DNA sequences necessary to code for the antigen.

IV. Summary

In summary, monoclonal antibodies have been extensively utilized in the study of parasitic diseases. The majority of the initial efforts have concentrated on the production of the monoclonal antibodies for the definition of antigens that are relevant in the induction of protective immunity or the mediation of pathology. Following the successful identification of these antigens, attempts have been made to utilize monoclonal antibodies and more highly purified antigens for vaccination and seroepidemiological studies. These latter studies have involved the measurement of antibody as well as circulating antigens in an attempt to document the presence of active infection and to begin truly quantitative evaluations. A number of *in vivo* and *in vitro* criteria for the biological activity of the monoclonal antibodies have been established and preliminary studies have begun to assess those intra- and extracellular mechanisms that are most relevant to resistance and morbidity. It is anticipated that monoclonal antibodies will become increasingly valuable in these and other modes of immunoparasitological study.

References

Aikawa, M., Rener, J., Carter, R., and Miller, L. H., 1981a, An electron microscopical study of the interactions of monoclonal antibodies with gametes of the malarial parasite *Plasmodium gallinaceum*, *J. Protozool.* **28**:383–388.

Aikawa, M., Yoshida, N., Nussenzweig, R. S., and Nussenzweig, V., 1981b, The protective antigen of malarial sporozoites (*Plasmodium berghei*) is a differentiation antigen, *J. Immunol.* **126**:2494–2495.

Anthony, R. L., Cody, T. S., and Constantine, N. T., 1981, Antigenic differentiation of *Trypanosoma cruzi* and *T. rangeli* by means of monoclonal-hybridoma antibody, *Am. J. Trop. Med. Hyg.* **30**:1192–1197.

Araujo, F. G., Handman, E., and Remington, J. S., 1980, Use of monoclonal antibodies to detect antigens of *Toxoplasma gondii* in serum and other body fluids, *Infect. Immun.* **30**:12–16.

Araujo, F. G., Scharma, S. D., Tsai, V., Cox, P., and Remington, J. S., 1982, Monoclonal antibodies to stages of *Tropanosoma cruzi:* Characterization and use for antigen detection, *Infect. Immun.* **37**:344–349.

Boyle, D. B., Newbold, C. I., Smith, C. C., and Brown, K. N., 1982, Monoclonal antibodies that protect *in vivo* against *Plasmodium chabaudi* recognize a 25,000-Dalton parasite polypeptide, *Infect. Immun.* **38**:94–102.

Campbell, G. H., Griswald, S., Kane, G., Giorgi, J. V., and Warner, N. L., 1981, *Res. Monogr. Immunol.* **3**:323.

Catty, D., Hassan, K., Mumo, J., Appleby, P., Hawkins, S., Adu, J., Das, P., Lavanchy, D., and Braun, D., 1983, Monoclonal antibodies and diagnosis of schistosomiasis in man, in: *30th Protides of Biological Fluids*, Brussels, in press.

Cochrane, A. H., Nussenzweig, R. S., and Nardin, E. H., 1980, Immunization against sporozoites, in: *Malaria*, Volume 3 (J. P. Kreir, ed.), Academic Press, New York, pp. 163–197.

Cochrane, A. H., Gwadz, R., Nussenzweig, A. S., and Nussenzweig, V., 1981, Monoclonal antibodies against surface antigen of sporozoites of simian malaria abolish parasite infectivity, *Fed. Proc.* **40**:1011 (abstract).

Cochrane, A. H., Santoro, F., Nussenzweig, V., Gwadz, R., and Nussenzweig, R. S., 1982, Monoclonal antibodies identify the protective antigens of sporozoites of *Plasmodium knowlesi*, *Proc. Natl. Acad. Sci. USA* **79**:5651–5655.

Colli, W., 1979, Chagas disease, in: *The Membrane Pathobiology of Tropical Diseases* (D. F. P. Wallach, ed.), Schwabe and Co., Basel, pp. 131–153.

Constantine, N. T., and Anthony, R. L., 1983, Antigenic differentiation of *Leishmania braziliensis* and *Trypanosoma cruzi* by means of monoclonal-hybridoma antibodies, *J. R. Soc. Trop. Med*, in press.

Cox, F. E. G., 1981, Hybridoma technology identifies protective malarial antigens, *Nature* **294**:612.

Cox, F. E. G., 1982, Vaccines for parasitic disease, in: *Parasites, Their World and Ours* (D. F. Mettrick and S. S. Desser, eds.), Elsevier Biomedical Press, Amsterdam, pp. 395–404.

Craig, P. S., Hocking, R. E., Mitchell, G. F., and Rickard, M. D., 1981, Murine hybridoma-derived antibodies in the processing of antigens for the immunodiagnosis of hydatid (*Echinococcus granulosus* infection in sheep, *Parasitology* **83**:303–317.

Cross, G., 1975, Identification, purification, and properties of clone-specific glycoprotein antigens constituting the surface coat of *Trypanosoma brucei*, *Parasitology* **71**:393–417.

Cruise, K. M., Mitchell, G. F., Garcia, E. G., and Anders, R. F., 1981a, Hybridoma antibody immunoassays for the detection of parasitic infection. Further studies on a monoclonal antibody with immunodiagnostic potential for *Schistosomiasis japonica*, *Acta Trop.* **38**:437–447.

Cruise, K. M., Mitchell, G. F., Tapales, F. P., Garcia, E. G., and Huang, S.-R., 1981b, Murine hybridoma-derived antibodies producing circumoval precipitation (COP) reactions with eggs of *Schistosoma japonicum*, *Aust. J. Exp. Biol. Med. Sci.* **59**:503–514.

Deedler, A. M., 1982, The application of monoclonal antibodies to studies of schistosomiasis, in: *Properties of the Monoclonal Antibodies Produced by Hybridoma Technology and Their Application to the Study of Diseases* (V. Houba and S. H. Chen, eds.), UNDP/WB/WHO, Geneva, pp. 93–103.

De Ibarra, A. A. L., Howard, J. G., and Snary, D., 1982, Monoclonal antibodies to *Leishmania tropica* major: Specificities and antigen location, *Parasitology*, **85**:523–531.

Des Moutis, I., Ouaissi, A., Grzych, J. M., Yarzabal, L., Hague, A., and Capron, A., 1983, *Onchocerca volvulus*: Detection of circulating antigens by monoclonal antibodies, *Am. J. Trop. Med. Hyg.* **32**:533–542.

Dissous, C., and Capron, A., 1982a, Characterization of potentially protective antigens from the surface of *Schistsoma mansoni* schistosomula, *Fed. Proc.* **41**:483 (abstract).

Dissous, C., and Capron, A., 1982b, Isolation of surface antigens from *S. mansoni* schistosomula, in: *Protides of the Biological Fluids* (H. Peeters, ed.), Proceedings of the 29th Colloquium, Pergamon Press, Oxford, pp. 179–182.

Dissous, C., Dissous, C., and Capron, A., 1981, Isolation and characterization of surface antigens from *Schistosoma mansoni* schistosomula, *Mol. Biochem. Parasitol.* **3**:215.

Dissous, C., Grzych, J. M., and Capron, A., 1982, *Schistosoma mansoni* surface antigen defined by a rat protective monoclonal IgG2a, *J. Immunol.* **129**:2232–2234.

Dresden, M. H., Sung, C. K., and Deedler, A. M., 1983, A monoclonal antibody from infected mice to a *Schistosoma mansoni* egg proteinase, *J. Immunol.* **130**:1–3.

Edwards, D. C., and Thorpe, P. E., 1981, Targeting toxins—The retiarian approach to chemotherapy, *TIBS* **6**:313–316.

Epstein, N., Miller, L. H., Kaushel, D. C., Udeinya, I. J., Rener, J., Howard, R. J., Asofsky, R., Aikawa, M., and Hess, R. L., 1981, Monoclonal antibodies against a specific surface determinant on malarial (*Plasmodium knowlesi*) merozoites block erythrocyte invasion, *J. Immunol.* **127**:212–217.

Esser, K. M., Schoenbechler, M. J., Gingrich, J. B., and Diggs, C. L., 1981, Monoclonal antibody analysis of *Trypanosoma rhodesiense* metacyclic antigen types, *Fed. Proc.* **40**:(3):1011.

Esser, K. M., Schoenbechler, M. J., and Gingrich, J. B., 1982, *Trypanosoma rhodesiense* blood forms express all antigen specificities relevant to protection against metacyclic (insect form) challenge, *J. Immunol.* **129**:1715–1718.

Freedman, R. F., Trejdosiewicz, A. J., and Cross, G. A. M., 1980, Protective monoclonal antibodies recognizing stage specific merozoite antigens of a rodent malaria parasite, *Nature* **284**:366–368.

Garcia, E. G., Tapales, F. P., Valdez, C. A., Mitchell, G. F., and Tiu, W. U., 1981, Attempts to standardize the circumoval precipitin test (COPT) for *Schistosomiasis japonica*, *Southeast Asian J. Trop. Med. Public Health* **12**(3):384–395.

Groot, M., Carrillo, P., and Espinol, C. A., 1982, Preparation of monoclonal antibodies with antisporozoite activity, in: *Proceeding of the International Atomic Energy Agency Research Coordination Meeting*, U. S. Naval Medical Research, Bethesda, Maryland.

Grzych, J. M., Capron, M., Bazin, H., and Capron, A., 1982, *In vitro* and *in vivo* effector function of rat IgG2a monoclonal anti-*S. mansoni* antibodies, *J. Immunol.* **129**:2739–2743.

Gwadz, R. W., and Greene, I., 1978, Malaria immunization in rhesus monkeys: A vaccine effective against both the sexual and asexual stages of *Plasmodium knowlesi J. Exp. Med.* **148**:1311–1323.

Hafez, S. K., Phillips, S. M., and Zodda, D. M., 1984, *S. mansoni*: Detection and characterization of schistosome derived antigens by enzyme–immunosorbent assay (IELISA) utilizing monoclonal antibodies, *Z. Parasitenkd.* **70**:105–117.

Hafez, S. K., Phillips, S. M., and Zodda, D. M., 1983b, *S. mansoni*: Detection of characterization of antigens and antigenemia by inhibition enzyme-linked immunosorbent assay (IELISA), *Exp. Parasitol.* **55**:219–232.

Handman, E., 1982, Characterization of *Leishmania tropica* antigens using hybridoma derived antibodies, in: *Molecular and Biochemical Parasitol.*, Supplement I (M. Muller, W. Gutteridge, and P. Kohler, eds.), Elsevier Biomedical Press, Amsterdam, p. 38.

Handman, E., and Hocking, E., 1982, Stage-specific, strain-specific, and cross-reactive antigens of *Leishmania* species identified by monoclonal antibody, *Infect Immunol.* **37**:28–33.

Handman, E., and Remington, J. S., 1980, Serological and immunochemical characterization of monoclonal antibodies to *Toxoplasma gondii, Immunology* **40**:579–588.

Handman, E., Goding, J. W., and Remington, J. S., 1980, Detection and characterization of membrane antigens of *Toxoplasma gondii, J. Immunol.* **124**:2578–2583.

Haque, A., des Moutis, I., Capron, A., Ouaissi, A., and Koumeni, L.-E., 1982, The application of monoclonal antibodies to studies of filariasis, in: *Properties of Monoclonal Antibodies Produced by Hybridoma Techonology and Their Application to the Study of Disease* (V. Houba and S. H. Chan, eds.), UNDP/WB/WHO, Geneva pp. 111–120.

Hauser, W. E., and Remington, J. S., 1981, Effect of monoclonal antibodies on phagocytosis and killing of *Toxoplasma gondii* by normal macrophages, *Infect. Immun.* **32**:637–640.

Hillyer, G. V. and Pelley, R. P., 1980, The major serological antigen (MSA$_1$) from *Schistosoma mansoni* eggs is a "circumoval" precipitinogen, *Am. J. Trop. Med. Hyg.* **29**(4):582–585.

Holder, A. A., and Freeman, R. R., 1981, Immunization against blood-stage rodent malaria using purified parasite antigens, *Nature* **294**:361–364.

Hollingdale, M. R., 1982, Entry of *Plasmodia berghei* sporozoites into cultured cells, in: *Molecular and Biochemical Parasitology* Supplement I (M. Muller, W. Gutteridge, and P. Kohler, eds.), Elsevier Biomedical Press, Amsterdam, p. 94.

Kasper, L. H., Crabb, J. H., and Pfefferkorn, E. R., 1983, Isolation and characterization of a monoclonal antibody resistant antigenic mutant of *Toxoplasma gondii, J. Immunol.* **129**:1694.

Krolick, K. A., Villemez, C., Isakson, P., Uhr, J. W., and Vitteta, E. S., 1980, Selective killing of normal or neoplastic B-cells by antibodies coupled to the A chain of ricin, *Proc. Natl. Acad. Sci. USA* **77**:5419–5423.

Lyon, J. A., Pratt, J. M., Travis, R. W., Doctor, B. P., and Olenik, J. G., 1981, Use of monoclonal antibody to immunochemically characterize variant-specific surface coat glycoprotein from *Trypanosoma rhodesiense, J. Immunol.* **126**:134–137.

Mansfield, J. M., 1981, The immunology of parasites, in: *Parasitic Diseases*, Volume 1 (J. M. Mansfield, ed.), Marcel Dekker, New York, p. 167–234.

McBride, D., Walliker, D., and Morgan, G., 1982, Antigenic diversity in human malaria parasite *Plasmodium falciparum Science* **217**:253–257.

McMahon-Pratt, D. M., Bennett, E., and David, J. R., 1982, Monoclonal antibodies that distinguish subspecies of *Leishmania braziliensis, J. Immunol.* **129**:926–927.

Mendis, K. N., and Targett, G. A. T., 1979, Immunization against gametes and asexual erthyrocytic stages of a rodent malaria parasite, *Nature* **277**:389–391.

Mitchell, G. F., Curtis, K. M., Garcia, E. G., and Anders, R. F., 1981, Hybridoma-derived antibody with immunodiagnostic potential for *Schistosomiasis japonicum, Proc. Natl. Acad. Sci. USA* **78**(5):3165–3169.

Mitchell, G. F., Garcia, E. G., Cruise, K. M., Tiu, W. U., and Howking, R. E., 1982, Lung granulomatous hypersensitivity to eggs of *S. japonicum* in mice analyzed by a radioisotopic assay and effects of hybridoma (idiotype sensitization), *Aust. J. Exp. Biol. Med. Sci.* **60**:401–416.

Mitchell, G. F., Garcia, E. G., and Cruise, K. M., 1983, Competitive radioimmunoassays using hybridoma and anti-idiotype antibodies in identification of antibody response to and antigens of *S. japonicum, Aust. J. Exp. Biol. Med. Sci.* **61**:27–36.

Myler, P. J., Saul, A. J., Mangan, T. L., and Kidson, C., 1982, Monoclonal antibodies against *Plasmodium falciparum* inhibiting merozoite invasion of erythrocytes, in *Molecular and Biochemical Parasitology*, Supplement I (M. Müller, W. Gutteridge, and P. Köhler, eds.), Elsevier Biomedical Press, Amsterda p. 95.

Naot, Y., and Remington, J. S., 1981, Use of enzyme-linked immunosorbant assays (ELISA) for detection of monoclonal antibodies: Experience with antigens of *Toxoplasma gondii, J. Immunol. Methods* **43**:333–341.

Nardin, E. H., Nussenzweig, V., Nussenzweig, R. S., Collins, W. E., Harinausta, K. T., Tapchaisri, P., and Chomcharn, Y., 1982, Circumsporozoite proteins of human malaria parasites *P. falciparum* and *P. vivax, J. Exp. Med.* **156**:20–30.

Nussenzweig, R. S., 1982, The application of monoclonal antibodies to studies of malaria, in: *The Properties of Monoclonal Antibodies Produced by Hybridoma Technology and Their Application to the Study of Diseases* (V. Houba and S. H. Chan, eds.), UNDP/WB/WHO, Geneva pp. 63–69.

Nussenzweig, V., 1982, Circumsporozoite (C.S.) proteins: A family of protective malarial antigens, *Fed. Proc.* **41B:**483 (abstract).

Pearson, T. W., and Anderson, L., 1980, Analytical techniques for cell fractions XXVIII. Dissection of complex antigenic mixtures using monoclonal antibodies and two-dimensional gel electrophoresis, *Anal. Biochem.* **101:**377–386.

Pearson, T. W., Kar, S. K., McGuire, T. C., and Lundin, L. B., 1981, Trypanosome variable surface antigens: Studies using two-dimensional gel electrophoresis and monoclonal antibodies, *J. Immunol.* **126:**823–828.

Perrin, L. H., 1982, Monoclonal antibodies in malarial research, in: *Parasites, Their World and Ours* (D. F. Mettrick and S. S. Desser, eds.), Elsevier Biomedical Press, Amsterdam pp. 13–16.

Perrin, L. H., and Dayal, R., 1982, Immunity to asexual erythrocytic stages of *Plasmodium falciparum:* Role of defined antigens in the humoral response, *Immunol. Rev.* **61:**245–269.

Perrin, L. H., Ramirez, E., Er-Hsiang, L., and Lambert, P. H., 1980, *Plasmodium falciparum:* Characterization of defined antigens by monoclonal antibodies, *Clin. Exp. Immunol.* **41:**91–96.

Perrin, L. H., Ramirez, E., Lambert, P. H., and Miescher, P. A., 1981, Inhibition of *P. falciparum* growth in human erythrocytes by monoclonal antibodies, *Nature* **289:**301–303.

Phillips, S. M., 1982, Monoclonal antibodies and mechanisms of immunogenesis, in: *Molecular and Biochemical Parasitology*, Supplement II (D. F. Mettrick and S. S. Desser, eds.), Elsevier Biomedical Press, Amsterdam, pp. 25–27.

Phillips, S. M., and Colley, D. G., 1978, Immunologic aspects of host responses to schistosomiasis: Resistance, immunopathology, and eosinophil involvement, *Prog. Allergy* **24:**49–182.

Potocnjak, P., Yoshida, N., Nussenzweig, R. S., and Nussenzweig, V., 1980, Monovalent fragments (Fab) of monoclonal antibodies to a sporozoite surface antigen (Pb44) protect mice against malarial infection, *J. Exp. Med.* **151:**1504–1513.

Potocnjak, P., Zavala, F., Nussensweig, R. S., and Nussensweig, V., 1982, Inhibition of idiotype–anti-idiotype interaction for detection of a parasite antigen: A new immunoassay, *Science* **215:**1637–1639.

Pratt, D. M., and David, J. R., 1981, Monoclonal antibodies that distinguish between New World species of *Leishmania, Nature* **291:**581–583.

Pratt, D. M., and David, J. R., 1982, Application of monoclonal antibodies to studies of leishmaniasis, in: *Properties of the Monoclonal Antibodies Produced by Hybridoma Technology and Their Applications to the Study of Diseases,* (V. Houba and S. H. Chen, eds.), UNDP/WB/WHO, Geneva, pp. 75–85.

Ramsey, J., and Charoenvit, Y., 1982, International Atomic Energy Agency Research Coordination Meeting, U.S. Naval Medical Research Institute, Bethesda, Maryland.

Rener, J., Carter, R., Rosenberg, Y., and Miller, L. H., 1980, Anti-gamete monoclonal antibodies synergistically block transmission of malaria by preventing fertilization in the mosquito, *Proc. Natl. Acad. Sci. USA* **77:**6797–6799.

Sacks, D. L., Esser, K. M., and Sher, A., 1982, Immunization of mice against African trypanosomiasis using anti-idiotypic antibodies, *J. Exp. Med.* **155:**1108–1119.

Santoro, F., Bandemeulebroucke, B., and Capron, A., 1978, The use of radio-immunoprecipitation–PEG assay (RIPEGA) to quantify circulating antigens and human experimental schistosomiasis, *J. Immunol. Methods* **24:**229–237.

Santoro, F., Cochrane, A. H., Gwadz, R., Nussenzweig, R. S., Nussenzweig, V., and Ferreira, A., 1982, Circumsporozoite (CS) proteins: A family of protective malaria antigens, in: *Molecular and Biochemical Parasitology*, Supplement I (M. Müller, W. Gutteridge, and P. Köhler, eds.), Elsevier Biomedical Press, Amsterdam, p. 22.

Schofield, D. L., Saul, S. J., Myler, P. G., and Kidson, C., 1982, Antigenic differences among isolates of *P. falciparum* demonstrated by monoclonal antibodies, *Infect. Immun.* **38:**893–897.

Sethi, K. K., 1982, Monoclonal antibodies against *Toxoplasma gondii*, in: *International Meeting: Immunology in Toxoplasmosis, Lyon, France*, Merieux Foundation, Paris.

Sethi, K. K., and Brandis, H., 1981, Generation of hybridoma cell lines producing monoclonal antibodies against *Toxoplasma gondii* or rabies virus following fusion of *in vitro* immunized spleen cells with myeloma cells, *Ann. Immunol. (Paris)* **132C:**29–41.

Sethi, K. K., Endo, T., and Brandis, H., 1980, Hybridoma secreting monoclonal antibodies with specificity for *Toxoplasma gondii, J. Parasitol.* **66:**192–196.

Sethi, K. K., Endo, T., and Brandis, H., 1981, *Toxoplasma gondii* trophozoites precoated with specific monoclonal antibodies cannot survive within normal murine macrophages, *Immunol. Lett.* **2:**343–346.

Simpson, A. J. G., Singer, D., Sher, A., and McCutchan, T. M., 1982, Investigation of possible homologies between the genome of *Schistosoma mansoni* and of its hosts, *Fed. Proc.* **241**(3):729 (abstract).

Smith, M. A., Clegg, J. A., Snary, D., and Trejdosiewicz, A. J., 1982, Passive immunization of mice against *Schistosoma mansoni* with an IgM monoclonal antibody, *Parasitology* **84:**83–91.

Snary, D., 1980, *Tropanosoma cruzi:* Antigenic invariance of the cell surface glycoprotein, *Exp. Parasitol.* **49:**68–77.

Snary, D., and Hudson, L., 1979, *Tropanosoma cruzi,* cell surface proteins: Identification of one major glycoprotein, *FEBS Lett.* **100:**166–170.

Snary, D., Ferguson, M. A. J., Scott, M. T., and Allen, A. K., 1981, Cell surface antigens of *Tropanosoma cruzi:* Use of monoclonal antibodies to identify and isolate an epimastigote specific glycoprotein, *Mol. Biochem. Parasitol.* **3:**343–356.

Taylor, D. W., and Butterworth, A. E., 1982, Monoclonal antibodies against the surface antigens of schistosomula of *Schistosoma mansoni, Parasitology* **84:**65–82.

Taylor, D. W., Jin Kim, K., Munoz, P. A., Evans, C. B., and Asofsky, R., 1981, Monoclonal antibodies to stage-specific, species-specific, and cross-reactive antigens of the rodent malarial parasite *Plasmodium yoelii, Infect. Immun.* **32**(2):563–570.

Verwaerde, C., Grzych, J. M., Bazin, H., Capron, M., and Capron, A., 1979, Production d'anticorps monoclonaux anti-*Schistosoma mansoni,* Étude préliminaire de leurs activités Biologigues, *C. R. Acad. Sci. Paris D* **289:**725–727.

Wood, J. N., Hudson, L., Jessell, T. M., and Yamamoto, M., 1982, A monoclonal antibody defining antigenic determinants on subpopulations of mammalian neurones and *Tropanosoma cruzi* parasites, *Nature* **296:**34–38.

Yoshida, N., Nussenzweig, R. S., Potocnjak, P., Nussenzweig, V., and Aikawa, M., 1980, Hybridoma produces protective antibodies directed against the sporozoite stage of malaria parasite, *Science* **270:**71–73.

Yoshida, N., Potocnjak, P., Nussenzweig, V., and Nussenzweig, R. S., 1981, Biosynthesis of Pb44, the protective antigen of sporozoites of *Plasmodium berghei, J. Exp. Med.* **154:**1225–1236.

Zodda, D. M., and Phillips, S. M., 1982, Monoclonal antibody-mediated resistance to *Schistosoma mansoni* infection in mice *J. Immunol.* **129:**2326–2329.

Zodda, D. M., Abdel-Hafez, S. K., and Phillips, S. M., 1983, Characterization of monoclonal antibodies against *Schistosoma mansoni, Am. J. Trop. Med. Hyg.* **32:**69–77.

PART V
DEVELOPING AREAS OF
BIOTECHNOLOGY

11

Production of Human Monoclonal Antibodies

David W. Buck, James W. Larrick,
Andrew Raubitschek, Kenneth E. Truitt,
G. Senyk, J. Wang, and Bradley J. Dyer

I. Introduction

The need to obtain human monoclonal antibodies has not been overshadowed by the immense success of mouse monoclonal antibody technology. Human monoclonal antibodies will be less antigenic for human *in vivo* studies and therapy; they will be more likely to recognize antigenic subtleties not easily detected by xenogeneic antibodies, and they will have less rapid catabolism *in vivo*. The study of human B-cell differentiation and development will be furthered by the availability of human hybridomas. These hybridomas also will be useful to dissect the human humoral immune response in autoimmune disease, cancer, and allergy.

Table I presents a list of conditions for which passively administered human antibodies are known to have therapeutic usefulness. Human monoclonal antibodies recognizing these targets will have therapeutic potential within a few years. A list of conditions for which human monoclonal antibodies are conceptually attractive is given in Table II. Clearly, much more basic research in animal models will be required before these anticipated therapeutic applications can be fulfilled.

In this chapter we will review the attempts by various groups to obtain human monoclonal antibodies. There are at least four potentially rewarding approaches:

David W. Buck, James W. Larrick, Andrew Raubitschek, Kenneth E. Truitt, G. Senyk, J. Wang, and Bradley J. Dyer • Cetus Immune Research Laboratories, Palo Alto, California 94303. Present address for D. W. B.: Becton Dickinson Monoclonal Center, Inc., Mountain View, California 94043.

1. Cell fusion, i.e., using mouse/human or human/human combinations of malignant cells and B cells, as have been used for production of mouse hybridomas.
2. Viral transformation, i.e., using Epstein–Barr virus or other oncogenic viruses to transform human B cells.
3. Lymphokines, i.e., using B-cell growth and differentiation factors, as in IL-2-promoted growth of T cells.
4. Recombinant DNA, i.e., directly cloning and expressing immunoglobulin genes or using transfection of cloned B-lineage oncogenes into B cells.

TABLE I

Targets for Which Human Antibodies Are Known to Be Useful

Passively administered antibody
1. Red cell antigens: Rh (hemolytic disease of newborn)
2. White cell antigens: anti-lymphocyte/thymocyte globulin
3. Viral antigens: hepatitis, rabies, CMV, HSV
4. Bacterial antigens: tetanus, endotoxins, pneumococcus
5. Anti-snake venom
6. Elimination of circulating drugs (i.e., overdoses)
7. Fertility control (e.g., β-hCG)

In vitro uses
1. Blood group typing antisera
2. HLA, Dr typing reagents

TABLE II

Future Prospects for Therapy with Human Monoclonal Antibodies

Cancer diagnosis and treatment
Imaging
  Tumors
  Cardiac, e.g., infarction, ischemia
  Emboli
  Vascular disease
  Location of parasites, abscesses, etc.
Immunological manipulation
  Immunodeficiency, dysfunction
  Transplantation
  Allergy
  Autoimmunity
  Infertility
Pharmacological uses
  Drug, toxin elimination (e.g., digoxin toxicity)
  Targeting of directly attached drugs, directly attached toxins,
    liposomes
Receptor modulation

II. Cell Fusion

Since Kohler and Milstein's original description of mouse hybridomas (Kohler and Milstein, 1975), investigators have recognized the potential of a hybridoma system for the generation of human monoclonal antibodies of pre-defined specificity. Schwaber and Cohen (1973) first demonstrated the possibility of immortalizing human immunoglobulin secretion by fusion of a mouse plasmacytoma with human peripheral blood lymphocytes. However, the specificity of the secreted human antibody was not demonstrated and the potential for this procedure was not recognized. Several laboratories have now demonstrated the feasibility of producing specific human monoclonal antibodies by fusion of immune human lymphocytes with mouse or human parental cell lines.

A. Mouse/Human Hybridomas

The most widely used mouse fusion parents are derivatives of the plasmacytoma P3/X63-Ag8 described by Cotton and Milstein (1973). With human lymphocytes, these plasmacytomas have relatively high fusion frequencies, and the resulting hybrids are capable of secreting high levels of human immunoglobulin. The selection of stable antigen-specific hybrids has been difficult because of rapid human chromosome loss in these interspecies hybrids (Ruddle, 1974). The human immunoglobulin heavy-chain genes are located on chromosome 14 (Croce et al., 1979) and the light-chain genes are located on chromosomes 2 (κ) (Malcom et al., 1982) and 22 (λ) (Erikson et al., 1981). Therefore, at least two human chromosomes must be retained in mouse/human hybrids for continued production and secretion of intact human immunoglobulin molecules. Although Croce has shown preferential retention of human chromosome 14 in mouse/human hybrids, the loss of other human chromosomes is rapid and random, generally resulting in unstable immunoglobulin secretion.

Nowinski et al., (1980) reported the production of human monoclonal antibodies to the Forssman antigen. Human spleen cells were immunized in vitro against influenza virus and the resulting blast cells were fused with a derivative of the mouse plasmacytoma NS-1 (Kohler et al., 1976). One hybrid clone reacted with three of five strains of influenza virus tested, but the antibody was cross-reactive with the Forssman antigen. Extensive subcloning of this hybrid was necessary before a stable clone of antibody-secreting cells was obtained. The secretion level of this hybrid was approximately 8 μg/ml of spent culture supernatant, which is comparable to that obtained with most murine hybridomas.

Schlom et al. (1980) fused NS-1 with lymphocytes from draining lymph nodes taken from breast tumor-bearing patients. Wells containing hybrids secreting immunoglobulin were screened on fixed sections of breast tumor tissue. Although moderate numbers of positively reacting hybrids were obtained, most were unstable. After approximately 7 months in culture, only one hybrid clone retained its original pattern of reactivity, and antibody secretion was reported to be 0.1–20 μg/ml of spent culture medium.

Sikora and Phillips (1981) reported human monoclonal antibodies to human glioma cells. Infiltrating lymphocytes obtained from a tumor mass obtained at craniotomy were fused with NS1. Out of 48 seeded wells, 18 secreted human immunoglobulin, and four of these 18 antibodies bound specifically to the patient's own tumor membrane preparations and not to normal tissue. All hybrids had ceased production of human immunoglobulin by 8 weeks postfusion, and no attempts to rescue antibody secretion by subcloning were reported. Sikora and Wright (1981) have also described production of human monoclonal antibodies to lung cancer antigens. Lymphocytes from draining lymph nodes obtained from a tumor patient were prepared as a single-cell suspension and fused with NS-1 mouse plasmacytoma cells or the Y3-Ag1.2.3. rat myeloma cell line described by Cotton and Milstein (1973). Secretion rates of greater than 100 μg/ml of culture medium were reported, but the hybrids ceased immunoglobulin production by 10 weeks postfusion.

Human monoclonal antibodies to keyhole limpet hemocyanin (KLH) were reported by Lane et al. (1982). Peripheral blood lymphocytes from a donor immunized with KLH 10 days previously were fused with mouse NS-1 plasmacytoma cells. Numerous antigen-specific hybridomas were produced, most of which were unstable due to segregation of human chromosomes. One IgM hybrid specific for KLH was reportedly stable for 10 months and produced 30 μg/ml of culture supernatant. Butler et al. (1983a) reported an increase in the frequency of tetanus toxoid-specific mouse/human hybridomas when peripheral blood lymphocytes from an immunized donor were boosted with specific antigen in vitro prior to fusion with NS-1 cells. Hybrid clones stably produced antibody specific for tetanus toxoid for 8 months after selection by repeated subcloning.

Kozbor et al. (1982b) also described the production of human monoclonal antibodies to tetanus toxoid (TT). They fused an antitetanus-producing, EBV-transformed lymphoblastoid line B6 (Kozbor and Roder, 1981) with the non-secreting and 8-azaguanine-resistant plasmacytoma line P3/X63-Ag8.653 (Kearny et al., 1979). Hybridomas were selected in HAT medium (Littlefield, 1964) and 10^{-5} M ouabain. Unlike human cells, mouse cells are resistant to relatively high concentrations of ouabain (10^{-3} M), and as ouabain resistance is inherited in a dominant fashion, mouse/human hybrid cells are able to survive this form of selection. Hybrid colonies were cloned by limiting dilution at 3 weeks postfusion, and of 100 clones examined, 70 secreted antibody specific for TT. In all cases, secreted immunoglobulin was the same IgMk as secreted by the lymphoblastoid parent. Four hybrid clones that secreted 10-fold more specific antibody than the parent lymphoblastoid cell line were selected for further study. Karyotypic analysis of these hybrids revealed a full complement of mouse chromosomes and a mean number of 24 human chromosomes. These hybrids were reportedly stable for greater than 6 months in continuous culture.

Gigliotti et al. (1982) have also described a mouse/human fusion system that resulted in secretion of human monoclonal antibodies to both tetanus toxoid and diphtheria toxoid. Peripheral blood lymphocytes (PBLs) from volunteers immunized 6 or 7 days previously with tetanus or diphtheria toxoids were fused with the nonsecreting mouse plasmacytoma P3x63Ag8.653 using standard techniques. Hybrids secreting antibody specific for tetanus or diphtheria toxoids were obtained and the percentage of antibody-secreting cells in these populations was increased by several cycles of an enrichment procedure which involved plating hybrid cells at 10 cells/well and subsequent expansion of wells producing high levels of antibody to TT. After several such cycles, a hybrid population, 9F12, was derived that produced an IgGk antibody. Modal chromosome number was shown to be 108, which included six to seven human chromosomes. Specific antibody secretion after approximately 6 months in culture was 5–10 μg/ml of spent culture medium. Other hybrids were found to be unstable and ceased antibody production after 1 month. This group proceeded to demonstrate the protective effect of these human monoclonal antibodies to tetanus toxin in a mouse tetanus toxin neutralization assay.

B. Human/Human Hybridomas

An alternative approach to the production of specific human monoclonal antibodies is the development of a human myeloma cell line or other human cell line capable of (1) fusing with human lymphocytes with high frequency, (2) permitting the synthesis and secretion of adequate amounts of specific antibody, and, (3) forming karyotypically stable hybrids. Human × human somatic cell hybrids have been shown to be chromosomally stable (Bengtsson et al., 1975; Stanbridge et al., 1982), with only 5–7% of the total chromosome complement being segregated after prolonged growth in vitro. Unfortunately, one of the limiting factors in producing human × human myeloma hybrids is the limited availability of human myeloma cell lines. Mouse plasmacytomas are easily induced by the injection of mineral oil, and the resulting cells are only moderately difficult to adapt to in vitro culture (Potter et al., 1972). On the other hand, human myelomas have proved to be exceedingly difficult to adapt to in vitro culture. Consequently, there are probably only four true human myeloma cell lines in existence at the present time. These are U266 (Nilsson et al., 1970), RPMI 8226 (Matsuoka et al., 1967), KARPAS 707 (Karpas et al., 1982), and KMM1 (Togawa et al., 1982). These cells are distinguished by their aneuploidy, by their production of monoclonal immunoglobulins, identical to those present in the patient's circulation, an abundant rough endoplasmic reticulum (RER), and relative lack of free polyribosomes, a well-developed Golgi apparatus, and many mitochondria. In addition, myeloma cells do not carry surface receptors for Epstein–Barr virus (EBV). Lymphoblastoid cell lines, in contrast to myeloma cells, are EBV-transformed and Epstein–Barr nuclear antigen (EBNA)-positive. They are polyclonally derived and have a poorly developed RER and Golgi apparatus. They are usually diploid or pseudodiploid, and generally secrete small amounts of immunoglobulin, generally <1 μg/ml. On the basis of their phenotypic characteristics, one might expect that a true myeloma would prove to be an ideal fusion partner. Perhaps, because of unknown differences in the states if differentiation between myelomas and plasmacytomas, the presently available human myelomas seem not to be equivalent to the mouse plasmacytomas in their ability to fuse and produce antibody-secreting hybridomas.

As a consequence, the majority of confirmed reports of human hybridomas have used EBNA-positive lymphoblastoid parents. Kozbor *et al.* (1983) have recently characterized most of the presently available fusion partners and reached the same conclusion.

Olsson and Kaplan (1980) utilized the IgE-secreting myeloma U266, first described by Nilsson *et al.* (1970), to make human anti-DNP antibodies. A faster growing subline was selected for resistance to 8-azaguanine and designated SKO-007. Patients with Hodgkin disease were immunized with dinitrochlorobenzene prior to staging laparotomy. Spleen cells were fused with SKO-007 and culture supernatants were shown to secrete specific anti-DNP antibody. Secretion rate was stated to be between 3 and 11 μg/ml per day, though the number of cells required to secrete these levels was not stated. The line SKO-007 was subsequently found to be heavily contaminated with *Mycoplasma orale* (Lewin, 1981), an arginine-depleting mycoplasma. This fact may account for the relative paucity of confirming reports using SKO-007.

Croce *et al.* (1980) used an 8-azaguanine-resistant derivative of the lymphoblastoid line GM1500 (GM1500 6TG-A11) as a fusion parent; when PBLs were fused from a patient with subacute sclerosing panencephalitis, a disease characterized by an aberrant and persistent measles virus infection, antibodies reacting with measles virus nucleocapsids were obtained. Secretion rates and the fusion index of the line were not specifically mentioned. The GM1500 line is EBNA-positive and has been shown to shed EB virus. It is therefore possible for direct transformation of the donor's lymphocytes to occur when using this cell line and other EBV-positive lymphoblastoid cell lines for fusions.

Edwards *et al.* (1982) made an 8-azaguanine-resistant derivative of ARH-77 (LICR-LON-HMy2). The ARH-77 was originally reported to be a human plasmacytoma cell line (Burk *et al.*, 1978), but recent derivatives are EBNA-positive and it is probably an unusual type of lymphoblastoid line. Azaserine replaced aminopterin in the culture system because others had shown this to be less toxic than conventional HAT medium (Buttin *et al.*, 1978; Foung *et al.*, 1982). The HMy2 line had a high cloning efficiency and a fairly low fusion frequency, but hydrids did produce up to 8 μg antibody/ml culture medium when fused to tonsil lymphocytes. Chromosome stability of the hybrids, as judged by secretion patterns, remained good after several months in culture, although the stated modal chromosome number was between 50 and 60, indicating a degree of chromosome instability in these particular hybrids. No specific monoclonal antibodies were described.

Sikora *et al.* (1982) also used LICR-LON-HMy2 to produce human antibodies. By fusing with lymphocytes extracted from tumor biopsies, they obtained antibodies reacting with a glioma cell line, but not with normal tissues. Fusion index in their system was reported to be low, and antibody secretion rates were not reported.

Human hybridomas secreting antibodies specific for tetanus toxoid were described by Chiorazzi *et al.* (1982). Two lymphoblastoid lines were employed as fusion parents, a subclone of GM467 (Sato *et al.*, 1972) and an HPRT⁻ derivative of WI-L2 (Lever *et al.*, 1974). Appearance of hybrids was late (3–6 weeks). One hybrid made by fusion of GM467-3 with tonsillar lymphocytes obtained from a patient immunized with tetanus toxoid 7 days prior to tonsillectomy secreted an IgM antibody specific for tetanus toxoid. This hybrid was stable over a 9-month period. The cloning efficiency of these hybrids was high. Secretion levels were 0.01–5.0 μg antibody/ml culture medium in 48 hr; however, the number of cells needed to secrete this level of antibody was not stated.

Schoenfeld *et al.* (1982) have fused PBLs and spleen cells from a patient with immunothrombocytopenic purpura with GM4672, a derivative of Croce's GM1500 line, to obtain autoantibodies directed against ssDNA and blood platelets. Fusion efficiency was low, with 2.5% of wells producing growth after a 4-week period. Sixteen of 108 growing hybrids produced autoantibodies, all of the IgM class. Light-chain data were not presented, and no evidence was presented to support the hybrid nature of the cells obtained from these fusions. The authors described the GM4672 parent cell line as being EBNA-negative. A later report (Schoenfeld *et al.*, 1983) describes the production of monoclonal antibodies derived by fusion of GM4672 with PBLs from patients with systemic lupus erythematosus. A total of 288 growth positive wells were obtained from seven fusions. Of these, 28 contained autoantibodies that bound to ssDNA. The human monoclonal antibodies reacted with a variety of nuclear antigens, and the authors suggested their polyspecificity was due to their recognition of a common epitope. To distinguish true hybrid cells from spontaneous EBV transformants, cultures were subjected to (1) biosynthetic labeling to demonstrate production of human IgG and IgM, (2) HLA typing with mouse monoclonal antibodies to HLA-A2 and B5 (neither parent expressed both antigens), and (3) karyotypic analysis. However, one puzzling aspect of these hybrid cells was the presence of large numbers of subdiploid cells (<46 chromosomes) in every hybrid examined. Hyperdiploid cells (52–92 chromosomes) represented 6–41% of all cells examined. This type of result has not been described by other investigators.

Handley and Royston (1982) have also developed a hybridoma system based on the use of a HAT-sensititve derivative of the human lymphoblastoid line WI-L2 (Levy *et al.*, 1968) designated UC729-6. The UC729-6 cells were fused with cells from a chronic lymphocytic leukemia (CLL) patient, using standard techniques. Cells from the fusion mixture were plated at 5×10^5 cells/well in 24 well culture plates in HAT medium. At 5 weeks postfusion, 12 wells (12.5%) were positive for hybrid growth. Four of these wells contained secreted human IgM antibody. Secretion rates were stated to be in the range 3–9 μg IgM antibody/ml culture medium. Evidence for hybrid production was provided by the presence of both membrane-bound κ and λ light chains, a tetraploid karyotype with a 21p$^+$ marker chromosome donated by the parent UC729-6, and the presence of the T65 antigen, which is normally present on CLL cells but not on UC729-6. In other studies (Handley *et al.*, 1983; Glassy *et al.*, 1983), lymphocytes obtained from the regional draining lymph nodes of tumor patients were fused with both UC729-6 and NS-1. Three antibodies were selected for in-depth study. MGH-7 is a mouse/human hybrid, which secretes an IgM antibody recognizing an antigen present on the prostate carcinoma cell lines Ln-Cap and PC-3. This antibody also reacted with paraffin and frozen sections of prostate carcinomas. The hybrids LNH5 and WLNA6, derived by fusion of lymph node cells with UC729-6, also secreted IgM antibodies that recognized the cervical carcinoma cell lines HeLa and Caski, and lung carcinoma cells, respectively. The LNH5 antibody also reacted with melanoma cell line SK-MEL-28. These antibodies did not react with normal foreskin fibroblasts, but their reactivity with other normal tissues was not reported.

Kozbor *et al.* (1982a) have produced human intraspecies hybrids that secrete antibody to TT by fusing a thioguanine- and ouabain-resistant derivative of GM1500 to the anti-TT-secreting lymphoblastoid line B6 (Kozbor and Roder, 1981). Surviving hybrid clones arose at a frequency of 10^{-5}, and 372 of 395 growing wells were positive for antibody to TT. Seven clones derived by limiting dilution continued to produce 3–6 µg/ml of specific antibody at 7 months postfusion, but the parent line B6 had ceased production of specific antibody at 10 months. Secretion rates in these hybrids were judged to be 15-fold higher than that obtained with the parent B6. In more recent work, these authors have fused the parent line KR4 to EBV-stimulated peripheral blood lymphocytes from lepromatous leprosy patients and patients with small cell carcinoma of the lung (Kozbor and Roder, 1983). These fusions resulted in hybrid clones secreting antibodies to *Mycobacterium leprae* antigens, and others that reacted to fixed monolayers of tumor cells in an ELISA assay.

In an extensive study by Cote *et al.* (1983), two human fusion partners, SKO-007 (Olsson and Kaplan, 1980) and LICR-LON-HMy2 (LICR-2) (Edwards *et al.*, 1982), were compared with the mouse plasmacytoma NS-1. In a series of over 75 fusions, each parent was fused with human lymphocytes from peripheral blood, spleen, lymph node, or tumor specimens. SKO-007 exhibited the lowest fusion frequency, with LICR-2 giving a fusion frequency approximately four times higher. NS-1 cells had a fusion frequency 5–20 times that of either human parent. In general, the source of human lymphocytes exerted a marked effect on the success of the fusions, with spleen cells giving the greatest number of hybrid clones and peripheral blood lymphocytes the lowest. The percentage of wells containing hybrids producing human immunoglobulin, secretion rates, and the proportion of clones producing IgG, IgA, or IgM were not significantly different when hybrids made with each of the three parents were compared. Seventy to seventy-five percent of human immunoglobulin-secreting clones produced between 1 and 10 µg/ml of culture medium, and 25–30% produced between 11 and 100 µg/ml. Surprisingly, NS-1 × lymphocyte hybridomas were reported to be as stable as human/human hybridomas over a 2–3 month period of subculture. However, only one to two subcultures took place during this period. This result is contrary to other published reports of mouse/human hybridomas, where extreme instability has generally been observed. Thirty-eight hybridomas secreting antibodies that recognized cytoplasmic, cytoskeletal, perinuclear, or nuclear antigens in cultured human cells were described. One IgG antibody, produced by a hybrid between NS-1 and draining lymph node cells from a breast cancer patient (Ri37), identified a cell surface antigen on some human tumor cell lines and peripheral blood mononuclear cells. The hybrid contains human and mouse chromosomes, has been subcloned five times by limited dilution, secretes 2–5 μg/ml of specific human IgG, and was reported stable for a 12-month period. Eleven of 87 tumor cell lines tested expressed the Ri37 antigen. These authors conclude that human hybridomas secreting antibodies to cell surface antigens are rare, whereas a significantly higher frequency of antibodies recognize intracellular antigens.

In a parallel and similar fusion study from the same laboratory, Houghton *et al.* (1983) have compared the results obtained with SKO-007 (Olsson and Kaplan, 1980), LICR-LON-HMy2 (LICR-2) (Edwards *et al.*, 1982), GM4672 (Croce *et al.*, 1980), and the mouse plasmacytoma NS-1. A total of 79 fusions were performed with these parent cell lines and lymph node cells or infiltrating lymphocytes from 33 patients with malignant melanoma. A further series of 79 fusions were performed by fusing LICR-2, SKO-007, and mouse NS-1 plasmacytoma parents to T-depleted peripheral blood lymphocytes obtained from 25 patients with melanoma. Combinations of parental cells and lymphocytes were fused using standard techniques. Fused cells were plated in HAT medium over feeder layers of mouse splenocytes or peritoneal macrophages. Outgrowth of hybrid cells was delayed, human/human hybrids appearing 3–8 weeks after fusion, and mouse/human hybrids appearing 2–6 weeks after fusion. The reasons for this late appearance, and the fact that hybrid cells were subcultured only twice after a 3–4 month culture period, were not discussed. Wells positive for hybrid growth were assayed for human immunoglobulin heavy chains using an ELISA inhibition assay, and 50–80% of wells contained 0.3–40 μg/ml of μ, γ, or α immunoglobulin chains. No correlation between secretion rates or class of immunoglobulin with parental cells or source of lymphocytes was found. Stability of the human/human hybridomas after two subcultures (61%) was found to be better than than of mouse/human hybrids (30%). This result is in contrast to that reported by Cote *et al.* (1983), but is in keeping with the majority of reports reviewed in this chapter. Of 771 Ig[+] wells tested for reactivity with cytoplasmic components of 20 different tumor cell lines, 24 antibodies reacted by immunofluorescence to nuclei, nucleoli, cytoskeletal elements, or Golgi complex. Five of these hybrids were stable for IgM production over a 5- to 8-month period. The 771 hybrid supernatants were also screened for reactivity to cell surface antigens, against a panel of cell lines including melanomas, gliomas, and epithelial cancers. Six hybrid wells produced antibodies reactive with cell surface antigens, and from these a cell line designated Ma4 was established. Ma4 is a hybrid derived from a fusion between LICR-2 and draining lymph node cells from a male patient with malignant melanoma. This hybrid was subcloned four times and stably produced 5 and 2 μg/ml of IgM and IgG, respectively. Karyotypic analysis revealed only human chromosomes, and flow cytometry showed a tetraploid chromosome number. The IgM antibody secreted by this hybrid was highly reactive with a human renal cancer cell line (SK-RC-9), and also reacted with 19 out of a total of 61 tumor cell lines tested. This pattern of reactivity did not appear to be differentiation related; however, no exhaustive screening of the antibodies on normal tissues was reported. This study and that of Cote *et al.* (1983) represent the first attempts to elucidate the nature of the human immune response to tumor antigens, using human hybridoma-derived monoclonal antibodies.

Dwyer *et al.* (1983) have very briefly described a human monoclonal anti-idiotype antibody, SR11, derived from a fusion between the parent line GK-5 (a derivative of Croce's GM1500 line), which produced only a κ light chain, and peripheral blood cells from a patient with myasthenia gravis. The antibody had specificity for the ACR-24 antibody, a mouse monoclonal antibody to the nicotinic acetylcholine receptor, and matched the binding of antiidiotype antibodies in the serum of patients with myasthenia gravis. Details of this fusion were not given. However, the line fuses well and will usually produce hybrid growth in every well, provided a mouse peritoneal macrophage feeder layer is used. SR11 secretes 60 μg of specific antibodies per milliliter of spent culture medium (J. F. Kearney, personal communication).

Eisenbarth *et al.* (1982) fused the GM1500 6TG-2 line of Croce with PBLs from a patient with type 1 diabetes mellitus. Twenty-two of 24 wells produced hybrid growth, and supernatants from these wells were tested by immunofluorescence for reactivity with either the surface of viable rat insulinoma cells or islets of Bouin's fixed human pancreas. One hybrid, B6, produced approximately 400 ng specific IgM/ml spent medium, which reacted with islets of fixed pancreas. Hybrid cells were subcloned by limiting dilution, and the resulting clones have stably maintained specific IgM production for over 1 year. The cells studied were shown to be hybrids by HLA typing studies.

C. Results with Lymphoblastoid Line LTR228

1. Development and Fusion with LTR228

We have studied most of the available human B-lineage cell lines described above. When it was apparent that these worked with only limited success, we set about the development of a new cell fusion parent. We chose a spleen-derived B-lymphoblastoid cell line because of its robust growth characteristics and long time in culture (Levy *et al.*, 1968). This line is EBNA-positive and produces small quantities of IgMk immunoglobulin. The line was initially cloned in soft agar and rendered free of mycoplasma. Following EMS mutagenesis, a 6TG-resistant (20 μg/ml) mutant was isolated. A series of minifusions permitted us to select a high-fusion subclone (LTR228). Cytogenetic characterization of LTR228 revealed a hyperdiploid modal chromosome number of 48. Trypsin-Giemsa banding studies showed that all cells had extra copies of chromosomes 13 and 20. All cells had a Robertsonian translocation between 14 and 21 and a copy of chromosome 8 with an enlarged short arm composed of a homogeneously staining region. Finally, there is a marker 21, which has a translocation from the distal end of chromosome 11. The karyotype (see Figure 1), performed by Dr. B. S. Emanuel, Children's Hospital of Philadelphia, is thus: 48,XY,+13, +20,−14, +t(14q;21q), −21,+der(21),t(11;21) (q13;p11),8p+.

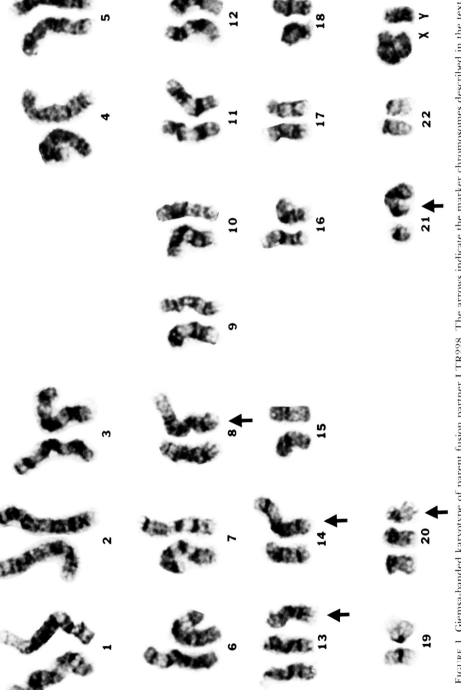

FIGURE 1. Giemsa-banded karyotype of parent fusion partner LTR228. The arrows indicate the marker chromosomes described in the text.

LTR228 and its sister clones are described in the work that follows. Typically fusions are performed as follows (Larrick et al., 1983). Heparinized peripheral blood is separated by Ficoll–Hypaque density gradient centrifugation, and T cells are removed by AET–SRBC rosetting and irradiated with 1500 R (Madsen and Johnson, 1979). An equal mix of nonrosetting cells and T cells is cultured in Iscove's DMEM + 15% fetal calf serum in the presence of pokeweed mitogen (PWM) (GIBCO 1 : 200) for 3 days. Viable cells are isolated on a Ficoll–Hypaque density gradient, mixed 1 : 1 with LTR228, and fused with PEG4000 in Hank's balanced salt solution (HBSS) without calcium, supplemented with 5 μg/ml poly-L-arginine and 10% DMSO. A modified plate fusion technique is used (Brahe and Serra, 1981). Basically, 2×10^7 cells are centrifuged onto a 60-mm petri dish and medium is removed. PEG is added for 1 min and then gently diluted and removed. Previous work from our laboratory with mouse hybridomas showed the superiority of hypoxanthine–azaserine selection (Table III). Azaserine, a glutamine analogue, inhibits two steps in de novo purine synthesis, but because the medium is supplemented with 2 mM glutamine, its disruption of other cellular functions is much less severe than dihydrofolate reductase inhibition by aminopterin in conventional HAT medium. Therefore, we routinely add 100 μM hypoxanthine and 4–8 μg/ml azaserine for selection after a 24-hr postfusion recovery period. Growing clones usually appear in 10–14 days. When cells are plated at 10^5 cells/well in microtiter plates, at least one hybrid per well is growing at 25 days. This fusion frequency compares favorably to that routinely obtained with mouse plasmacytomas.

TABLE III

Comparison of Surviving Mouse/Mouse Hybrid Wells: Aminopterin versus Azaserine

Parental cell line	Fusion number	Hybrid wells	
		Aminopterin	Azaserine
SP2/0Ag14	1	16	40
	2	18	54
	3	56	141
	4	18	33
	5	196	204
F0	6	33	46
653	7	117	199
653 (CMV)[a]	8	149	304
Antigen-specific clones		14	21
653 (transferrin)[a]	9	135	191
Antigen-specific clones		1	2
Total		738	1212

[a]Mice immunized with cytomegalovirus or transferrin.

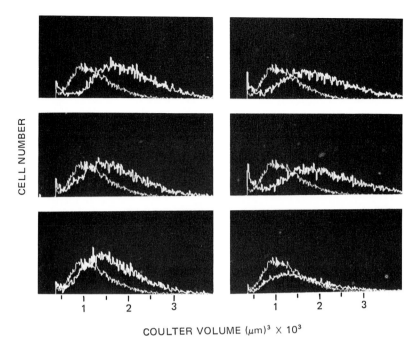

CELL NUMBER

COULTER VOLUME (μm)³ × 10³

FIGURE 2. Coulter volumes of the parent LTR228 (988 μm³) and six representative antitetanus-secreting hybridomas (mean 1611 μm).

2. Phenotype of Human Hybridomas

Hybrid cells were noted by light microscopy to be larger than the parent LTR228. Sizing of cells by a Coulter counter (Figure 2) and scanning EM studies (Figure 3) substantiated these results. The parent cell line mean volume is 988 μm³; that of six representative hybrids is approximately 1611 μm³. Examination of cells by transmission EM also demonstrated the larger size of the hybrids, but few cytoplasmic differences were seen (Figure 4). The marked proliferation of polyribosomes seen in plasma cells was not seen in any cell, although they synthesize 2–8 μg specific antitetanus antibody/10⁶ cells per 24 hr. These morphological results are in agreement with work by others (Kozbor *et al.*, 1983).

Because the parent line was known to express EBNA, we stained hybrid cells by the fluorescent anticomplement method (Reedman and Klein, 1973). Unlike the predominantly nuclear pattern of LTR228, hybrid cells have a perinuclear location of this antigen (Figure 5). The meaning of this altered staining pattern is unclear, although we have seen it in several clones.

We were also curious to know if the hybrid cells expressed any novel B-cell differentiation antigens and if any of these could be used to select for more "plasmacytoid" higher secreting clones. Two-dimensional EPICS V cell sorter

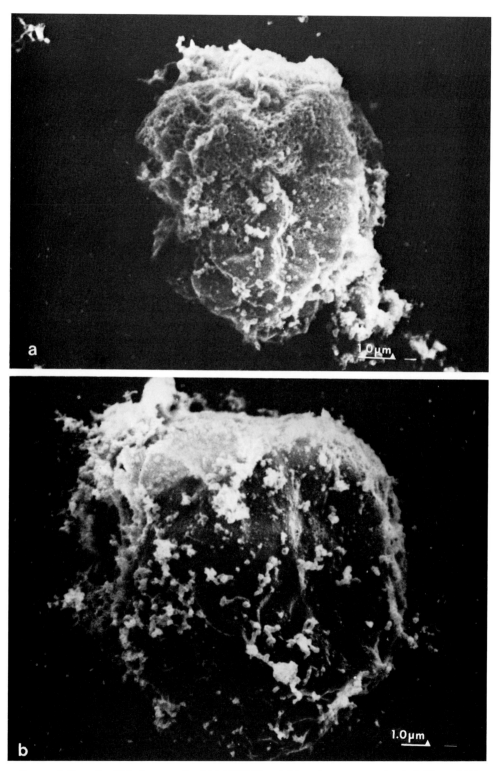

FIGURE 3. Scanning EM photograph of (a) LTR228 and (b) antitetanus-secreting hybridoma LD4.

histograms showed that the hybrids were larger (forward light scatter) and express somewhat less B1 antigen (Stashenko *et al.*, 1980) and surface μ and γ chains but equivalent amounts of surface chain DR and leu 10 antigens compared to the LTR228 parental cell line. (Figure 6) We were unable to correlate the expression of any of these antigens with the amount of immunoglobulin secreted.

3. Genotype of Human Hybridomas

To follow chromosome stability, we have periodically examined DNA histograms of cloned antibody-producing cell lines (Taylor and Milthorpe, 1980). Six representative clones are shown in Figure 7. Note that all are near-tetraploid 6 months after fusion. A representative chromosome spread of a hybrid cell line substantiates the near-tetraploid nature of the hybrids (average chromosome number 90–92) (Figure 8). We have examined 25 subclones from one of the original hybrids. One of these has lost chromosomes, the others have remained tetraploid.

4. Antibody Production by Human Hybridomas

We have studied the production of specific human monoclonal antibodies using a model antigen, tetanus toxoid. Eight to 10 days after an intramuscular tetanus toxoid boost, 50–100 ml of blood was prepared and stimulated with PWM as above. After hybridization, about 5% of the seeded wells produced specific antibody. For purposes of immunoglobulin and specific antibody quantitation, we have employed specific inhibition ELISA essays (Larrick *et al.*, 1983). The ELISA positive wells have been cloned twice by limiting dilution, in soft agar or by cell sorter. After the second cloning, all growing clones (over 200) have continued to secrete specific antitetanus antibody and maintain a near-tetraploid genotype.

To select for high-producer clones we have used a reverse plaque technique (Gronowicz *et al.*, 1976). Clones producing higher (Figure 9b) or lower (Figure 9a) amounts of antibody can be selected as early as 2–3 days after seeding in soft agar.

We have examined growth rates and secretion rates of hybrid clones maintained in culture for over six months. Figure 10 shows that LTR228 doubles every 16–18 hr and reaches densities of 4×10^6 cell/ml. Three hybrids are shown to double every 20 hr and secrete specific antibody at a rate of 3–8 μg/10^6 cells per 24 hr.

5. Biochemical Analysis of Secreted Antibody

SDS PAGE (18%) of the purified antibody shows the novel γ chains, a novel κ chain, and a small amount of parent κ light chain (Figure 11). Light-chain mixing has also been shown in mouse hybridomas (Kohler and Shulman, 1978). We recently selected a nonsecreting parent line (LTR228LS) by the reverse

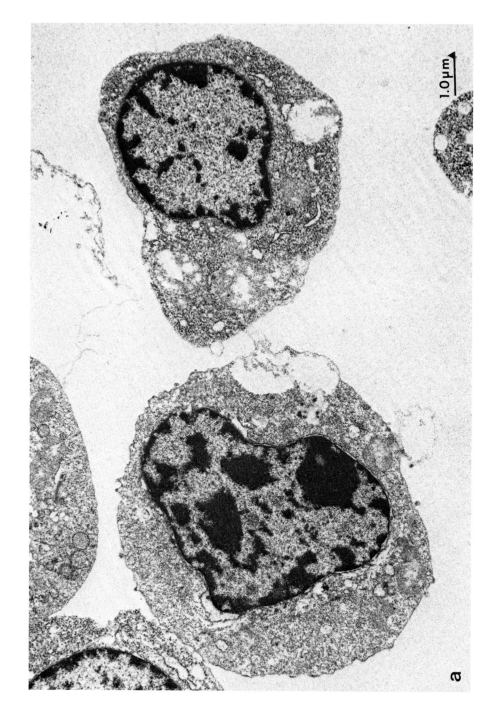

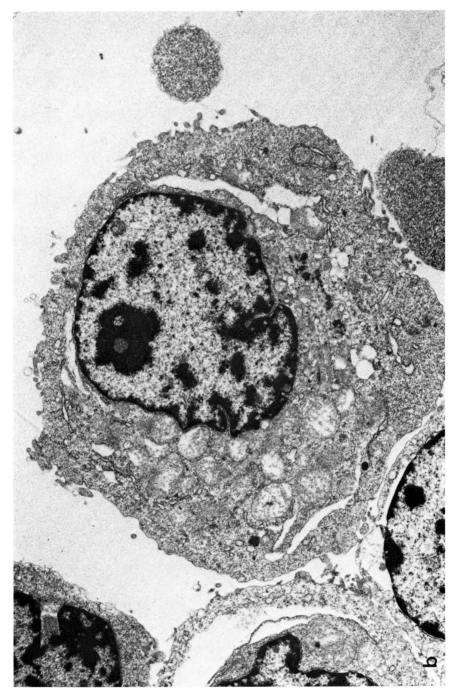

FIGURE 4. Transmission EM photographs of (a) LTR228 and (b) antitetanus-secreting hybridoma LD4.

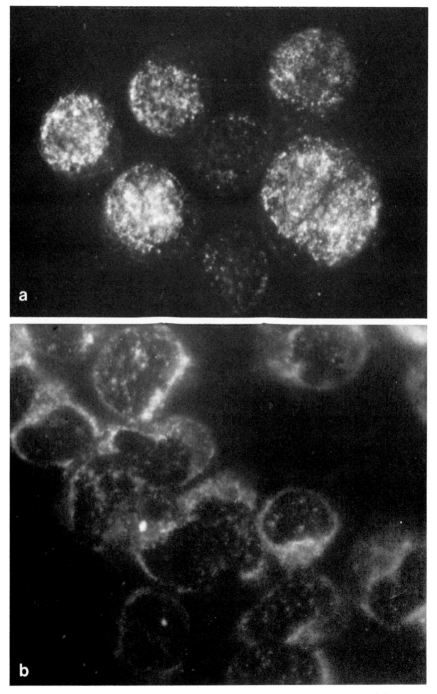

FIGURE 5. Epstein–Barr nuclear antigen (EBNA) staining of (a) parent LTR228 and (b) antitetanus-secreting hybridoma SA13.

plaque technique, and it appears to form immunoglobulin-secreting hybrids as well as the parent.

One-half milliliter of culture supernatant containing antitetanus human monoclonal antibody neutralized tetanus toxin when incubated with it prior to injection into mice. The preincubation with these anti-TT antibodies protected mice given up to 1000 times the LD_{50} of tetanus toxin given i.p. (Larrick *et al.*, 1983).

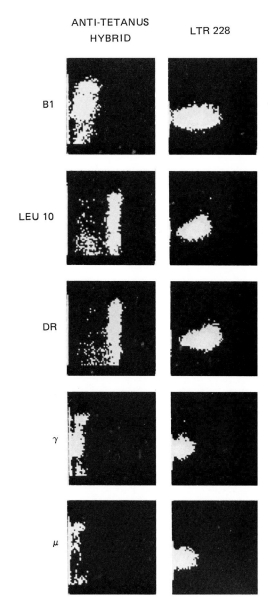

FIGURE 6. Surface phenotype of parent LTR228 and an antitetanus-secreting hybridoma clone. Cells were incubated with FITC-labeled monoclonal antibodies and analyzed on an EPICS V cell sorter. Fluorescence intensity (antigen density) is on the abscissa. Cell size is on the ordinate. [For technical details see Loken and Stall (1982).]

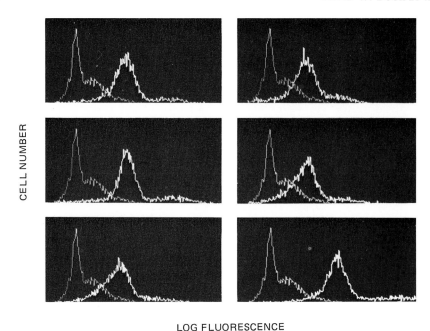

LOG FLUORESCENCE

FIGURE 7. DNA histograms of the parent LTR228 (left peak in each frame) and six representative hybrids.

6. Large-Scale Production of Human Monoclonal Antibodies

The antitetanus clones have been grown in 5-liter spinner cultures without apparent loss of antibody production, and the hybridomas have been adapted to growth in serum-free Iscoves DMEM supplemented with 10 μg/ml transferrin, 500 μg/ml BSA, and 0.2 unit/ml insulin, although their proliferation rate is diminished by 30%. Milligram quantities of monoclonal IgG from these cultures have been purified on Staph-A Sepharose columns. A sister clone of LTR228 and hybridomas made with it have successfully been adapted to growth as solid tumors in nude mice (Figure 12). Antibody production and karyotype were stable in cells passaged several times through nude mice. Experiments are in progress to adapt these cells to ascites growth in mice, and we have yet to determine the maximum levels of human Ig that can be harvested from such an *in vivo* system.

Thus it appears that LTR228 and its derivatives can stably produce sizeable quantities of monoclonal human immunoglobulins over long periods of time in large-scale cultures. Fusions are in progress to produce human monoclonal antibodies to some of the other targets outlined in Table I.

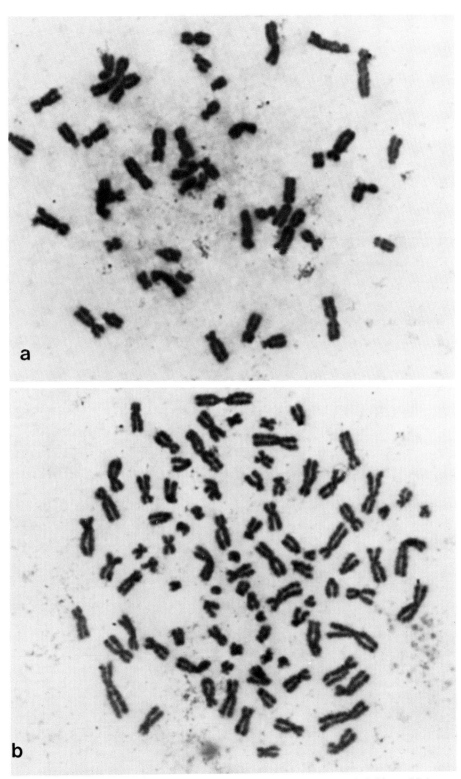

FIGURE 8. Representative metaphase spreads of (a) LTR228 and (b) hybridoma LD4.

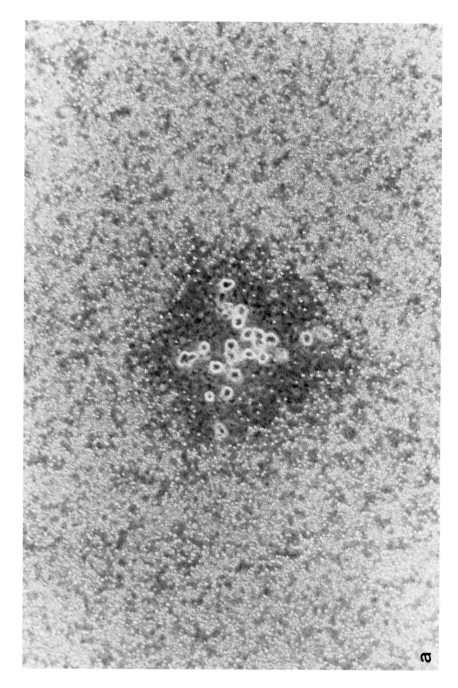

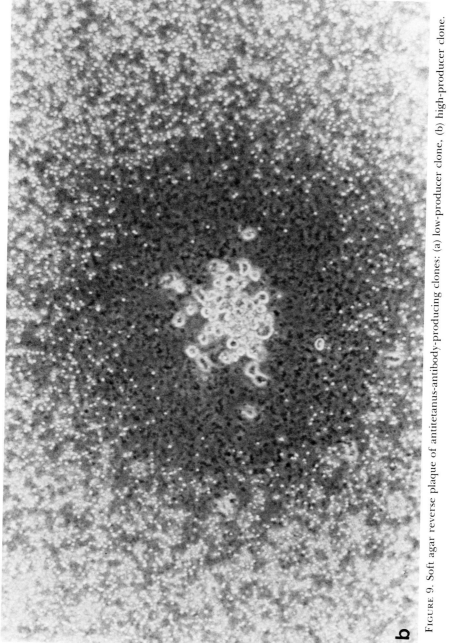

FIGURE 9. Soft agar reverse plaque of antitetanus-antibody-producing clones: (a) low-producer clone, (b) high-producer clone.

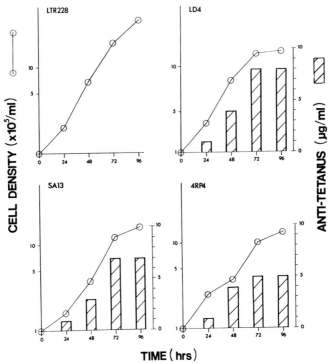

FIGURE 10. Growth rates and specific antitetanus-antibody produced by parent LTR228 and three representative antitetanus-antibody-producing clones.

D. Summary

The successful use of a mouse/human fusion system for the generation of human monoclonal antibodies has been described by several authors. These hybridomas are easily generated, provided sources of human immune lymphocytes are available; secretion rates are comparable to murine hybridomas, generally in the range 2–20 µg/ml. The chromosome instability of these mouse/human hybridomas is probably the major problem at the present time and will most likely limit their usefulness in the future.

The paucity of suitable human myeloma lines has forced investigators to employ lymphoblastoid lines as fusion partners. Surprisingly, these have proven to be superior to the available myelomas for production of hybridoma cells. These hybridomas generally secrete up to 10 µg of Ig/ml spent culture medium, and according to most reports, have relatively stable production. Successful fusions have used lymphocytes from a variety of tissues, including peripheral blood cells, tonsil, lymph node, spleen, and malignant tissue. In spite of these successes, potential difficulties still remain, most notably a ready source of immune lymphocytes for fusion purposes and the development of nonsecreting parental lines that will sustain production of high levels of specific immunoglobulins.

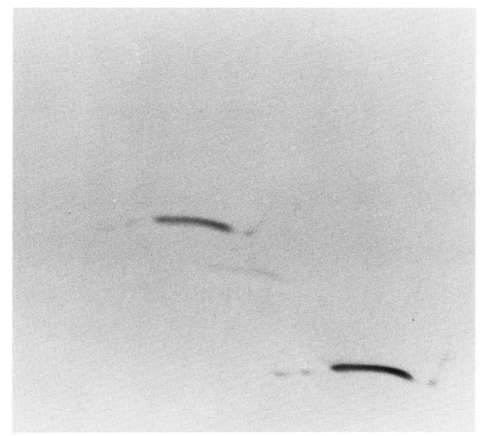

FIGURE 11. SDS polyacrylamide gel-separation of Staph protein A affinity-purified antitetanus antibody. Note the presence of a single γ chain and a major κ light chain, and a small amount of the parent κ light chain. The sample was run on a two-dimensional 18% SDS PAGE gel.

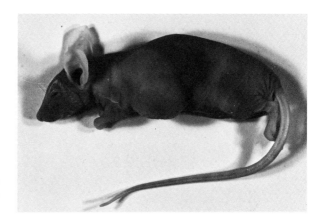

FIGURE 12. A nude mouse with a human/human hybridoma growing as a 1.5-g tumor.

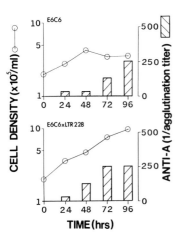

FIGURE 13. Growth rates and specific anti-A antibody titer produced by EBV-transformed line E6C6 (top) and a human/human hybridoma of E6C6 and a ouabain-marked LTR228 line (bottom).

III. EBV Transformation

Various groups have reported the establishment of antigen-specific EBV-transformed B-cell lines produced by *in vitro* EBV infection (Miller and Lipman, 1973). The specificities have included antibodies to Rh, tumor antigens, tetanus toxoid, synthetic haptens, influenza virus, streptococal carbohydrate, human Ig complexes, acetylcholine receptor, and diphtheria toxoid (Zurawski *et al.*, 1980; Tsuchiya *et al.*, 1980; Steinitz and Tamir, 1982; Steinitz *et al.*, 1979; Steinitz, 1981; Steinitz *et al.*, 1977; Kozbor *et al.*, 1979; Koskomies, 1980; Irie *et al.*, 1982; Hirohashi and Shimosato 1982; Crawford *et al.*, 1983a; Boylston *et al.*, 1980; Crawford *et al.*, 1983b; Kamo *et al.*, 1982). In most cases the antibody was of the IgM class, but in some cases IgGs were also found.

Problems with this technique have been twofold. First, in general only low levels of antibody have been produced, and second, the level of antibody production has not been stable. These problems could result from either uncloned cell lines in which nonproducers gradually overgrow producers, or cloned lines that are phenotypically unstable in their antibody production.

Work in our laboratory has confirmed the possibility of EBV lines making specific antibody and we have produced antibodies against the major blood group antigens as well as both an IgG and IgM anti-Rh.

Initially, we had difficulty cloning EBV lines in soft agar at low density with high efficiency (Brown and Miller, 1982). As one decreased agarose concentration, cells would clone at higher efficiency but they would also migrate through the agarose, making the clonal nature of a given colony questionable. Anti-Rh clones selected in this way secreted antibody for several months but then either lost antibody secretion or else ceased to grow.

EBV clones appear to be stable at the antibody-encoding loci (Heiter *et al.* 1982). This raised the possibility that antibody secretion could be rescued by agents that would modulate the suppressed genes. We therefore set out to look at the effect of various drugs on antibody secretion and found, like Ralph and Kishimoto (1981), that TPA, as well as other factors, could increase antibody levels in the medium. However, any agent that increased antibody levels also slowed cell replication and in some cases stopped cells from dividing completely. Initial trials using 8-mercaptoguanosine (Goodman and Weigel, 1983) showed neither an increase in antibody levels nor an effect on cell growth.

In our laboratory an exceptional cell line, E6C6, has continued to secrete an IgM anti-blood group A antibody over a 6-month period without decrease in level (approximately 1 μg/ml spent 7-day medium at 10^6 cells/ml). This antibody shows reactivity against A_1, A_2, and A_3 cells (data to be published elsewhere).

At the moment we are in the process of fusing this cell line to human myelomas LTR228, mouse plasmacytomas (e.g., SP2/o), and mouse/human hybrids to look for increased antibody levels as well as stability (mouse fusions performed by S. Foung, Stanford University Medical Center). Using standard fusing procedures, we found a high rate of specific hybrids in all cases (see Table IV). However, expanded wells of the human/mouse hybrids failed to secrete antibody, while a low percentage of the human/human–mouse hybrids secreted antibody. In contrast, a high percentage of originally positive human/human hybrids continued to secrete antibody. Levels of antibody produced and growth rates are compared in Figure 10. Previously, other workers (Kozbor et al., 1982a) have demonstrated the feasibility of this approach and showed increased antibody levels as well as one tetanus-specific clone that was stable for 12 months.

Even if EBV-transformed cells do not produce antibodies at significant levels, they may be useful as a source of DNA for cloning of these Ig genes. It is also possible that variants may be selected that secrete enough antibody to allow for in vivo immunotherapy. Infectious virus or DNA may be released into culture, but EB virus can be easily inactivated by organic solvents. Furthermore, transfection with EBV DNA has been extremely difficult except on placental cells (Miller et al., 1981). It is somewhat ironic that although EB-virus-transformed B cells have been available for more than a decade, it took the discovery of mouse hybridomas to rekindle interest in lymphoblastoid cell lines as a source of human monoclonal antibodies.

TABLE IV
Hybrid Stability: Specific Positive Wells (Percent)

	Initial fusion	First cloning	Second cloning
E6C6 × LTR228	60	90	100
E6C6 × SP2/oAg14	90	0[a]	Not done
E6C6 × human/mouse	90	4	95

[a]Expanded positive wells had already become negative prior to cloning.

IV. B-Cell Growth and in Vitro Immunization

The identification and use of T-cell growth factor (TCGF) raised the hope that lymphokines could be found for B cells that would allow their continued growth in tissue culture. Expanded antigen-reactive clones could then be used for the purpose of fusion or transformation.

Howard *et al.* (1982), in the murine system, identified a specific factor that promoted [^{3}H]thymidine incorporation of anti-µ stimulated murine B cells. However, long-term growth of murine B cells has never been easily accomplished (Howard *et al.*, 1981; Wetzel *et al.*, 1982; Whitlock and Witte, 1982). To date only one antigen-specific murine B-cell clone has been reported (Aldo-Benson and Scheiderer, 1983).

In the human system, B-cell growth factor (BCGF) has also been identified (Maizel *et al.*, 1982; Muraguchi *et al.*, 1983; Muraguchi and Fauci, 1982) and Kishimoto's laboratory (Okada *et al.*, 1983) has isolated two distinct BCGFs that, as in the murine system, allow for thymidine incorporation of anti-µ stimulated B cells. Except for the isolated report of Sredni (1981), no one has yet been able to grow human B cells in long-term culture, even when purified BCGFs from T-cell hybrids were available (Butler *et al.*, 1983b; Okada *et al.*, 1983). Either human B cells are not capable of expansion like T cells, or else the correct mixture of lymphokines has not yet been identified.

Although long-term human B-cell growth is not presently possible, short-term growth is possible and, as such, is useful in expanding small numbers of antigen-reactive cells for subsequent transformation or fusion. For example, the polyclonal stimulation of early EBV infection may provide sufficient expansion of antigen-specific clones for its own transformation or for subsequent fusion (Rosen *et al.*, 1977; Kozbor and Roder, 1983). Our feeling, however, is that an antigen-driven step will be necessary to increase the low precursor frequency of specific clones available from human peripheral blood. The point is well borne out by Crawford's recent work on the influenza virus system (Crawford *et al.* 1983b), where antigen-specific lymphoblastoid lines were established only if lymphocytes from immune individuals were cultured 3–6 days with antigen prior to transformation.

The primary human *in vitro* immune responses have not been as successful as primary murine immune responses (Mishell and Dutton, 1967; Zurawski *et al.*, 1980). Since the publication of the first volume of this series on monoclonal antibodies, at least three *in vitro* systems have been reported. The first is a complex system described by Hoffman (1980) involving multiple nonspecific as well as specific mitogens. Antigen used was the standard TNP and SRBC. Human serum was needed, but only at 24 hr after culture initiation. Although the system worked well for the described antigens, we have had difficulty eliciting responses to more conventional antigens using these methods.

Morimoto *et al.* (1981) have also described a human system using DNP-KLH as antigen. In this case, suppressor T-cell subsets were removed with monoclonal antibodies, and antigen was removed after 5 days with the culture period proceeding for an additional 4 days.

The most recent study comes from Cavagnaro and Osband (1983), who report primary *in vitro* responses against a variety of antigens, including rabbit Ig, dog serum albumin, tumor extracts, sheep erythrocytes, allogeneic lymphocytes, and Rh(D) erythrocytes. These authors remove suppressor cells on cimetidine-coated plates and perform cultures with autologous serum added at day 0 along with conditioned media from a 48-hr mixed lymphocyte culture. Not only did these cultures produce antibody, but the cells could be used for fusion. Most antibodies were IgMs, consistent with a primary response. If cells can be represented with antigen and IgGs selected, this system may be useful for the generation of B cells for transformation or fusion, as well as for dissecting immune dysfunction syndromes.

In many cases, primary immunizations are not necessary, as patients are available who have been immunized to appropriate targets, i.e., tetanus, hepatitis, and Rh(D). Whether the above system will be useful for an *in vitro* boost prior to fusion remains to be explored. A note of caution arises from antiinfluenza studies, where both peripheral blood and spleens were available. Callard *et al.* (1982) was able to show lack of responses *in vitro* with PBL, while spleen tissue responded well. The defect was apparently due to the lack of circulating memory B cells in the peripheral blood.

It is clear from our own work on tetanus that B cells are present in PBLs that can fuse to make hybrids. Now that there is the potential to rescue these rare cells by fusion, *in vitro* primary and secondary responses can begin to be used not only for the small amount of antibody they produce, but rather as a source of cells for the production of relevant human monoclonal antibodies.

V. Recombinant DNA

Human and mouse immunoglobulin genes of all major classes have recently been mapped and cloned (Heiter *et al.*, 1980, 1981, 1982; Matthyssens and Rabbitts, 1980; Rabbitts *et al.*, 1981; Ellison and Hood, 1982; Ravetch *et al.*, 1981; Nishida *et al.*, 1982) and the relative roles of rearrangements and somatic mutation in the generation of immunoglobulin diversity has been defined (Tonegawa, 1983). Oi *et al.* (1983) and Ochi *et al.* (1983) have demonstrated successful transfection of light chains into plasmacytomas, and within a short period whole immunoglobulins will be produced by recombinant DNA methods.

Are there any advantages to this technology?

1. Large-scale stable production of human monoclonal antibodies will be facilitated by genetically engineered molecules under the control of amplifiable, selectable genes.
2. Mutagenesis of variable regions will permit antibody affinity to be engineered and it will be possible to exchange constant regions to change antibody function. Finally, F(ab) fragments of antibodies will be easily engineered.

3. Specifically reactive side chains, spacer arms, and similar factors for the attachment of toxins and imaging molecules can easily be added to antibodies by genetic manipulation.

Korsmeyer et al. (1981) have recently shown that the gene rearrangments in B cells transformed by EBV are stable. This suggests that clones of specific antibody-producing lymphoblastoid cell lines would provide a suitable source from which to clone human antibodies. The precise cloning strategies are beyond the scope of this chapter, but many laboratories are pursuing this marriage of monoclonal antibody and recombinant DNA technology.

A final use of recombinant DNA is just on the horizon. Many laboratories have recently reported the existence of cell lineage-specific oncogenes. For example, c-Myc is translocated from chromosome 8 to regions active in immunoglobulin transcription, i.e., chromosomes 2, 14, and 22 in Burkitt lymphoma (Dalla-Favera et al., 1982). Whether similar B-lineage or myeloma-specific genes can be used to transform B cells more stably and efficiently than EBV is also under active investigation in our laboratory as well as others. One laboratory (R. H. Kennett's) has immortalized mouse spleen cells by transfecting them with human cancer cell DNA. However, the applicability of this method requires further investigation.

ACKNOWLEDGMENTS

The authors gratefully acknowledge the excellent technical help of Hanna Hutchins, David Lippman, Timothy Culp, and Howard Weintraub, and the efforts of Joan Murphy and Dianne Jacobs in the preparation of this manuscript. The electron micrographs were generously provided by Dr. John Kosek, Veterans' Administration Hospital, Palo Alto, California.

References

Aldo-Benson, M., and Scheiderer, L., 1983, Long term growth of lines of murine dinitrophenyl-specific B lymphocytes in vitro, J. Exp. Med. **157:**342–347.

Bengtsson, B. O., Nabholz, M., Kennett, R. H., and Bodmer, W. F., 1975, A genetic and karyotypic analysis of crosses between lymphocytes and D98/AH-2, Somatic Cell Genet. **1:**41–64.

Boylston, A. W., Gardner, B., Anderson, R. L., and Hughes-Jones, W. C., 1980, Production of human IgM anti-D in tissue culture by EB-virus transformed lymphocytes, Scand. J. Immunol. **12:**355–358.

Brahe, C., and Serra, A.,1981, A simple method for fusing human lymphocytes with rodent cells in monolayer by polyethylene glycol, Somatic Cell Genet. **7:**109–115.

Brown, N. A., and Miller, G., 1982, Immunoglobulin expression by human B lymphocytes clonally transformed by Epstein–Barr virus, J. Immunol. **128:**24–29.

Burk, K. M., Drewinko, B., Trujillo, J. M., and Ahearn, M. J., 1978, Establishment of a human plasma cell line in vitro, Cancer Res. **38:**2508–2513.

Butler, J. L., Lane, H. C., and Fauci, A. S., 1983a, Delineation of optimal conditions for producing mouse/human heterohybridomas from human peripheral blood B cells of immunized subjects, *J. Immunol.* **130:**165–168.

Butler, J. L., Muraguchi, A., Lane, H. C., and Fauci, A. S., 1983b, Development of a human T-T cell hybridoma secreting B cell growth factor, *J. Exp. Med.* **157:**60–68.

Buttin, G., LeGuern, G., Phalente, L., Lin, E. C. C., Medrano, L., and Cazenave, P. A., 1978, Production of hybrid lines secreting monoclonal anti-idiotypic antibodies by cell fusion on membrane filters, in: *Lymphocyte Hybridomas* (F. Melchers, M. Potter, and N. I. Warner, eds.), Springer-Verlag, Berlin, pp. 27–36.

Callard, R., McCaughan, G., Babbage, J., and Souhami, R., 1982, Specific *in vitro* antibody responses by human blood lymphocytes: Apparent nonresponsiveness of PBL is due to a lack of recirculating memory B cells, *J. Immunol.* **129:**153–156.

Cavagnaro, J., and Osband, M., 1983, Successful *in vitro* primary immunization of human peripheral blood mononuclear cells and its role in the development of human derived monoclonal antibodies, *Biotechniques* **1:**31–36.

Chiorazzi, N., Wasserman, R. L., and Kunkel, H. G., 1982, Use of Epstein–Barr virus transformed B cell lines for the generation of immunoglobulin-producing human B cell hybridomas, *J. Exp. Med.* **156:**930–935.

Cote, R. J., Morrissey, D. M., Houghton, A. N., Beattie, Jr., E. J., Oettgen, H. F., and Old, L. J., 1983, Generation of human monoclonal antibodies reactive with cellular antigens, *Proc. Natl. Acad. Sci. USA* **80:**2026–2030.

Cotton, R. G. H., and Milstein, C., 1973, Fusion of two immunoglobulin producing myeloma cells, *Nature* **244:**42–43.

Crawford, D. H., Barlow, M. J., Harrison, J. F., Winger, L., and Huehns, E. R., 1983a, Production of human monoclonal antibody to rhesus D antigen, *Lancet* **1983** (February 19)**:**386–388.

Crawford, D., Callard, R. E., Muggeridge, M. I., Mitchell, D. M., Zanders, E. D., and Beverley, P. C. L., 1983b, Production of human monoclonal antibody to X31 influenza virus nucleoprotein, *J. Gen. Virol.* **64:**697–700.

Croce, C. M., Shander, M., Martinis, J., Cicurel, L., D'Ancona, G. G., Dolby, T. W., and Koprowski, H., 1979, Chromosomal location of the genes for human immunoglobulin heavy chains, *Proc. Natl. Acad. Sci. USA* **76:**3416–3419.

Croce, C. M., Linnenbach, A., Hall, W., Steplewski, Z., and Koprowski, H., 1980, Production of human hybridomas secreting antibodies to measles virus, *Nature* **288:**488–489.

Dalla-Favera, R., Breeni, M., Erikson, J., Patterson, D., Gallo, R. C., and Croce, C., 1982, Human *c-myc* oncogene is located on the region of chromosome 8 that is translocated in Burkitt's lymphoma cells, *Proc. Natl. Acad. Sci. USA* **79:**7824–7827.

Dwyer, D. S., Bradley, R. J., Urguhart, C. K., and Kearney, J. F., 1983, Naturally occurring anti-idiotypic antibodies in myasthenia gravis patients, *Nature* **301:**611–614.

Edwards, P. A. W., Smith, C. M., Neville, A. M., and O'Hare, M. J., 1982, A human/human hybridoma system based on a fast growing mutant of the ARH-77 plasma cell leukemia derived line, *Eur. J. Immunol.* **12:**641–648.

Eisenbarth, G. S., Linnenbach, A., Jackson R., Scearce R., and Croce, C. M., 1982, Human hybridomas secreting anti-islet antibodies, *Nature* **300:**264–267.

Ellison, J., and Hood, L., 1982, Linkage and sequence homology of two human immunoglobulin gamma heavy chain constant region genes, *Proc. Natl. Acad. Sci. USA* **79:**1984–1988.

Erikson, J., Martinis, J., and Croce, C. M., 1981, Assignment of the genes for human immunoglobulin chains to chromosome 22, *Nature* **294:**173–175.

Foung, S. K. H., Sasaki, D., Grumet, F. C., and Engleman, E. G., 1982, Production of functional human T/T hybridomas in selection medium lacking aminopterin and thymidine, *Proc. Natl. Acad. Sci. USA* **79:**7484–7488.

Gigliotti, F., and Insel, R. A., 1982, Protective human hybridoma antibody to tetanus toxin, *J. Clin. Invest.* **70:**1306–1309.

Glassy, M. C., Handley, H. H., Royston, I., and Lowe, D. H., 1983, Human monoclonal antibodies to human cancers, in: *Proceeding of the 4th Arm and Hammer Cancer Symposium* (B. D. Boss, R. Langman, I. S. Trowbridge, and R. Dulbecco, eds.), Academic Press, New York, pp. 163–170.

Goodman, M., and Weigel, W., 1983, Activation of lymphocytes by a thiol-derivatized nucleoside:

Characterization of cellular parameters and responsive subpopulations, *J. Immunol.* **130:**552–557.

Gronowicz, E., Coutinho, A., and Melchers, F., 1976, A plaque assay for all cells secreting Ig of a given type or class, *Eur. J. Immunol.* **6:**588–590.

Handley, H. H., and Royston, I., 1982, A human lymphoblastoid B cell line useful for generating immunoglobulin secreting human hybridomas, in: *Hybridomas in Cancer Diagnosis and Treatment* (M. S. Mitchell and H. F. Oettgen, eds.), Raven Press, New York, pp. 125–132.

Handley, H., Royston, I., and Glassy, M. C., 1983, The production of human monoclonal antibodies to human tumor associated antigens, in: *Proceedings of the 15th International Leucocyte Conference* (J. W. Parker and R. L. O'Brien, eds.), Wiley Interscience, New York, pp. 617–620.

Heiter, P. A., Max, E. E., Maizel, J. V., and Leder, P., 1980, Cloned human and mouse kappa immunoglobulin constant and J region genes conserve homology in functional segments, *Cell* **22:**197–207.

Heiter, P. A., Hollis, G. F., Korsmeyer, S. J., Waldman, T. A., and Leder, P., 1981, Clustered arrangement of immunoglobulin lambda constant region genes in man, *Nature* **294:**536–540.

Heiter, P. A., Korsmeyer, S. J., Waldman, T. A., and Leder, P., 1981, Human immunoglobulin k light-chain genes are deleted or rearranged in λ-producing B cells, *Nature* **290:**368–372.

Hirohashi, S., and Shimosato, Y., 1982, *In vitro* production of tumor-related human monoclonal antibody and its immunohistochemical screening with autologous tissue, *Gann* **73:**345–347.

Hoffman, M., 1980, Antigen-specific induction and regulation of antibody synthesis in cultures of human peripheral blood mono-nuclear cells, *Proc. Natl. Acad. Sci. USA* **77:**1139–1143.

Houghton, A. N., Brooks, H., Cote, R. J., Taormina, M. C., Oettgen, H. F., and Old, L. J., 1983, Detection of cell surface and intracellular antigens by human monoclonal antibodies: Hybrid cell lines derived from lymphocytes of patients with malignant melanoma, *J. Exp. Med.* **158:**53–65.

Howard, M., Kessler, S., Chused, T., and Paul W., 1981, Long term culture of normal mouse B lymphocytes, *Proc. Natl. Acad. Sci. USA* **78:**5788–5792.

Howard, M., Farrar, J., Hilfiker, M., Johnson, B., Takatsu, K., Hamaoka, T., and Paul, W., 1982, Identification of a T cell-derived B cell growth factor distinct from interleukin-2, *J. Exp. Med.* **155:**914–923.

Irie, R. F., Sze, L. L., and Saxton, R. E., 1982, Human antibody to OFA-1, a tumor antigen produced *in vitro* by Epstein–Barr virus-transformed human B-lymphoid cell lines, *Proc. Natl. Acad. Sci. USA* **79:**5666–5670.

Kamo, I., Furukawa, S., Tada, A., Mano, Y., Iwasaki, Y., and Furuse, T., 1982, Monoclonal antibody to acetylcholine receptor: Cell line established from thymus of patient with myasthenia gravis, *Science* **215:**995–997.

Karpas, A., Fischer, P., and Swirsky, D., 1982, Human myeloma cell line carrying a Philadelphia chromosome, *Science* **216:**997–999.

Kearney, J. F., Radbruch, A., Liesegang, B., and Rajewsky, K., 1979, A new mouse myeloma line that has lost immunoglobulin expression that permits the construction of antibody secreting hybrid cell lines, *J. Immunol.* **123:**1548–1550.

Kohler, G., and Milstein, C., 1975, Continuous cultures of fused cells secreting antibody of pre-defined specificity, *Nature* **256:**495–497.

Kohler, G., and Shulman, M. J. L., 1978, Cellular and molecular restrictions of the lymphocyte fusion, in: *Lymphocyte Hybridomas* (F. Melchers, M. Potter, and N. I. Warner, eds.), Springer-Verlag, Berlin, pp. 143–148.

Kohler, G., Howe, C. S., and Milstein, C., 1976, Fusion between immunoglobulin secreting and non-secreting lines, *Eur. J. Immunol.* **6:**292–295.

Korsmeyer, S. J., Hieter, P., Ravetch, J. V., Poplack, D. G., Waldmann, T. A., and Leder, P., 1981, Developmental hierarchy of immunoglobulin gene rearrangements in human leukemic pre-B-cells, *Proc. Natl. Acad. Sci. USA* **78:**7096–7100.

Koskimies, S., 1980, Human lymphoblastoid cell line producing specific antibody against Rh-antigen D, *Scand. J. Immunol.* **11:**73–77.

Kozbor, D., and Roder, J., 1981, Requirements for the establishment of high titred human monoclonal antibodies against tetanus toxoid using the Epstein–Barr virus technique, *J. Immunol.* **127:**1275–1280.

Kozbor, D., and Roder, J. C., 1983, *In vitro* stimulated lymphoocytes as a source of human hybridomas, *Eur. J. Immunol.*, in press.

Kozbor, D., Steinitz, M., Klein, G., Koskimies, S., and Makela, O., 1979, Establishment of anti-TNP antibody-producing human lymphoid lines by preselection for hapten binding followed by EBV transformation, *Scand. J. Immunol.* **10**:187–194.

Kozbor, D., Lagarde, A. E., and Roder, J. C., 1982a, Human hybridomas constructed with antigen-specific EBV transformed lines, *Proc. Natl. Acad. Sci. USA* **79**:6651–6655.

Kozbor, D., Roder, J. C., Chang, T. H., Steplewski, Z., and Koprowski, H., 1982b, Human anti-tetanus toxoid monoclonal antibody secreted by EBV-transformed human B cells fused with murine myeloma, *Hybridoma* **1**(3):323–328.

Kozbor, D., Dexter, D., and Roder, J. C., 1983, A comparative analysis of the phenotypic characteristics of available fusion partners for the construction of human hybridomas, *Hybridoma* **2**(1):7–16.

Lane, H. C., Shelhamer, J. H., Mostowski, H. S., and Fauci, A. S., 1982, Human monoclonal anti-KLH antibody-secreting hybridoma produced from peripheral blood B lymphocytes of a KLH-immune individual, *J. Exp. Med.* **155**:333–338.

Larrick, J. W., Truitt, K. E., Raubitschek, A. A., Senyk, G. S., Wang, J. C. N., 1983, Characterization of human hybridomas secreting antibody to tetanus toxoid, *Proc. Natl. Acad. Sci. USA* **80**:6376–6380.

Lever, J. E., Nuki, G., and Seegmiller, J. E., 1974, Expression of purine overproduction in a series of 8-azaguanine resistant diploid human lymphoblast lines, *Proc. Natl. Acad. Sci. USA* **71**:2679–2683.

Levy, J. A., Virolainen, M., and Defendi, V., 1968, Human lymphoblastoid lines from lymph node and spleen, *Cancer* **22**:517–524.

Lewin, R., 1981, An experiment that had to succeed, *Science* **212**:767–769.

Littlefield, J. W., 1964, Selection of hybrids from matings of fibroblasts *in vitro* and their presumed recombinants, *Science* **145**:709–710.

Loken, M. R., and Stall, A. M., 1982, Flow cytometry as an analytical and preparative tool in immunology, *J. Immunol. Methods* **50**:R85–R112.

Madsen, M., and Johnson, H. E., 1979, A methodological study of E-rosette formation using AET treated sheep red blood cells, *J. Immunol. Methods* **27**:61–74.

Maizel, A., Sahasrabuddhe, C., Mehta, S., Morgan, J., Lachman, L., and Ford, R., 1982, Biochemical separation of a human B cell mitogenic factor, *Proc. Natl. Acad. Sci. USA* **79**:5998–6002.

Malcom, S., Barton, P., Murphy, C., Ferguson-Smith, M. A., Bentley, D. L., and Rabbitts, T. H., 1982, Localization of human immunoglobulin K light chain variable region genes to the short arm of chromosome 2 by *in situ* hybridization, *Proc. Natl. Acad. Sci. USA* **79**:4957–4961.

Matsuoka, Y., Moore, G. E., Yagi, Y., and Pressman, D., 1967, Production of free light chains of immunoglobulin by a haematopoietic cell line derived from a patient with multiple myeloma, *Exp. Biol. N. Y.* **125**:1246–1250.

Matthyssens, G., and Rabbitts, T. H., 1980, Structure and multiplicity of human immunoglobulin heavy chain variable region genes, *Proc. Natl. Acad. Sci. USA* **77**:6561–6565.

Miller, G., and Lipman, M., 1973, Release of infectious Epstein–Barr virus by transformed marmoset leukocytes, *Proc. Natl. Acad. Sci. USA* **70**:190–194.

Miller, G., Grogan, E., Heston, H., Robinson, J., and Smith, D., 1981, Epstein–Barr viral DNA: Infectivity for human placental cells, *Science* **212**:452–455.

Mishell, R., and Dutton, R., 1967, Immunization of dissociated spleen cells cultures from normal mice, *J. Exp. Med.* **126**:424–442.

Morimoto, C., Reinherz, E., and Schlossman, S., 1981, Regulation of *in vitro* primary anti-DNP antibody production by functional subsets of T lymphocytes in man, *J. Immunol.* **127**:69–73.

Muraguchi, A., and Fauci, A., 1982, Proliferative responses of normal human B lymphocytes: Development of an assay system for human B cell growth factor (BCGF), *J. Immunol.* **129**:1104–1108.

Muraguchi, A., Butler, J., Kehrl, J., and Fauci, A., (1983), Differential sensitivity of human B cell subsets to activation signals delivered by anti-μ antibody and proliferative signals delivered by a monoclonal B cell growth factor, *J. Exp. Med.* **157**:530–546.

Nilsson, K., Bennich, H., Johansson, S. G. O., and Ponten, J., 1970, Established immunoglobulin producing myeloma (IgE), Clin. Exp. Immunol. 7:477–489.

Nishida, Y., Miki, T., Hisajima, H., and Honjo, T., 1982, Cloning of human immunoglobulin epsilon chain genes: Evidence for multiple C epsilon genes, Proc. Natl. Acad. Sci. USA 79:3833–3837.

Nowinski, R., Berglund, C., Lane, J., Lostrom, M., Bernstein, I., Young, W., and Hakomori, S., 1980, Human monoclonal antibody against Forssman antigen, Science 210:537–539.

Ochi, A., Hawley, R. G., Shulman, M. J., and Hoyuni, N., 1983, Transfer of a cloned immunoglobulin light chain gene to mutant hybridoma cells restores specific antibody production, Nature 302: 340–342.

Oi, V. T., Morrison, S. L., Herzenberg, L. A., and Berg, P., 1983, Immunoglobulin gene expression in transformed lymphoid cells, Proc. Natl. Acad. Sci. USA 80:825–829.

Okada, M., Sakaguchi, N., Yoshimura, N., Hara, H., Shimizu, K., Yoshida, W. Shizaki, K., Kishimoto, S., Yamamura, Y., and Kishimoto, T., 1983, B cell growth factors and B cell differentiation factor from human T hybridomas, J. Exp. Med. 157:538–590.

Olsson, L., and Kaplan, H. S., 1980, Human/human hybridomas producing monoclonal antibodies of predefined antigenic specificity, Proc. Natl. Acad. Sci. USA 77:5429–5431.

Potter, M., Humphrey, J. G., and Walters, J. L., 1972, Growth of primary plasmacytomas in the mineral oil conditioned periotoneal environment, J. Natl. Cancer Inst. 49:305–308.

Rabbitts, T. H., Bentley, D. L., and Milstein, C. P., 1981, Human antibody genes: V gene variability and CH gene switching strategies, Immunol. Rev. 59:69–91.

Ralph, P., and Kishimoto, T., 1981, Tumor promoter phorbol myristir oretak stimulates immunoglobulin secretion correlated with growth cessation in human B lymphocyte cell lines, J. Clin. Invest. 68:1093–1096.

Ravetch, J. V., Siebenlist, U., Korsmeyer, S., Waldmann, T., and Leder, P., 1981, Structure of the human immunoglobulin μ locus: Characterization of embryonic and rearranged J and D genes, Cell 27:583–591.

Reedman, B., and Klein, G., 1973, Cellular localization of an Epstein–Barr virus (EBV)-associated complement fixing antigen in producer and non-producer lymphoblastoid cell lines, Int. J. Cancer 11:499–520.

Rosen, A. S., Britton, B., Gergely, P., Jondal, M., and Klein, G., 1977, Polyclonal Ig production after Epstein–Barr virus infection of human lymphocytes in vitro, Nature 267:52–54.

Ruddle, F. H., 1974, Human genetic linkage and gene mapping by somatic cell genetics, in: Somatic Cell Hybridization (R. L. Davidson and F. F. de la Cruz, eds.), Raven Press, New York, pp. 1–12.

Sato, K., Slesinski, R. S., and Littlefield, J. W., 1972, Chemical mutagenesis at the phosphoribosyltransferase locus in cultured human lymphoblasts, Proc. Natl. Acad. Sci. USA 69:1244–1248.

Schlom, J., Wunderlich, D., and Teramoto, Y. A., 1980, Generation of monoclonal antibodies reactive with human mammary carcinoma cells, Proc. Natl. Acad. Sci. USA 77:6841–6845.

Schoenfeld, Y., Hsu-Lin, S., Gabriels, J., Silberstein, L., Furie, B. C., Furie, B., Stollar, B., and Schwartz, R., 1982, Production of autoantibodies by human–human hybridomas, J. Clin. Invest. 70:205–208.

Schoenfeld, Y., Rauch, J., Massicotte, H., Datta, S., Schwartz, J., Stollar, D., and Schwartz, R. S., 1983, Polyspecificity of monoclonal lupus autoantibodies produced by human/human hybridomas, New Engl. J. Med. 308(8):414–420.

Schwaber, J., and Cohen, E. P., 1973, Human/mouse somatic cell hybrid clone secreting immunoglobulin of both parental types, Nature 244:444–447.

Sikora, K., and Phillips, J., 1981, Human monoclonal antibodies to glioma cells, Br. J. Cancer 43:105–107.

Sikora, K., and Wright, R., 1981, Human monoclonal antibodies to lung cancer antigens, Br. J. Cancer 43:696–700.

Sikora, K., Alderton, T., Phillips, J., and Watson, J., 1982, Human hybridomas from malignant gliomas, Lancet i:11.

Sredni, B., Sieckmann, D., Kumagai, S., House, S., Green, I., and Paul, W., 1981, Long term culture and cloning of nontransformed human B lymphocytes, J. Exp. Med. 154:1500–1516.

Stanbridge, E. J., Der, C. J., Doerson, C. J., Nishimi, R. Y., Peehl, D. M., Weissman, B. E., and Wilkinson, J. E., 1982, Human cell hybrids: Analysis of transformation and tumorigenicity, *Science* **215**:252–259.

Stashenko, P., Nadler, L. M., Hardy, R., and Schlossman, S. F., 1980, Characterization of a human B lymphocyte-specific antigen, *J. Immunol.* **125**:1678–1685.

Steinitz, M., 1981, Human monoclonal antibodies produced by Epstein–Barr virus-immortalized cell lines, in: *Monoclonal Antibodies and T-Cell Hybridomas Perspectives and Technical Advances* (G. J. Hammerling, U. Hammerling, and J. F. Kearney, eds.), Elsevier/North-Holland Biomedical Press, New York, pp. 447–452.

Steinitz, M., and Tamir, S., 1982, Human monoclonal autoimmune antibody produced *in vitro:* Rheumatoid factor generated by Epstein–Barr virus-transformed cell line, *Eur. J. Immunol.* **12**:126–133.

Steinitz, M., Klein, G., Koskimies, S., and Makela, O., 1977, EB virus-induced B lymphocyte cell lines producing specific antibody, *Nature* **269**:420–22.

Steinitz, M., Koskimies, S., Klein, G., and Makela, O., 1979, Establishment of specific antibody producing human lines by antigen preselection and Epstein–Barr virus (EBV) transformation, *J. Clin. Lab. Immunol.* **2**:1–7.

Taylor, I. W., and Milthorpe, B. K., 1980, An evaluation of DNA fluorochrome, staining techniques, and analysis for flow cytometry, *J. Histochem. Cytochem.* **28**:1224–1232.

Togawa, A., Inoue, N., Myamoto, K., Hyodo, H., and Namba, M., 1982, Establishment and characterization of a human myeloma cell line, *Int. J. Cancer* **29**:495–500.

Tonegawa, S., 1983, Somatic generation of antibody diversity, *Nature* **302**:575–581.

Tsuchiya, S., Yokoyama, S., Yoshie, O., and Ono, Y., 1980, Production of diphtheria antitoxin antibody in Epstein–Barr virus induced lymphoblastoid cell lines, *J. Immunol.* **124**:1970–1976.

Wetzel, G. D., Swain, S. L., and Dutton, R. W., 1982, A monoclonal T cell-replacing activity can act directly on B cells to enhance clonal expansion, *J. Exp. Med.* **156**:306–311.

Whitlock, C. A., and Witte, O. N., 1982, Long-term culture of B lymphocytes and their precursors from murine bone marrow, *Proc. Natl. Acad. Sci. USA* **79**:3608–3612.

Zurawski, V., Black, P., and Haber, E., 1980, Continuously proliferating human cell lines synthesizing antibody of predetermined specificity, in: *Monoclonal Antibodies. Hybridomas: A New Dimension in Biological Analyses* (R. H. Kennett, T. J. McKearn, and K. Bechtol, eds.), Plenum Press, New York, pp. 19–33.

12

Monoclonal Antibodies and Molecular Genetics
Oncogenes and Oncogene Products

Roger H. Kennett, Zdenka L. Jonak,
and Naohiko Ikegaki

I. Introduction

Two developing disciplines, recombinant DNA and monoclonal antibodies, have been at the forefront of the rapid expansion in biotechnology during the past few years. These techniques are, in fact, complementary with regard to the detailed information on the structure of biological macromolecules that they provide. The application of recombinant DNA techniques has given details of gene structure, including the existence of introns (intervening sequences), the recombination taking place during the rearrangement of genes in B-lymphocyte ontogeny, and the structure of specific transcription, RNA splicing, and translation signal sequences that were, for all practical purposes, previously unobtainable (Leder *et al.*, 1982). On the other hand, monoclonal antibodies have made it possible to detect, isolate, and characterize new gene products as well as provide ways to study individual antigenic determinants (epitopes) on specific macromolecules in more detail (Kennett, 1981). It is evident that a more complete understanding of the relationships between gene structure and function will come more quickly as a combination of these technologies is applied to a variety of questions in cell and molecular biology. We will review applications in which monoclonal antibodies are being used to analyze details of molecular structure

Roger H. Kennett, Zdenka L. Jonak, and Naohiko Ikegaki • Department of Human Genetics, University of Pennsylvania School of Medicine, Philadelphia, Pennsylvania 19104.

and how this technology interacts with recombinant DNA technology. We will then discuss in more detail how the investigators in our own and other laboratories have begun to study oncogenes and oncogene-related gene products using monoclonal antibody and DNA technologies. Although we cannot hope to include references to all the published work even in this somewhat restricted area of monoclonal antibody application, we will attempt to include examples that illustrate the usefulness of these reagents in this context.

II. Analysis of Molecular Structure with Monoclonal Antibodies

A. Analysis of Protein and Carbohydrate Epitopes

Monoclonal antibodies have been used in a variety of ways to characterize the fine antigenic structure of biological macromolecules. These procedures take advantage of the fact that monoclonal antibodies react with a single epitope, rather than having a reactivity representing the additive binding of a heterogeneous population of antibodies against a variety of antigenic determinants as is the case with conventional antisera. Even though a given monoclonal antibody may react with closely related "cross-reactive" epitopes (Lane and Koprowski, 1982; Kennett *et al.*, 1982b), these cross-reactions can be kept constant by maintaining consistent assay conditions. This makes possible an epitope-by-epitope comparison of the structure of proteins that are the products of "different" genes, i.e., either allelic forms of the same gene or genes for products with structural homology. Part II, Chapters 2–4 of this volume discuss this type of application in detail for three different systems. In Chapter 2, Dr. Richman describes the analysis of the nicotine acetylcholine receptor. Such an analysis allows one to identify antigenic determinants that are associated with the binding sites of receptors and to determine the relationship between one binding site and another on the same complex molecule. Dr. Harris discusses, in Chapter 3, the use of monoclonal antibodies to detect polymorphic variation in the structure of the enzyme alkaline phosphatase. He describes ways in which monoclonal antibodies can be combined with conventional electrophoretic methods to detect variation in the structure of proteins. Monoclonal antibodies have also been used as reagents for fine structure analysis of carbohydrate molecules that are present on glycolipids and glycoproteins, as described by Dr. Hakomori in Chapter 4. Dr. Lin *et al.* and Dr. Lampson discuss in their respective chapters how the detection of similar epitopes on molecules that are, by other criteria, distinctly different can be used to detect structural homologies and in some cases define "families" of molecules that were previously unknown. In each of these cases the reaction of monoclonal antibodies to a single epitope or a group of cross-reactive epitopes of similar structure has made it possible to detect structural variation and in some cases structural homologies that would not be detectable and certainly not consistently reproducible from batch to batch if one were using conventional antisera.

Methods similar to those used by Harris for enzymes have been applied to protein without enzymatic activity, such as myoglobin, fibronectin, and α_2-macroglobulin. Berzofsky *et al.* (1980, 1982), taking advantage of the detailed information available on the structure of myoglobins from different species, have used monoclonal antibodies to define the actual array of amino acids making up the epitopes recognized by individual antibodies. Their analyses indicate that these antibodies recognize determinants composed of amino acids that, although removed from each other in the primary sequence, come together to form an epitope in the three-dimensional structure of the myoglobin molecule. Investigators in several laboratories have prepared monoclonal antibodies against fibronectin. These have been used to compare epitopes present on fibronectin from different species (Koteliansky *et al.*, 1982), to detect variation in fibronectin structure within a species (Kennett *et al.*, 1982a), and to define functional regions of the fibronectin molecules, such as the cell attachment site of plasma fibronectin (Atherton *et al.*, 1981; Pierschbacher *et al.*, 1981). Monoclonal antibodies that distinguish two conformational forms of the protease inhibitor α_2-macroglobulin and others that detect polymorphic variation in this molecule have been reported (Marynen *et al.*, 1981; Eager and Kennett, 1980).

Another useful application of monoclonal antibodies resulting from their ability to detect a single determinant has been the analysis of viral protein structure and variation (Gerhard *et al.*, 1980). Several investigators have used panels of monoclonal antibodies to distinguish between viral strains. Antibodies against a single determinant have also been used to study the variation of viral protein structure. By analysis of the influenza virus proteins one epitope at a time, it is possible to estimate the mutation rate of the determinant detected by the antibody (Laver *et al.*, 1979). Niman and Elder (1982) have recently described in detail work in which they make a comprehensive analysis of the envelope glycoproteins (gp70s) of the murine retroviruses using a combination of monoclonal antibody and biochemical techniques. They define and localize 19 different domains using a panel of antibodies and peptide fragments of the proteins. Their work provides a good example of the structural information that can be derived by using these epitope-specific reagents.

Besides being useful for detecting variation in viral protein structure, monoclonal antibodies have also been used to select for cultured cells expressing variant histocompatibility antigens. Variants of H-2 had previously been selected with conventional antisera; however, most of those variants no longer expressed any H-2 molecules and specific mutants could be obtained only when one could select against one epitope at a time with monoclonal antibodies. Rajan (1980) has used cytotoxic antibodies against specific epitopes on H-2 molecules to select populations of cells. Cells expressing variant molecules lacking the specific determinant survive the selection and these variant molecules can then be characterized. This procedure has been used to select a variety of H-2 mutants, which can then be compared to the original H-2 structure, and opens the way to studies on the effects that variation in specific regions of the molecule have on particular functions of the H-2 molecules.

B. *Analysis of Immunoglobulin Structure Using Monoclonal Antibodies*

The ways in which monoclonal antibodies have contributed to the analysis of immunoglobulin structure are well beyond the scope of this brief overview. The ability to generate a large number of monoclonal antibodies against specific haptens (well-defined molecules of low molecular weight acting as antigenic determinants) has made it possible to relate the amino acid structure of the antibody binding site to previously defined idiotypic determinants (structural variations in antibody binding sites detected by antigenic differences between one antibody variable region and another) (Clevinger *et al.,* 1980). This type of analysis was previously dependent upon the chance detection of myeloma proteins that showed binding to a given hapten or the isolation of serum antibodies that represented one of a few predominant idiotypes of antibodies made in response to a given hapten. Rauch *et al.* (1982), in their discussion of autoimmunity and monoclonal antibodies, discuss ways in which monoclonal antibodies have contributed to the analysis of idiotypes, including the details of and references to recent work on cross-reactive idiotypes and idiotype networks and the implications with regard to the structure of germ-line genes and the control of their expression. Denis *et al.* (1980) had previously described how the production of hybridomas from neonatal spleen cells provides insight into the development of the murine B-cell repertoire. Each of these analyses was made possible by the ability to immortalize a specific B cell making an antibody of predefined specificity so the specific monoclonal antibodies could be isolated in sufficient quantity to be analyzed in detail.

III. *Monoclonal Antibodies and DNA Technology*

A. *Monoclonal Antibodies Reacting with Nucleic Acids*

Just as it has been possible to detect structural variation in proteins and carbohydrates using monoclonal antibodies, it has been possible to make similar reagents against nucleic acids. While some of these antibodies detect variations in primary nucleotide sequence, i.e., provide the same order of information as supplied by nucleic acid sequencing, other antibodies are able to discriminate conformational differences and thus provide information in addition to that obtained from the primary sequence. There have been several reports of monoclonal antibodies that react with various forms of nucleic acids. Eilat *et al.* (1980) reported a monoclonal antibody produced from an unimmunized autoimmune mouse that binds ribosomal RNA with high affinity but does not bind DNA, tRNA, or synthetic single- or double-stranded polynucleotides. Klotz *et al.* (1981) describe antibodies that react with denatured DNA but not with native DNA. These antibodies were also made by producing hybridomas from autoimmune animals. Rauch *et al.* (1982), in reviewing the use of monoclonal antibodies in the study of autoimmunity, include an informative discussion of monoclonal antibodies that react with nucleic acids and the basis of their cross-reactions with glycolipids. This is an analysis made possible by the ability to consider these antigenic relationships on an epitope-by-epitope basis. Monoclonal antibodies reacting specifically with aflatoxin B_1-modified DNA (Haugen *et al.*, 1981) and antibodies and DNA into which 5-bromodeoxyuridine or 5-iododeoxyuridine has been incorporated (Gratzner, 1982) have been reported. The usefulness of antibodies against forms of DNA is well illustrated by the report that affinity-purified antibodies from mice or rabbits immunized with brominated poly(dG-dC)-poly(dG-dC) can detect Z-DNA in *Drosophila* polytene chromosomes (Nordheim *et al.*, 1981). Each of these specific antibodies allows the detection of a particular form of nucleic acid sequence or conformation even when it is present in small quantities within a mixture of other molecules. It is possible that antibodies with specificities similar to these may eventually be useful for the analysis of changes in the conformation of nucleic acid molecules during processes of transcription or DNA replication at a chromosomal level.

B. Useful Combinations of Monoclonal Antibody and DNA Technology

The literature contains several examples of ways in which the technologies of recombinant DNA and monoclonal antibody production can in principle be effectively combined. One of the best examples is the use of monoclonal antibodies to define specific "immunodominant" determinants on infectious organisms such as parasites (see Phillips and Zodda, Chapter 10, this volume), followed by the cloning of the corresponding gene and its insertion into a vector that facilitates its expression in bacteria. Large amounts of this antigen can then be produced and used as an effective vaccine. This procedure is likely to eventually replace the use of attenuated organisms as vaccines. By defining the molecules that elicit antibodies that are the most effective in providing protection, and removing this antigen from the potentially dangerous context of the whole organism, these procedures provide a very effective way of producing large quantities of a well-characterized vaccine of consistent quality.

Many such vaccines against a variety of infectious organisms are in various stages of preparation by several biotechnology companies. The success of such an approach depends, of course, on several factors. It is necessary first of all that the antigenic determinant detected by the monoclonal antibodies be a protein determinant rather than on a carbohydrate or glycolipid determinant. The latter are synthesized by enzymatic addition of specific moieties to a receptor molecule and thus are at least one step removed from the structure of a primary gene product. Second, once the gene product of interest is identified by a monoclonal antibody it is necessary to identify the cloned gene in a library of cloned DNA molecules or to obtain a population of messenger RNA enriched for the mRNA corresponding to the gene product of interest.

In either case the availability of antisera or monoclonal antibodies that can be used to identify the gene product in an *in vitro* translation system facilitates the isolation of the cloned gene by recombinant DNA techniques (Maniatis *et al.*, 1982). In the case where one must isolate an enriched population of mRNA prior to the synthesis and cloning of cDNA, the antibody allows one to assay mRNA fractions by immunoprecipitation after *in vitro* translation. Precipitation of the specific gene product indicates that the corresponding mRNA is present in a given fraction (Ricciardi *et al.*, 1979; Ploegh *et al.*, 1979). In the case where one is attempting to identify the cloned gene in a library of cloned DNAs one can assay by determining whether or not a particular clone or pool of cloned DNAs can inhibit the *in vitro* translation of the mRNA for the specific gene product (because the mRNA hybridizes with the corresponding DNA and thus its translation is inhibited) as detected by immunoprecipitation of the product from the *in vitro* translation system (Peterson *et al.*, 1977). In both of these cases it is not essential that the precipitation be done with a monoclonal antibody. There may be, in fact, an advantage in using a conventional antiserum that contains antibodies against a variety of determinants, since some of these determinants may be more readily detectable on the *in vitro* translation product. The advantage that monoclonal antibody technology has provided in this respect is that, even in the case where there may be an advantage in using a polyvalent antiserum, the production of monoclonal antibodies against the antigen provides a way to isolate the antigen in a form pure enough and in large enough quantities that a monospecific polyvalent antiserum can be produced. An alternative that is perhaps even more effective is to pool a collection of monoclonal antibodies against different determinants on the antigen of interest to produce a synthetic polyvalent "antiserum." One advantage of such a mixture of monoclonal antibodies is that if one or more of the antibodies cross-reacts with *in vitro* translation products other than the one of interest, one can simply remove the cross-reactive antibody from the mixture and thus remove this "background."

Another way in which antibodies can be used in conjunction with gene cloning techniques is by using the antibodies to purify enough of the antigen to permit microsequencing of the amino acids so that the corresponding nucleotide probes can be synthesized. These synthetic nucleotide probes can then be used to detect and isolate the piece of genomic DNA or a cDNA clone corresponding to the gene of interest (Rossi *et al.*, 1982). Conversely, in cases where a gene has been isolated and sequenced but the gene product not identified, the amino acid sequence can be deduced and antibodies made against the corresponding peptides (Sutcliffe *et al.*, 1980). Making antibodies against the defined peptides has the advantage of producing antibodies against a defined region of the protein antigen and will undoubtably become an important procedure as antibodies are used more and more for the analyses of protein structure/function relationships.

In addition to being applied to the detection of immunodominant proteins and isolation of the corresponding genes, or going from gene to protein, the above combination of techniques can be applied to a variety of different types of molecules. Another particularly useful application will certainly be the analysis of differentiation antigens and their expression. Monoclonal antibodies have been used to detect a large number of differentiation antigens that had not been previously detectable with conventional antisera (Kennett, 1981). By using the above methods or those described in the following section to obtain the corresponding genes, one may begin to study the control of the expression of this gene product. One would have the capacity to detect both the mRNA and the gene product as it is synthesized and processed within the cell. It would thus be possible to study the control of synthesis and the turnover rate of both the mRNA and the specific gene product. The monoclonal antibody also allows one to isolate the molecule and thus obtain more information on the molecular function of the gene product. This type of procedure is especially useful in the case where a molecule of particular biological interest is present in only very small quantities. The most striking example of this is the case of leukocyte interferon, in which a monoclonal antibody was prepared and used to purify and characterize the product of a recombinant DNA clone (Staehelin *et al.*, 1981).

Similar procedures are likely to be important in the study of other effector molecules, such as lymphokines, that are synthesized in relatively small quantities. In this context, the ability to produce monoclonal antibodies by *in vitro* immunization with very small amounts of material (Luben and Mohler, 1980; Jonak and Kennett, Appendix of this volume) will be particularly important.

Another useful application of antibodies in the context of gene cloning is for the detection of the gene product produced in colonies of bacteria containing a mixture of DNA sequences cloned in expression vectors. By screening with antibodies for the specific gene product, it is possible to determine whether there are any clones producing at least a portion of the gene product from the cloned DNA (Broome and Gilbert, 1978; Young and Davis, 1983). In this case it is especially important to use an antiserum or a collection of monoclonal antibodies reacting with as many of the antigenic determinants on the molecule as possible, because in some cases only a portion of the gene product may be produced by a given clone. This again emphasizes the fact that the real advantage of monoclonal antibodies in this context is the ability to make a specific molecular probe that can be used to detect and sometimes even make the initial identification of a specific molecule of interest even when it is present in a complex mixture of molecules. Once the antibody is available one can isolate sufficient antigen in pure enough form to either make a conventional antiserum or other monoclonal antibodies against other determinants on the molecule (Berthold, Chapter 9, this volume). These antibodies are then useful for assaying for the presence of the molecule in complex mixtures and in *in vitro* translation systems, and for detecting the expression of the product in clones of producing bacteria or yeast. Once this source of the gene product is available, the antibodies can be used for affinity purification of the molecule prior to its analysis or application.

C. Monoclonal Antibodies, Transfection, and Gene Cloning

One of the most useful potential application of monoclonal antibodies that react with cell surface antigens is likely to be as reagents for detecting the expression of genes that have been transfected into eukaryotic cells. Pellicer *et al.* (1980) reported that transfer of genomic DNA into Daudi cells that do not express β_2-macroglobulin resulted in the expression of the antigen in the recipient cells. After transfer of DNA from the leukemic cell line HL60 into mouse fibroblasts [the LTA cell line lacking thymidine kinase (TK$^-$) and phosphoribo-syl transferase], Chang *et al.* (1982) used immunofluorescence with monoclonal antibodies to detect the transient expression of the differentiation antigens MY-1 and OKT 3. Barbosa *et al.* (1982) screened a large number of isolated human genomic clones that hybridized to cloned cDNA probes for the human major histocompatibility antigens (HLA) for the ability to direct the synthesis of HLA antigens when transfected into mouse L cells. The recipient cells were screened for the expression of HLA with the mouse monoclonal antibody W6/32. Kavathas and Herzenberg (1983) transfected mouse L cells (TK$^-$) with a mixture of human cellular DNA and the cloned herpes simplex virus thymidine kinase gene. The recipient cells were selected for the expression of the TK gene and the surviving TK$^+$ cells were screened by a flourescence-activated cell sorter (FACS) for cells expressing T-cell differentiation antigens, HLA, and β_2-micro-globulin. These transfectants appeared to be stable and express antigens of the same molecular size as the corresponding antigens on human cells.

These transfection procedures, if they can be applied in general to cell surface antigens, can be considered a first step toward cloning of the genes for the protein antigens defined by monoclonal antibodies. If cells expressing these gene products can be isolated, one could then use a probe for a human repetitive sequence that is not present in the mouse genome as an aid to identification and isolation of the human DNA sequence containing the gene for the antigen. One could produce secondary transfectants (take DNA from the first transfectants and produce a second series of transfectants that contains much less human DNA that is not associated with the selected gene sequence) and then detect the human DNA sequence using a probe such as the cloned Alu sequence. This is a highly conserved sequence of 300 base pairs that appears on the average approximately once for every few thousand base pairs (Jelinek *et al.*, 1980). It is not found in the mouse genome, so the BLUR8 probe carrying the Alu sequence is a useful marker for the presence of human DNA in the mouse context. In this case the techniques of cell culture, monoclonal antibodies, and DNA tansfection may make it possible to isolate the gene sequences for a large number of important cell surface differentiation antigens.

In addition to these procedures, one can expect to see reports of combining monoclonal antibodies with what have come to be known as "shuttle vectors." The bovine papilloma virus (BPV) transforms mouse cells with high efficiency and exists in the cells as multiple copies of extrachromosomal DNA. Several investigators have constructed hybrid molecules by combining regions of BPV with regions of bacterial plasmids to form a vector that can be introduced into either mammalian cells or bacteria and in both cases exist as multiple copies of extrachromosomal DNA (Sarver *et al.*, 1981,1982; DiMaio *et al.*, 1982; Binetruy *et al.*, 1982; Sekiguchi *et al.*, 1983). The cloned genes for β-globin (DiMaio *et al.*, 1982) and hepatitis B surface antigen (Wang *et al.*, 1983) and a clone in which the structural sequence of the human growth hormone was fused to the promotor and control regions of the mouse metallothionein-I gene (Pavlakis and Hamer, 1983) have been inserted into the BPV "shuttle vectors" and expression of these genes detected in eukaryotic cells. As ways are developed to allow this system to incorporate larger pieces of genomic DNA in a stable extrachromosomal state,

BPV vector libraries can be transfected and recipients expressing specific gene products can be detected and isolated on the FACS. The extrachromosomal DNA can be isolated and transferred to bacteria for production of large amounts of the cloned DNA so that the genomic DNA corresponding to the antigen can be isolated and analyzed. Again the ability to detect the antigen with antibodies enhances the system and makes it valuable for studying a variety of molecules at the level of the gene and gene product.

An additional and somewhat different application of recombinant DNA methods to monoclonal antibody production is the possibility of cloning immunoglobulin-chain genes from specific hybridomas and having these genes expressed in bacteria or yeast. The limiting factor in applying this procedure could be the need to have the heavy and light chains assembled into an active immunoglobulin molecule. Apparently Genentech has made some initial progress in this area (Klausner, 1983), but the practicability of such a procedure remains to be determined.

Although there are many other present and potential applications that could be mentioned specifically, the above discussion is intended to stress the point that the two technologies considered are complementary in their applications and in the information and capabilities they provide. To understand the total spectrum of gene structure and regulation and gene product synthesis and function will require that these technologies be integrated effectively.

IV. Oncogenes and Oncogene Products

A. Detection of Oncogenes by Transfection with Tumor DNA

One rapidly developing area of research that will necessarily involve the combined application of monoclonal antibody and DNA technology is the study of oncogenes and oncogene products. The term oncogene refers, in general, to any gene involved in determining the oncogenic, i.e., malignant, phenotype of a tumor cell. It has recently come to be applied more specifically to the genes that have been detected by transfection of DNA from tumor cells into cells that do not express characteristics of the transformed phenotype, i.e., lack of contact inhibition, growth in semisolid agarose, and growth as a tumor in syngeneic mice. This transfection assay provides a way to identify sequences of DNA that are responsible for expression of the oncogenic phenotype (Weinberg, 1981). It is clear that this is only one aspect of the problem of understanding transformation to malignancy, the others being detection and characterization of the gene products produced from or affected by the presence of this transforming DNA, and understanding the molecular changes that take place in the tumor cell. By understanding the function and the localization of the gene products involved, it is more likely that effective protocols for tumor cell detection and therapy can be devised.

Our own interest in the oncogene transfection system developed from our interest in using monoclonal antibodies to detect gene products that are altered in structure or expression as a result of malignant transformation of human cells (Kennett and Gilbert, 1979; Kennett *et al.*, 1981). We will review here the oncogene transfection system and ways in which we have begun to combine it with monoclonal antibody production to detect oncogene-related products as a prelude to determining their structure and functions within transformed cells. The fact that DNA from human cells can transfect mouse cells provides a situation where products from the "human oncogenes" may be expressed in the mouse cells transfected with the DNA. If these human gene products are different in structure from mouse gene products, they will be recognized as antigenic when the transfectants are injected into mice. Mouse gene products synthesized in the transfectants but not in the nontransformed recipient cells may also be detected, particularly if they are altered gene products or oncofetal antigens not normally seen by the immune system. Three different laboratories have recently reported that immunization of mice with mouse cells transfected with tumor DNA results in the production of antisera that detect antigens present on the transfectants but not detectable on the cells used as a recipient of the transfected DNA (Hopkins *et al.*, 1981; Padhy *et al.*, 1982; Becker *et al.*, 1982). Production of such antisera is likely to be an efficient first step in identifying a variety of antigenic differences that may exist. This can be followed by production of monoclonal antibodies against each of the components, i.e., by *in vitro* immunization with each of the immunoprecipitation bands present in the transfectants but not in the recipient cells. These monoclonal antibodies can then be used to localize the antigen in the cells, to detect whether the same gene product is produced in the tumor from which the transfecting DNA was derived, and to isolate the antigen from the tumor cells in sufficient quantity to determine its structure and function and compare it to similar molecules that may be expressed in normal cells. The usefulness of monoclonal antibodies against oncogene products has been well illustrated by the use of anti-p21 antibodies against the Harvey sarcoma *ras* oncogene product. These monoclonal antibodies have been useful in isolating the product, localizing it in the cells, and comparing the Harvey-*ras* product to the Kirsten-*ras* protein (Furth *et al.*, 1982).

1. Transfection of Fibroblasts with Tumor DNA

The transfer of genetic information by transfection of calcium phosphate–DNA coprecipitate (Graham and van der Eb, 1973a,b) has been applied to viral genomes, selectable markers such as thymidine kinase, and oncogenic DNA from tumor cells (reviewed in Kucherlapati, 1982; Weinberg, 1981). In most cases, the recipient cells were cultured fibroblast lines, such as L-cell derivatives, that could be used in drug selection systems, or the mouse fibroblast line NIH/3T3. Murine bone marrow cells have reportedly been transfected with DNA conferring resistance to methotrexate. These cells were then detectable *in viro* under selective conditions (Cline *et al.*, 1980).

There has been much interest and activity recently because of the ability to transfect oncogenic sequences from tumors to recipient fibroblasts that, prior to the transfection, exhibit a nontransformed phenotype (Weinberg, 1981; Lane *et al.,* 1981, 1982; Perucho *et al.,* 1981; Shih *et al.,* 1981; Der *et al.,* 1982; Parada *et al.,* 1982; Shilo and Weinberg, 1981; Krontiris and Cooper, 1981). These "transformed" fibroblasts appear as foci of cells in a background of contact-inhibited cells. The transfected cells can be cloned in semisolid agarose and grow as tumors in nude mice. In cases where human tumor DNA has been transfected into cells of other species, specific human DNA sequences can be detected in the transformed cells (Krontiris and Cooper, 1981; Perucho *et al.,* 1981; Shih *et al.,* 1981). The oncogenic DNA sequences from tumors of the same type have the same restriction endonuclease sensitivity and the restricted DNA shows the same pattern as detected with a human DNA probe such as the BLUR8 probe containing the human Alu sequence. Three different oncogene sequences from four different types of tumor (bladder carcinoma, lung carcinoma, and a neuroblastoma) that have been transfected into NIH/3T3 have been well characterized. They are present as a single piece of DNA containing a nucleotide sequence homologous to the *ras* family of oncogenes originally identified as retroviral oncogene sequences (Der *et al.,* 1982; Parada *et al.,* 1982; Shimizu *et al.,* 1983).

The initial results from the characterization of oncogenes detected by fibroblast transfection assays that relate these genes to the previously identified retroviral oncogenes provide some encouragement that it may soon become possible to understand the molecular mechanisms by which cells are transformed to a malignant phenotype. There have recently been excellent reviews on the topic of retroviral oncogenes (Bishop, 1983; Weiss *et al.,* 1982) so that we will provide here only a brief overview and refer the reader to those sources for more detailed references.

Analyses of retroviral oncogenes have indicated that these viral transforming genes (v-*onc* genes) are actually altered forms of cellular genes referred to as c-*onc* genes or proto-oncogenes. These c-*onc* genes are present in very similar if not identical forms in all vertebrate species and have even been detected in *Drosophila* (Hoffman-Falk *et al.,* 1983) and yeast. The relatively conserved nature of these loci and the evidence that there is differential expression of these c-*onc* loci in different tissues during normal ontogeny (Müller *et al.,* 1982) have been taken to imply that these genes may play an important role in mechanisms of normal cellular differentiation.

There are apparently various ways in which a c-*onc* gene can be activated to produce an active oncogene that contributes to the transformation of a cell. There is evidence that DNA rearrangement of various kinds can result in c-*onc* activation. Recent results indicate that the certain c-*onc* genes are located near breakpoints of chromosomal translocations that are characteristic of certain types of human and mouse tumors and that in other types of tumors the level of c-*onc* gene expression is increased by either gene amplification or increased levels of transcription (Bishop, 1983). An alternative mechanism that could possibly alter c-*onc* gene activity is the presence of a mutation in the c-*onc* gene itself. Comparison of the oncogene detected by transfection of NIH/3T3 by bladder carcinoma DNA to the normal, nontransforming cellular analog of the Harvey *ras* gene (c-Ha-*ras*) indicates that the only difference detectable is the change from a glycine residue to a valine at position 12 of the amino acid sequence in the first exon of the protein (Reddy *et al.,* 1982). Yuasa *et al.* (1983) have recently reported that the c-Ha-*ras* gene detected by transfecting NIH/3T3 with DNA from Hs242, a lung carcinoma cell line, also differs from the corresponding nononcogenic c-*onc* gene by only a single amino acid. This protein is altered by the substitution of a leucine for a glutamine at amino acid 61 in the second exon of the gene in these tumor cells. The implication is that these minimal structural changes are responsible for the normal *onc* gene product being changed into an active oncogene product responsible in some way for transformation of NIH/3T3 to a malignant phenotype.

The identification of oncogenic sequences by transfection is a significant contribution toward understanding the genetic basis of malignancy. At this point, however, the general conclusions that can be drawn are somewhat limited. Although DNA from several tumor types can mediate transformation (approximately 10% of those tried), there are many others that do not produce foci in the fibroblast transfection assay. Several investigators have discussed the observation that NIH/3T3 cells have characteristics that bring into question the assumption that they are representative of a "normal cell." It may, in fact, have already undergone one or more of the steps necessary for malignant transformation, and the introduction of the tumor DNA provides the final step (Littlefield, 1976, 1982). Smith *et al.* (1982) have reported that the hamster fibroblast line CHEF/18 can be transformed by DNA from the human bladder carcinoma EJ. The hamster cell line is in fact more "normal" in its phenotype than the usual recipient NIH/3T3. Whereas NIH/3T3 has a heteroploid karyotype and a high frequency of spontaneous transformation, the CHEF/18 line has a diploid karyotype and requires a multistep process requiring several selection steps for transformation by means other than transfection. One question that cannot be answered using the systems currently available concerns the extent to which the differentiated state of the recipient cells affects whether DNA from a given tumor is able to produce transformed foci. This question is particularly relevant in light of the observations that some retroviruses can actively infect several cell types but often show a more restricted host range when it comes to transformation (Durban and Boettiger, 1981). To what extent does this reflect differences in the recipient genome resulting in alterations due to cell differentiation? Is the observation that DNA from several human tumors will not produce foci with NIH/3T3 an indication that genetic mechanisms for the production of malignancy are basically different in different tumor types, is or is it because DNA from these tumors will not transform the fibroblasts? Will the DNA sequences that transform fibroblasts, such as NIH/3T3 or CHEF/18, also transform other types of cells, or do these tumors contain other DNA sequences that will transform cells other than fibroblasts?

2. Transfection of Mouse Primary Lymphocytes with Tumor DNA

In order to begin to ask questions concerning the possible relationships between cell differentiation and malignancy, we decided to attempt transfection of cells other than fibroblasts. Having an interest in lymphoid tumors and experience in growing hybridomas, we set out to transfect primary mouse spleen cells with DNA from the human acute lymphocytic leukemia cell line Reh (Rosenfeld *et al.*, 1977). Based on our observations that cells recently stimulated are more likely to produce hybridomas (Kennett *et al.*, 1978), and that the transforming activity of viruses is often dependent on cell proliferation or DNA replication (Varmus *et al.*, 1978), we assumed that spleen cells that were recently stimulated with antigen would be more likely to be transformed with transfected DNA. We also postulated that if our assumptions were valid, a certain portion of the transfectants produced should be producing antibodies against the antigen with which the mouse had been immunized.

With the purpose of developing a system for further analysis of transfecting DNA, and on the basis of the above assumptions, we began a series of experiments demonstrating that primary mouse spleen cells can be transformed with human tumor DNA and that some of these transfectants do produce monoclonal antibodies reacting with the antigens used to stimulate the spleen cells.

a. Transfection of NIH/3T3 with Reh DNA. Parallel with our initial lymphocyte transfection experiments, we transfected NIH/3T3 with the same Reh DNA preparation so that we could eventually compare the transfecting DNA in NIH/3T3 and in transfected lymphocytes. Procedures for the transfections and the growth of transfectants are included in the Appendix to this volume. Using DNA introduced by our PEG–DMSO treatment, we were able to obtain NIH/3T3 transfection frequencies (Table I) that were in the "higher" range compared to those for other human tumor DNAs (Weinberg, 1981; Perucho *et al.*, 1981; Shih *et al.*, 1981). These foci appeared within 10–20 days. Each had a morphology distinct from NIH/3T3 cells. Three of these foci were chosen at random and cloned in semisolid agarose. Cells from the same foci were injected subcutaneously into nude mice (10^6 cells/mouse), and large tumors were formed within 2 weeks. These initial results confirmed that Reh DNA was effective in producing transformed foci in NIH/3T3 fibroblasts as reported for several other human tumor cell lines, including lymphoid tumors of comparable phenotype (Lane *et al.*, 1982). From the transfections included in Table I, we saved five transfectants for further analysis.

b. Transfection of Mouse Lymphocytes with Reh DNA. Table II shows the results of two separate lymphocyte transfections done with the same Reh DNA preparation used to transfect NIH/3T3. In each lymphocyte transfection, more than 100 of the 288 wells plated showed clumps of dividing lymphocytes. In the control

TABLE I

Focus Formation by NIH/3T3 Cells Transfected with Reh DNA

DNA	Total foci/total dishes	Foci per μg DNA per 10^6 cells
Placental	0/6	—
Reh	20/6	0.6
Harvey sarcoma	18/3	9

TABLE II
Transformation of Mouse Lymphocytes with Reh DNA

DNA	Total "foci"/ total wells	Lines passaged/ total "foci"[a]	"Foci" per μg DNA/10^6 cells	Number making specific Ab/number tested
Placental	4/288	0/4	—	0/4
Reh 1	105/288	35/105	0.07	3/4 (3/4)[b]
Reh 2	157/288	47/157	0.1	11/35 (2/5)

[a]These were chosen because they grew well under the conditions in culture at the time. It is not clear how many would have been successfully passaged now that initial culture conditions have been optimized.
[b]Number of cell lines producing specific antibody/stable lines derived from transfection.

transfection done with human placental DNA, only four wells showed any sign of lymphocyte growth and attempts to passage these cells were unsuccessful. On the other hand, cells from 30% of the wells with lymphocytes growing after transfection with Reh DNA could be passaged. From these initial experiments, we chose four lymphocyte transfectants on the basis of their growth rate and concentrated on their further analysis. These have been in culture for more than 1 year, and have cloned in semisolid agarose.

Figure 1 shows a culture of one of these cell lines and Figure 2 shows a chromosome spread of one of the lines. These cells contain only acrocentric chromosomes and have a modal number of 40. Whether there are subtle variations from the apparently normal mouse chromosomes that will be detectable by chromosome banding techniques remains to be determined. Whether, as the cells grow in culture or are passaged in mice, there will be an evolution to a heteroploid karyotype is a question that is of considerable interest to those interested in the "clonal evolution" of tumor cells.

c. Detection of Human DNA in Transfectants. As described above, human DNA can be detected in the mouse cells by using radioactively labeled human DNA sequences that do not hybridize to mouse DNA sequences. We used the cloned Alu sequence to detect the human DNA sequences in the transfectants. Figure 3 shows the Southern blot analysis of three Reh–NIH/3T3 transfectants and one Reh–lymphocyte transfectant. Each contains a large amount of human DNA. As reported previously by others, these primary transfectants contain not only the DNA containing the transforming oncogene, but a large amount of other human DNA that was transfected into the cells. By extracting DNA from these primary transfectants and using it to produce a second round of transfectants (secondary transfectants), one can obtain cells that contain a limited number of human DNA sequences that have been selected for by the transfection assay. Figure 4 shows that the first of the secondary lymphocyte transfectants that we have analyzed does contain a limited number of human DNA bands. This DNA presumably contains the oncogene that is responsible for conferring the property of unlimited proliferation on the mouse primary lymphocytes. The relationship between this DNA and the DNA responsible for the transformation of the NIH/3T3 cells remains to be determined.

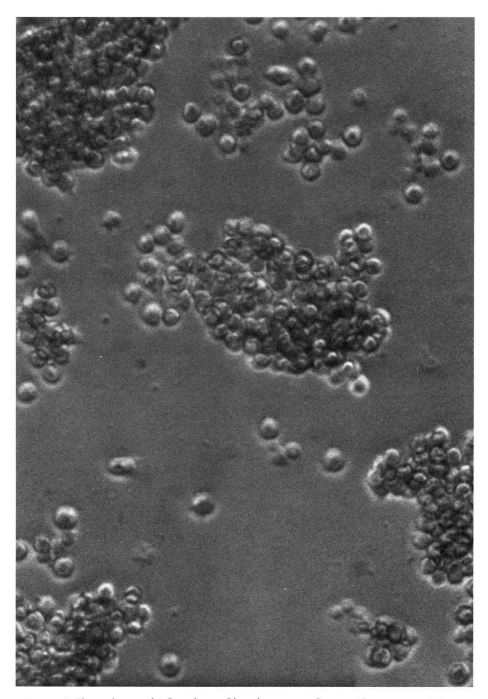

Figure 1. Photomicrograph of a culture of lymphocyte transfectants. Phase contrast 125×.

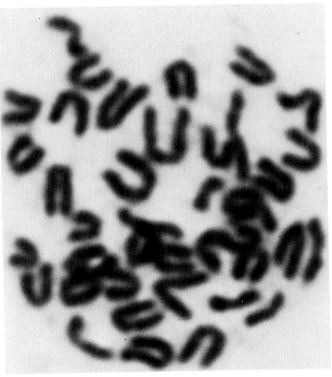

FIGURE 2. Chromosome spread of lymphocyte transfectant 16-91L. Note that the modal chromosome number is diploid and contains only acrocentric chromosomes. This spread contains 40 chromosomes.

    d. Immunoglobulin Production by the Lymphocyte Transfectants. Each of the four primary lymphocyte transfectants that we have studied in some detail produces immunoglobulin that can be detected by immunodiffusion and is produced in amounts comparable to that synthesized by cultures of hybridoma cells (Figure 5). Table III indicates the classes of immunoglobulin produced by these transfectants. Two of these cell lines produce antibodies that bind to the human cells used to immunize the mouse prior to transfection of the spleen cells. The cell line that was passaged through a BALB/c mouse has maintained the production of specific antibody for the past year. It appears that it is therefore possible to produce monoclonal antibodies against a predefined antigen without the production of hybrid plasmacytomas. Whether there may be any advantages in producing monoclonal antibodies by transfection methods rather than by cell fusion is not clear at this point, although it does present a possibility for the production of monoclonal antibodies from human cells and from the cells of other species if the lymphocytes are properly stimulated and if the lymphocytes can be immortalized by transfection with oncogenic DNA.

B. Production of Monoclonal Antibodies against Oncogene Products

In general one can conceive of at least two ways to obtain monoclonal antibodies against oncogene-related products expressed in mouse cells transfected with human DNA. In the first case, immunization of mice with the transfectants is likely to result in the production of antibodies against any human gene products expressed in the transfectants as well as antibodies against any murine

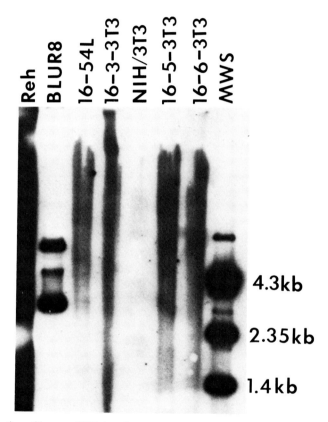

FIGURE 3. Detection of human DNA in primary transfectants. DNA was extracted, treated with *Bam* HI, and run on an agarose gel (20 μg/slot). After transfer to nitrocellulose paper, it was hybridized with 10⁸ cpm of BLUR8 probe nick-translated with all four (dXT³²P) bases. Hybridization was done at 62°C in the presence of 5% dextran sulfate. The washed and dried paper was autoradiographed and the X-ray film developed after 1 week of exposure. The source of DNA is indicated on the figure. 6-54L: Lymphocyte transfectant; 16-3-3T3, 16-5-3T3, 16-6-3T3: NIH transfectants. Reh: DNA from the human leukemia cell lines used as a source of transfecting DNA. NIH/3T3: DNA from parental mouse cells. BLUR8 hybridization to monomer, dimer, and partially restricted BLUR8 (pBR322-Alu) probe. MWS: Labeled DNA markers of indicated size. As reported, the primary transfectants contain a large amount of human DNA sequences containing the Alu sequence, whereas the mouse genome does not contain sequences hybridizing with the BLUR8 probe.

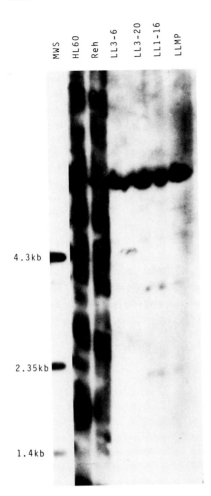

FIGURE 4. Detection of human DNA in secondary lymphocyte transfectants by Southern blot analysis. DNA from primary lymphocyte transfectants was used to produce secondary lymphocyte transfectants. DNA was extracted, treated with BamHI endonuclease, and run on an agarose gel (5 μg/slot). Human DNA was detected on the Southern blot with the cloned Alu probe. Each of the secondary transfectant clones contains the same human DNA sequence. LL3 clones were derived from transfection with one primary transfectant and LLI and LLMP form another primary transfectant.

antigens that are altered so as to make them antigenic. There will also be a response against any transplantation antigens present on the recipient mouse cells but not on the strain immunized. This is particularly relevant to the case of NIH/3T3 cells, which were not derived from an inbred strain of mice. Second, other separation methods, such as 2D electrophoresis, may be used to detect gene products in the transfectants that are not present, or are present in altered amounts compared to the recipient cells, and antibodies may then be made against these proteins by immunizing with the molecules extracted from the gel on which they are identified. Analogous to this second approach would be the production of conventional antisera against the transfectants followed by immunoprecitation of extracts from the transfectants and from the mouse cells used as recipients. This type of general screening of antigens has the advantage of possibly detecting a variety of antigenic differences. Monoclonal antibodies could then be made against each of the molecules showing variation in the transfectants.

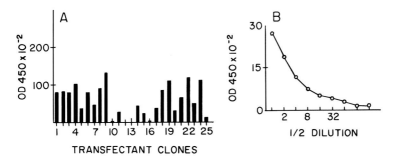

FIGURE 5. Detection of immunoglobulins secreted by lymphocyte transfectants. Supernatants from transfectants were incubated with human cells bound to microtiter plates. After washing, mouse immunoglobulin bound was detected with goat anti-mouse immunoglobulin conjugated with peroxidase. Orthophenylenediamine was used as a substrate and the OD_{450} was read on a multiscan spectrophotometer. (A) Assay of antibody produced by individual clones of transfectants. (B) Titration of the antibody in the supernatant of a dense culture of transfectant 16-21L.

There are some properties of retroviral oncogene products that should be taken into consideration when the immunization and screening protocols are designed for these attempts at antibody production. The first is that many of the products of these oncogenes are apparently present in the interior of the cell and so one should include in the assays either cell extracts or permeablized cells as targets. Also, if the difference between an oncogenic product and a nononcogenic gene product shows a high degree of conservation across species, the oncogene products may have minimal antigenicity with standard immunization protocols. It may also be significant that in most cases where the production of antisera against oncogene products has been reported, they were obtained from animals bearing tumors produced by transformation of cells by the oncogenic virus rather than by immunization of the animals with cell extracts. With these factors in mind we will present here our initial results on the production of monoclonal antibodies against oncogene-related gene products.

TABLE III

*Class of Mouse Antibody Secreted by
Transfectants as Assayed by Immunodiffusion[a]*

Transfectant	Class of Ig chains secreted
16-50L	μ, κ
16-54L	μ, $\gamma 1$, κ
16-21L	μ, κ
16-91L	$\gamma 1$, κ

[a]Note that supernatants showing more than one heavy-chain class were from cultures of uncloned transfectants.

1. *Monoclonal Antibodies against Transfectants*

For our initial experiments on the production of monoclonal antibodies against transfectants, we chose to use a transfectant cell line that was derived by transfecting NIH/3T3 fibroblasts with DNA from a primary lymphocyte transfectant. This lymphocyte transfectant was one of those described above that were obtained by transfecting spleen cells from an immunized mouse with DNA from the human lymphoblastic cell line Reh. In several initial experiments in which transfectant cells were injected into BALB/c mice and monoclonal antibodies produced, none of the hundreds of antibodies screened showed any specificity for the transfectant cells. We then decided to inject live transfectant cells subcutaneously into the mice and wait for a tumor to form. In the first mouse from which hybridomas were derived using this procedure only 30 hybridomas were obtained. Eleven of these antibodies reacted with the transfectants and with Reh (the cells from which the transfecting DNA was initially obtained), but showed only minimal binding with the NIH/3T3 cells. Screening of these antibodies against neuroblastoma cells and human fibroblasts showed a variety of reaction patterns (Figure 6). Each of these antibodies, which detect an antigen expressed

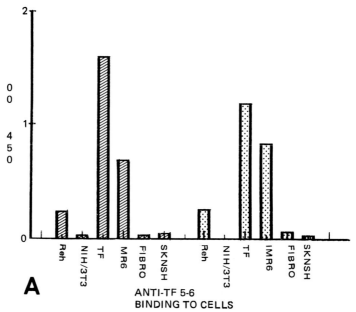

A   ANTI-TF 5-6
                         BINDING TO CELLS

FIGURE 6. Binding of antitransfectant monoclonal antibodies to NIH/3T3 and to human cells as detected by an enzyme-linked antibody assay (Kennett, 1980). Monoclonal antibodies were produced by fusing spleen cells, from a mouse bearing transfected cells growing as a tumor, to the plasmacytoma cell line SP2/o-Ag14. Antibodies were screened initially for binding the Reh, the human leukemia cell line used as the source of DNA for producing the transfectants. Those that bound to these cells were screened against NIH/3T3. Those antibodies binding to Reh and the transfectants (TF) but not to NIH/3T3 were tested for binding to other human cells: IMR6 and SKNSH are human neuroblastoma cell lines, FIBRO are human diploid fibroblasts. Each graph shows the binding of two of the antibodies to the cells. (A) Antibodies 5 and 6; (B) antibodies 7 and 9; (C) control antibodies PI153/3 (antineuroblastoma antibody that also binds to some leukemia cells,

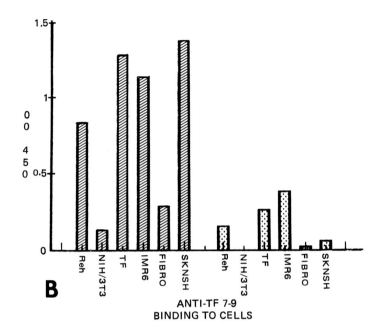

B

ANTI-TF 7-9
BINDING TO CELLS

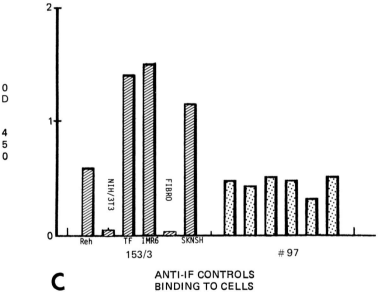

C

ANTI-IF CONTROLS
BINDING TO CELLS

including Reh) and #97 (a monoclonal antibody that binds to all mouse, rat, and human cells tested). These initial experiments indicate that it is possible, using the techniques of immunizing mice with mouse cells transfected with human tumor DNA, to produce monoclonal antibodies reacting with the transfectants and with human tumors but not with the mouse cells used as recipients of the tumor DNA. Note that the neuroblastoma cell lines IMR6 and SKNSH are different in one respect: DNA from SKNSH produces foci when transfected into NIH/3T3, whereas IMR6 (a clone of IMR32) does not produce a significant number of foci (Perucho *et al.*, 1981). The transfectant used in this experiment was derived by transfecting lymphocytes with Reh DNA and then producing secondary NIH/3T3 transfectants.

on the transfectants but not on NIH/3T3, is potentially useful for isolating an antigen that could possibly be related to the molecular changes taking place as NIH/3T3 is transformed to malignancy.

2. Production of Monoclonal Antibodies against Oncogene-Related Products Using In Vitro Immunization

We decided to produce monoclonal antibodies against the *myc* protein in order to determine the appropriate conditions for producing similar reagents against specific molecules that by other criteria, such as detection by standard antisera or 2D electrophoresis, may be oncogene-related. Although the v-*myc* and the c-*myc* genes from various species have been cloned and each characterized to some extent, attempts to isolate and to determine the cellular localization of the *myc* gene product have had to depend on the use of relatively indirect methods. Monoclonal antibodies against the *gag* portion of the *gag–myc* protein have been used to demonstrate that this fusion protein, produced by the combination of a portion of the viral protein *gag* and the *myc* oncogene, is localized in the nucleus in cells transformed with the myelocytomatosis virus MC29 (Abrams *et al.*, 1982). Donner *et al.*, 1982), using similar methods, again with anti-*gag* antibodies, demonstrated that the *gag–myc* protein binds DNA.

Although this type of information is useful and implies that the *myc* protein may play a significant role in some function within the nucleus, the use of the anti-*gag* antibodies does not make it possible to analyze the normal c-*myc* product. If anti-v-*myc* antibodies were available, on the other hand, the high degree of homology between the v-*myc* and the c-*myc* genes of various species makes it likely that some of the antibodies would cross-react with several of the *myc* products—both viral and those of various species—and would therefore be very useful reagents.

We began with the rationale that *in vitro* immunization would allow us to make antibodies against a relatively small quantity of protein, and also that possibly the mechanisms of tolerance that limit the *in vivo* response to a conserved protein such as *myc* would be relaxed *in vitro*. The procedure we used will be published in detail elsewhere (Ikegaki and Kennett, 1983), but was essentially the following. We obtained an anti-p19 monoclonal antibody from the laboratory of Dr. David Boettiger. Antibody was added to the Q8 cells (a nonproducing quail cell line transformed by MC29 virus) along with Sepharose beads conjugated with protein A and a rabbit anti-mouse κ antiserum. This mixture, which, in effect, produced a complex of beads coated with the antibodies and the *gag–myc* protein, was washed and added to the *in vitro* immunization mixture as described in the Appendix of this volume (Jonak and Kennett, 1983a). The monoclonal antibodies produced from these *in vitro*-stimulated cells were screened against Q8 nuclei and HL-60 nuclei for positive selection and against Rous sarcoma virus (RSV) for negative selection. HL-60 is a human leukemia cell line that has elevated expression of the *myc* gene (Favera *et al.*, 1982). Seven antibodies that reacted with the nuclei but not the virus (and therefore were not reacting with viral structural protein) were cloned and characterized. Figure 7

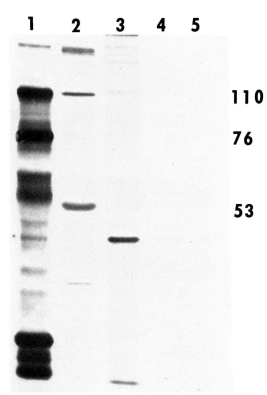

FIGURE 7. Immunoprecipitation of [³⁵S]methionine-labeled proteins from chick embryo fibroblasts infected with MC29 (RAV-61). Chick embryo fibroblasts were labeled for 4 hr with 150 Ci [³⁵S]methionine/ml, then subjected to immunoprecipitation with anti-p19 (lane 1), I-106-1 (lane 2), I-142-1 (lane 3), I-34-1 (lane 4), and P3 (lane 5). Anti-p19 monoclonal antibody precipitates the p110K *gag–myc* fusion protein as well as the *gag* precursor protein Pr76 and its processed products (brackets) synthesized by the helper virus. Monoclonal antibodies I-106-1 and I-142-1 precipitate the p110K protein but not Pr76. They also precipitate a protein with a molecular weight of 53,000 daltons, which could be either the processed p110K fusion protein or the cellular *myc* gene product. A monoclonal antibody, I-34-1, reacts in Western immunoblotting to a 51,000-dalton protein but is not effective in immunoprecipitating the corresponding 53,000-dalton protein. The antibodies I-106-1 and I-142-1 react in both assays. P3 is the supernatant from the plasmacytoma cell line P3/X63-Ag8 (γ₁k).

shows that when two of these antibodies are used to immunoprecipitate extracts of Q8 cells and quail cells infected with MC29 and a helper virus, they precipitate the *gag–myc* fusion protein p110 and a protein with an approximate molecular weight of 53,000, but do not react with the *gag*-related proteins p19 and Pr76. Each of the antibodies reacts with a band of approximately 51,000 mol. wt. in an immunoblot assay and shows bright immunofluorescence on the nuclei of Q8 cells.

We are currently analyzing the 53,000-dalton protein, which is likely to be either the processed product of the p110 fusion protein or the cellular *myc* gene product. For further analysis of the nature of the *myc* gene products, we need more detailed information concerning the properties of these anti-*myc* antibodies. Again the molecular cloning technology will provide an appropriate approach. Since the cloned *myc* genes, including the v-*myc*, human c-*myc* cDNA, and murine c-*myc* cDNA clones, are available, we will be able to construct a vector composed of a strong bacterial promoter and the *myc* gene sequence. This will allow expression of the *myc* products in large quantities. Similar vectors in which only part of the gene is expressed, i.e., one of the exons, can also be constructed. Using such serial expression vectors and the monoclonal antibodies, we will be able to determine the location of each of the epitopes detected by the monoclonal antibodies. By relating the epitope mapping data with the ability of the monoclonal antibodies to inhibit particular functions of the *myc* protein, such as DNA binding, we should be able to obtain information on the structure–function relationships of the *myc* gene product. This approach is now underway.

The above procedure demonstrates that even when only a small amount of protein can be obtained, and when the "antigen" may be very similar in structure to a mouse protein, use of the *in vitro* immunization protocol and the proper screening assay can make it possible to obtain monoclonal antibodies with high enough affinity to immunoprecipitate and to analyze the desired antigen.

V. Summary and Discussion

A. Some General Conclusions

We have attempted here to discuss and illustrate several points concerning the relationships between monoclonal antibody and molecular genetic techniques:

1. The two technologies provide complementary information on the structure and function of biological macromolecules.
2. Monoclonal antibodies have made it possible to analyze the antigenic structure of a variety of molecules on an epitope-by-epitope basis.
3. As the two techniques continue to be used together they will provide significant information on the structure and function of genes and gene products, and we can see by some recent developments that the two technologies will together make it possible to manipulate and analyze genes and their products in ways that would not be possible without combining these technologies.
4. Specifically related to our own interests, these two aspects of current biotechnology will make it possible to understand the molecular events that take place during oncogenic transformation and to isolate gene products that play some role in the molecular mechanisms of oncogenesis.

B. Transfection and Continuous Cell Lines

Our initial results on the transfection of primary mouse lymphocytes are an example of how combining current technologies to approach a basic question can lead to unexpected results with interesting implications. As we stated above, our original purpose was to introduce oncogenes from human tumors into a recipient cell type other than fibroblasts. Because of our interest in leukemias and our experience with hybridoma technology, our first choice was to use stimulated mouse spleen cells as recipients for the human DNA obtained from leukemia cells. Our initial hypothesis, that if transfectants grew, some of them might be making monoclonal antibodies against the antigen with which the mouse was immunized, was based on observations of the hybridoma system in conjunction with our understanding of the mechanism of viral infection and the possible relationship between cellular DNA replication and viral transformation.

Our results thus far indicate that DNA from the human leukemia cell line Reh transfected into stimulated spleen cells does induce proliferation of cells, which can be maintained in continuous culture. We have maintained four of the cell lines from our original lymphocyte transfection in culture for about 1 year. The cells have a normal number of acrocentric chromosomes (40) and this number has been maintained for the extended culture period. Even in the one line that we have passaged through a BALB/c mouse the cells obtained from the mouse have still maintained the some chromosome number. Each of these four original transfectant cell lines as well as several others that we have obtained from other primary and secondary transfection experiments produce immunoglobulin in amounts comparable to standard hybridoma cell lines. Transfectants passaged through mice continue to produce antibody with this specific binding activity.

The growth characteristics of the cell in culture and their apparently normal karyotype suggest that the transfected cells may be at a different stage of transformation than the plasma cell tumors normally grown in culture. The cell density of the transfectants can be decreased to the point where there are only a few cells per microwell without any obvious detrimental effects, except that a long lag period ensues followed by the resumption of growth. This lag period can be reduced by adding supernatant from short-term cultures of mouse spleen cells. The cells behave as if they may be producing a growth factor that that they themselves require. This is consistent with the suggestion that some early stages of leukemias may be cells that are stimulated by growth factors that they produce themselves. This suggests the possibility that these transfected cells may be a useful model system for studying the *in vitro* evolution of leukemic cells from a proliferative preleukemic state.

It is possible that the proliferating lymphocytes produced by transfection of stimulated spleen cells are comparable to the normal NIH/3T3 fibroblast line prior to its transfection with the oncogenes that have to this point been characterized as members of the *ras* family of retroviral oncogenes. This would imply that transfection of these proliferating lymphocytes with a second oncogenic sequence, perhaps one with a function complementary to the one that provides the lymphocytes with their proliferative capacity, would take these cells another step toward being a more malignant lymphoid tumor. If the model we have developed is correct, we would expect these cells to be independent of growth factors or to be producing excess amounts of the same growth factors. The karyotype would perhaps be heteroploid and the cells more malignant in terms of the number of cells needed to efficiently induce a tumor in syngeneic mice. We are currently carrying out studies based on this model as well as using the cells in an attempt to define gene products that are altered, or new products in the transfectants compared to the normal mouse spleen cells or spleen cells stimulated with mitogens.

The ability to induce cell proliferation and produce mouse lymphocyte cell lines synthesizing significant amounts of specific antibody was not previously possible without cell fusion. This has worked well for the mouse or rat systems in which there are plasmacytoma cell lines that can be used as efficient fusion partners. Some progress has been made with the human system, but it is still not clear that there is a human cell line that will be as effective a fusion partner as have the mouse and rat plasmacytomas. In fact, most of the lymphoblastoid lines used in human fusions do not produce as much immunoglobulin as the mouse cell lines. There are also many other species of animals, particularly those of economic value, for which it would be useful to produce monoclonal antibodies and other cell-specific products, such as lymphokines, but for which there are no parental cell lines to be used for hybridizations. It is possible that transfection of stimulated lymphocytes from these species will either provide continuous cell lines making specific monoclonal antibodies or alternatively provide a way to make a perental cell line that in turn can be used in hybridoma formation.

Finally, it is possible that by using procedures similar to those that we have described for lymphocytes it may be possible to produce cell lines from other differentiated tissues. These cells may then be used to produce specific differentiated products, such as hormones or growth factors. Alternatively, they may be used as cell lines for fusion and production of hybrid cell lines making such factors, or may be valuable sources of specific mRNA for these factors so that the corresponding genes may be cloned and the products may be produced in bacteria or yeast. Whether any or all of the possibilities mentioned in this chapter become realities may depend, as we have seen, on the degree to which a large number of investigators are able to combine their efforts and their expertise in a cooperative effort to understand and utilize the various biological systems available to us. Certainly there are many unforeseen possibilities that are present but will remain unrealized until various disciplines and techniques are brought together for one reason or another in the future.

ACKNOWLEDGMENTS

We would like to thank Virginia Braman, Lakshmi Kucherlapati, Barbara Meyer, and Sue Newberry for their excellent technical help. Thanks to Karen Flaherty for her excellent typing and continued patience. Our own work referred to and included here was supported by the following PHS grants: CA 24263, CA 14489, and GM 20138.

References

Abrams, H. D., Rohrschneider, L. R., and Eisenman, R. N., 1982, Nuclear location of the putative transforming protein of avian myelocytomatosis virus, *Cell* **29**:427–439.

Atherton, B. T., Taylor, D. M., and Hynes, R. O., 1981, Structural analysis of fibronectin with monoclonal antibodies, *J. Supramol. Struct. Cell. Biochem.* **17**:153–161.

Barbosa, J. A., Kamarck, M. E., Biro, P. A., Weissman, S. M., and Ruddle, F. H., 1982, Identification of human genomic clones coding the major histocompatibility antigens HLA-A2 and HLA-B7 by DNA-mediated gene transfer, *Proc. Natl. Acad. Sci. USA* **79:**6327–6331.

Becker, D., Lane, M., and Cooper, G. M., 1982, Identification of an antigen associated with the transforming genes of human and mouse mammary carcinomas, *Proc. Natl. Acad. Sci. USA* **79:**3315–3319.

Berzofsky, J. A., Hicks, G., Fedorko, J., and Minna, J., 1980, Properties of monoclonal antibodies specific for determinants of a protein antigen, myoglobin, *J. Biol. Chem.* **255:**11188–11191.

Berzofsky, J. A., Buckenmeyer, G. K., Hicks, G., Gurd, F. R. N., Feldmann, R. J., and Minna, J., 1982, Topographic antigenic determinants recognized by monoclonal antibodies to sperm whale myoglobin, *J. Biol. Chem.* **257:**3189–3198.

Binetruy, B., Meneguzzi, G., Breathnach, R., and Cuzin, F., 1982, Recombinant DNA molecules comprising bovine papilloma virus type 1 DNA linked to plasmid DNA are maintained in a plasmidial state both in rodent fibroblasts and in bacterial cells, *EMBO (Eur. Mol. Biol. Org.) J.* **1:**621–628.

Bishop, J. M., 1983, Cellular oncogenes and retroviruses, *Annu. Rev. Biochem.* **52:**301–354.

Broome, S., and Gilbert, W., 1978, Immunological screening method to detect specific translation products, *Proc. Natl. Acad. Sci. USA* **75:**2746–2749.

Chang, L. J.-A., Gamble, C. L., Izaquirre, M. D., Minden, M. D., Mak, T. W., and McCulloch, E. A., 1982, Detection of genes coding for human differentiation markers by their transient expression after DNA transfer, *Proc. Natl. Acad. Sci. USA* **79:**146–150.

Clevinger, B., Schilling, J., Griffith, R., Hansburg, D., Hood, L., and Davie, J., 1980, Antibody diversity patterns and structure of idiotypic determinants on murine anti-α-(1 → 3) dextran antibodies, in: *Monoclonal Antibodies. Hybridomas: A New Dimension in Biological Analyses.* (R. H. Kennett, T. J. McKearn, and K. B. Bechtol, eds.), Plenum Press, New York, pp. 37–48.

Cline, M. J., Stang, H., Mercola, K., Morse, L., Ruprecht, R., Browne, J., and Salser, W., 1980, Gene transfer in intact animals, *Nature* **284:**422–425.

Denis, K., Kennett, R. H., Klinman, N., Molinaro, C., and Sherman, L., 1980, Defining the B-cell repertoire with hybridomas derived from monoclonal fragment cultures, in: *Monoclonal Antibodies. Hybridomas: A New Dimension in Biological Analyses* (R. H. Kennett, T. J. McKearn, and K. B. Bechtol, eds.), Plenum Press, New York, pp. 49–59.

Der, C. J., Krontiris, T. G., and Cooper, G. M., 1982, Transforming genes of human bladder and lung carcinoma cell lines are homologous to the *ras* genes of Harvey and Kirsten sarcoma viruses, *Proc. Natl. Acad. Sci. USA* **79:**3637–3640.

DiMaio, D., Treisman, R., and Maniatis, T., 1982, Bovine papilloma virus vector that propagates as a plasmid in both mouse and bacterial cells, *Proc. Natl. Acad. Sci. USA* **79:**4030–4034.

Donner, P., Grieser-Wilke, I. and Moelling, K., 1982, Nuclear localization and DNA binding of the transforming gene product of avian myelocytomatosis virus, *Nature* **296:**262–266.

Durban, E. M., and Boettiger, D., 1981, Differential effects of transforming avian RNA tumor virus on avian macrophages, *Proc. Natl. Acad. Sci. USA* **78:**3600–3604.

Eager, K., and Kennett, R. H., 1980, Analysis of alpha-2-macroglobulin with monoclonal antibodies, *Am. J. Hum. Genet.* **32:**153A.

Eilat, D., Asofsky, R., and Laskov, R., 1980, A hybridoma from an autoimmune NZB/NZW mouse producing monoclonal antibody to ribosomal-RNA, *J. Immunol.* **124:**766–768.

Favera, R. D., Wong-Staal, F., and Gallo, R. C., 1982, *onc* gene amplification in promyelocytic leukemia cell line HL-60 and primary leukemic cells of the same patient, *Nature* **299:**61–63.

Furth, M. E., Davis, L. J., Fleurdelys, B. and Scolnick, E. M., 1982, Monoclonal antibodies to the p21 products of the transforming gene of Harvey sarcoma virus and of the cellular *ras* gene family, *J. Virol.* **43:**294–304.

Gerhard, W., Yewdell, J., Frankel, M. E., Lopes, A. D., and Staudt, L., 1980, Monoclonal antibodies against influenza virus, in: *Monoclonal Antibodies. Hybridomas: A New Dimension in Biological Analyses* (R. H. Kennett, T. J. McKearn, and K. B. Bechtol, eds.), Plenum Press, New York, pp. 317–333.

Graham, F. L., and van der Eb, A. J., 1973a, A new technique for the assay of infectivity of human adenovirus DNA, *Virology* **52:**456–467.

Graham, F. L., and van der Eb, A. J., 1973b, Transforming of rat cells by DNA of human adenovirus 5, *Virology* **54:**536–539.

Gratzner, H. G., 1982, Monoclonal antibody to 5-bromodeoxyuridine and 5-iododeoxyuridine: A new reagent for detection of DNA replication, Science 218:474–475.

Haugen, A., Groopman, J. D., Hsu, I.-C., Goodrich, G. R., Wogan, G. N., and Harris, C. C., 1981, Monoclonal antibody to aflatoxin B_1-modified DNA detected by enzyme immunoassay, Proc. Natl. Acad. Sci. USA 78:4124–4127.

Hoffman-Falk, H., Einat, P., Shilo, B.-Z. and Hoffman, F. M., 1983, Drosophila melanogaster DNA clones homologous to vertebrate oncogenes: Evidence for a common ancestor to the src and abl cellular genes, Cell 32:589–598.

Hopkins, N., Besmer, P., DeLeo, A. B., and Law, L. W., 1981, High frequency co-transfer of the transformed phenotype and a tumor-specific transplantation antigen by DNA for the 3-methylcholanthrene-induced Meth A sarcoma of BALB/c mice, Proc. Natl. Acad. Sci. USA 78:7555–7559.

Ikegaki, N., and Kennett, R. H., 1983, Monoclonal antibodies against the myc oncogene product produced by in vitro immunization, in preparation.

Jelinek, W. R., Toomey, T. P., Leinwand, L., Duncan, C. H., Biro, P. A., Choudary, P. V., Weissman, S. M., Rubin, C. M., Houck, C. M. Deininger, P. L., and Schmid, C. W., 1980, Ubiquitous, interspersed repeated sequences in mammalian genomes, Proc. Natl. Acad. Sci. USA 77:1398–1402.

Jonak, Z. L., Smith, A. A., Glick, M. C., Feder, M., and Kennett, R. H., 1983a, Wandering around the cell surface: Monoclonal antibodies against human neuroblastoma and leukemia cell surface antigens, in: Hybridomas and Cellular Immortality (J. P. Allison and B. H. Tom, eds.), Plenum Press, New York.

Jonak, Z. L., Braman, V., and Kennett, R. H., 1983b, Production of continuous mouse plasma cell lines by transfection with human leukemia DNA, Hybridoma, in press.

Kavathas, P., and Herzenberg, L. A., 1983, Stable transformation of mouse L cells for human membrane T-cell differentiation antigens, HLA and β_2-microglobulin: Selection by fluorescence-activated cell sorting, Proc. Natl. Acad. Sci. USA 80:524–528.

Kennett, R. H., 1980, Enzyme linked antibody assay with cells attached to polyvinyl chloride plates, in: Monoclonal Antibodies. Hybridomas: A New Dimension in Biological Analyses (R. H. Kennett, T. J. McKearn, and K. B. Bechtol, eds.), Plenum Press, New York, pp. 376–377.

Kennett, R. H., 1981, Hybridomas: A new dimension in biological analyses, In Vitro 17:1036–1049.

Kennett, R. H., and Gilbert, F., 1979, Hybrid myelomas producing antibodies against a human neuroblastoma antigen present on fetal brain, Science 203:1120–1121.

Kennett, R. H., Denis, K. A., Tung, A. S., and Klinman, N. R., 1978, Hybrid plasmacytoma production. Fusions with adult spleen cells, monoclonal spleen fragments, neonatal spleen cells, and human spleen cells, Curr. Top. Microbiol. Immunol. 81:77–94.

Kennett, R. H., Jonak, Z. L., Bechtol, K. B., and Byrd, R., 1981, Monoclonal antibodies as probes for cell surface changes in malignancy, in: Fundamental Mechanisms in Human Cancer Immunology (J. P. Saunders, J. C. Daniels, B. Serrou, C. Rosenfeld, and C. B. Denny, eds.), Elsevier/North-Holland, New York, pp. 332–348.

Kennett, R. H., Eager, K. B., Meyer, B., Braman, V., Newberry, S., and Buck, D. W., 1982a, Monoclonal antibodies in the analysis of the molecular basis of human genetic diseases, in: From Gene to Protein: Translation into Biotechnology (F. Ahmad, J. Schultz, P. E. Smith, and W. J. Whalen, eds.), Academic Press, New York, pp. 143–164.

Kennett, R. H., Jonak, Z. L., Momoi, M., Glick, M. C., and Lampson, L. A., 1982b, Analysis of cell surface molecules on human neuroblastoma cells and leukemia cells, in: Monoclonal Antibodies in Drug Development (T. August, ed.), American Society for Pharmacology and Experimental Therapeutics, Bethesda, Maryland, pp. 91–107.

Klausner, A., 1983, Monoclonals from E. coli, Biotechnology 1:396–397.

Klotz, J. L., Phillips, M. L., Miller, M. M., and Teplitz, R. L., 1981, Monoclonal autoantibody production by hybrid cell lines, Clin. Immunol. Immunopathol. 18:368–374.

Koteliansky, V. E., Arsenyeva, E. L., Bogacheva, G. T., Chernousov, M. A., Glukhova, M. A., Ibraghimov, A. R., Metsis, M. L., Petrosyan, M. N., and Rokhlin, O. V., 1982, Identification of the species-specific antigenic -eterminant(s) of human plasma fibronectin by monoclonal antibodies, FEBS Lett. 142:199–202.

Krontiris, T. G., and Cooper, G. M., 1981, Transforming activity in human tumor DNAs, *Proc. Natl. Acad. Sci. USA* **78:**1181–1184.

Kucherlapati, R., 1982, Introduction and expression of foreign DNA sequences in mammalian cells, in: *Advances in Cell Culture* (K. Maramorsch, ed.), Academic Press, New York, pp. 69–98.

Lane, D., and Koprowski, H., 1982, Molecular recognition and the future of monoclonal antibodies, *Nature* **296:**200–202.

Lane, M., Sainten, A., and Cooper, G. M., 1981, Activation of related transforming genes in mouse and human mammary carcinomas, *Proc. Natl. Acad. Sci. USA* **78:**5185–5189.

Lane, M., Sainten, A., and Cooper, G. M., 1982, Stage-specific transforming genes of human and mouse B- and T-lymphocyte neoplasms, *Cell* **28:**873–880.

Laver, W. G., Air, G. M., Webster, R. G., Gerhard, W., Ward, C. W., and Dopheide, T. A., 1979, Antigenic drift in type A influenza virus sequence differences in the hemagglutinin of Hong Kong (H3N2) variants selected with monoclonal antibodies, *Virology* **98:**226–237.

Leder, P., Hieter, P. A., Hollis, G. F., and Leder, A., 1982, Moving genes: Promises kept and pending, in: *From Gene to Protein: Translation into Biotechnology*, Miami Winter Symposium, Volume 19 (F. Ahmed, J. Schultz, E. E. Smith, and W. J. Whalen, eds.), Academic Press, New York, pp. 27–42.

Littlefield, J. W., 1976, *Variation, Sonescence, and Neoplasia in Cultured Somatic Cells*, Harvard University Press, Cambridge.

Littlefield, J. W., 1982, NIH/3T3 cell line, *Science* **218:**215–216.

Luben, R. A., and Mohler, M. A., 1980, *In vitro* immunization as an adjunct to the production of hybridomas producing antibodies against the lymphokine osteoclast activating factor, *Mol. Immunol.* **17:**635–639.

Maniatis, T., Fritsch, E. F., and Sambrook, J., 1982, *Molecular Cloning: A Laboratory Manual*, Cold Spring Harbor Laboratory, Cold Spring Harbor, New York.

Marynen, P., VanLeuven, F., Cassiman, J.-J., and Van Den Berghe, H., 1981, A monoclonal antibody to a neo-antigen on α_2-macroglobulin complexes inhibits receptor-mediated endocytosis, *J. Immunol.* **127:**1782–1786.

Müller, R., Slamon, D. J., Tremblay, J. M., Cline, M. J., and Verma, J. M., 1982, Differential expression of cellular oncogenes during pre- and postnatal development of the mouse, *Nature* **299:**640–644.

Niman, H. L., and Elder, J. H., 1982, mAbs as probes of protein structure: Molecular diversity among the envelope glycoproteins (gp 70s) of the murine retroviruses, in: *Monoclonal Antibodies and T-Cell Products* (D. H. Katz, ed.), CRC Press, Boca Raton, Florida, pp. 23–51.

Nordheim, A., Pardue, M. L., Lafer, E. M., Moller, A., Stoller, B. D., and Rich, A., 1981, Antibodies to left-handed Z-DNA bind to interband regions of *Drosophila* polytene chromosomes, *Nature* **294:**417–422.

Padhy, L. C., Shih, C., Cowing, D., Finkelstein, R., and Weinberg, R. A., 1982, Identification of a phosphoprotein specifically induced by the transforming DNA of rat neuroblastomas, *Cell* **28:**865–871.

Parada, L. F., Tabin, C. J., Shih, C., and Weinberg, R. A., 1982, Human EJ bladder carcinoma oncogene is homologous of Harvey sarcoma virus *ras* gene, *Nature* **297:**474–478.

Pavlakis, G. N., and Hamer, D. H., 1983, Regulation of metallothionein–growth hormone hybrid gene in bovine papilloma virus, *Proc. Natl. Acad. Sci. USA* **80:**397–401.

Pellicer, A., Robins, D., Wold, B., Sweet, R., Jackson, J., Lowy, I., Roberts, J. M., Sim, G. K., Silverstein, S., and Axel, R., 1980, Altering genotype and phenotype by DNA-mediated gene transfer, *Science* **209:**1414–1422.

Perucho, M., Goldfarb, M., Shimizu, K., Loma, C., Fogh, C., and Wigler, M., 1981, Human tumor-derived cell lines contain common and different transforming genes, *Cell* **27:**467–476.

Peterson, B. M., Roberts, B. E., and Kuff, E. L., 1977, Structural gene identification and mapping by DNA–mRNA hybrid arrested cell-free translation, *Proc. Natl. Acad. Sci. USA* **74:**4370–4374.

Pierschbacher, M. D., Hayman, E. G., and Rouslahti, E., 1981, Location of the cell-attachment site in fibronectin with monoclonal antibodies and proteolytic fragments of the molecule, *Cell* **26:**259–267.

Ploegh, H. L., Cannon, L. E., and Strominger, J. L., 1979, Cell-free translation of the mRNAs for the heavy and light chains of HLA-A and HLA-B antigens, *Proc. Natl. Acad. Sci. USA* **76:**2273–2277.

340										ROGER H. KENNETT *ET AL.*

Rajan, T. V., 1980, H-2 antigen variants on a cultured heterozygous mouse leukemia cell line. VII. Effect of selection with hybridoma antibody, *Immunogenetics* **10:**423–431.

Rauch, J., Schwartz, R. S., and Stollar, B. D., 1982, Applications of hybridoma technology to autoimmunity, in: *Monoclonal Antibodies and T-Cell Products* (D. H. Katz, ed.), CRC Press, Boca Raton, Florida, pp. 91–111.

Reddy, E. P., Reynolds, R. K., Santos, E., and Barbacid, 1982, A point mutation is responsible for the acquisition of transforming properties by the T24 human bladder carcinoma oncogene, *Nature* **300:**149–152.

Ricciardi, R. P., Miller, J. S., and Roberts, B. E., 1979, Purification and mapping of specific mRNAs by hybridization-selection and cell-free translation, *Proc. Natl. Acad. Sci. USA* **76:**4927–4931.

Rosenfeld, C., Goutner, A., Choquet, C., Venuat, A. M., Kayibanda, B., Pico, J. L., and Greaves, J. L., 1977, Phenotypic characterization of a unique non-T, non-B acute lymphoblastic leukemia cell line, *Nature* **267:**841–843.

Rossi, J. J., Kierzek, R., Huang, T., Walker, P., and Itakura, K., 1982, The role of synthetic DNA in the preparation of structural genes for proteins, in: *From Gene to Protein: Translation into Biotechnology,* Miami Winter Symposium, Volume 19 (F. Ahmed, J. Schultz, E. E. Smith, and W. J. Whalen, eds.), Academic Press, New York, pp. 213–234.

Sarver, N., Gruss, P., Law, M.-F., Khoury, G., and Howley, P. M., 1981, Bovine papilloma virus deoxyribonucleic acid: A novel eucaryotic cloning vector, *Mol. Cell. Biol.* **1:**486–496.

Sarver, N., Byrne, J. C., and Howley, P. M., 1982, Transformation and replication in mouse cells of a bovine papilloma virus-pML2 plasmid vector that can be rescued in bacteria, *Proc. Natl. Acad. Sci. USA* **79:**7147–7151.

Sekiguchi, T., Nishimoto, T., Kai, R., and Sekiguchi, M., 1983, Recovery of a hybrid vector, derived from bovine papilloma virus DNA, pBR322 and the HSV tk gene, by bacterial transformation with extra chromosomal DNA from transfected rodent cells, *Gene* **21:**267–272.

Shih, C., Padhy, L. C., Murray, M., and Weinberg, R. A., 1981, Transforming genes of carcinomas and neuroblastomas introduced into mouse fibroblasts, *Nature* **290:**261–264.

Shilo, B., and Weinberg, R. A., 1981, Unique transforming gene in carcinogen-transformed mouse cells, *Nature* **289:**607–609.

Shimizu, K., Goldfarb, M., Suard, Y., Perucho, M., Li, Y., Kamata, T., Feramisco, J., Stavnezer, E., Fogh, J., and Wigler, M. H., 1983, Three human transforming genes are related to the viral *ras* oncogenes, *Proc. Natl. Acad. Sci. USA* **80:**2112–2116.

Smith, B. L., Anisowicz, A., Chodosh, L. A., and Sager, R., 1982, DNA transfer of focus- and tumorforming ability into non-tumorigenic CHEF cells, *Proc. Natl. Acad. Sci. USA* **79:**1964–1968.

Staehelin, T., Hobbs, D. S., Kugn, H., Lai, C. Y., and Pestka, S., 1981, Purification and characterization of recombinant human leukocyte interferon (IFLrA) with monoclonal antibodies, *J. Biol. Chem.* **256:**9750–9754.

Sutcliffe, J. G., Shinnick, T. M., Green, N., Liu, F. T., and Lerner, R. A., 1980, Chemical synthesis of a polypeptide predicted from nucleotide sequence allows detection of a new retroviral gene product, *Nature* **287:**801–805.

Varmus, H. E., Shank, S. E., Hughes, H. J., Kung, S., Majors, J., Vogt, P. K., and Bishop, J. M., 1978, Synthesis, structure and integration of the DNA of RNA tumor viruses, *Cold Spring Harbor Symp. Quant. Biol.* **43:**851–864.

Wang, Y., Stratowa, C., Schaefer-Ridder, M., Doehmer, J., and Hofschneider, P. H., 1983, Enhanced production of hepatitis B surface antigen in NIH/3T3 mouse fibroblasts by using extra chromosomally replicating bovine papilloma virus vector, *Mol. Cell. Biol.* **3:**1032–1039.

Weinberg, R. A., 1981, Use of transfection to analyze genetic information and malignant transformation, *Biochem. Biophys. Acta* **651:**161–169.

Weiss, R., Teich, N., Varmus, H., and Coffin, J. (eds.), 1982, *RNA Tumor Virus,* Cold Spring Harbor Laboratory, Cold Spring Harbor, New York.

Young, R. A., and Davis, R. W., 1983, Efficient isolation of genes by using antibody probes, *Proc. Natl. Acad. Sci. U.S.A.* **80:**1194–1198.

Yuasa, Y., Srivastava, S. K., Dunn, C. Y., Rhim, J. S., Reddy, E. P., and Aaronson, S. A., 1983, Acquisition of transforming properties by alternative point mutations within *c-bas/has* human proto-oncogene, *Nature* **303:**775–779.

13

Functional Murine T-Cell Clones

FRANK W. FITCH AND ANDREW L. GLASEBROOK

I. Introduction

Many important immunological phenomena can be characterized only in operational terms, and this leads often to circular reasoning. For example, antigens are identified and characterized in terms of the biological responses, antibody formation or cell-mediated reactions, that are induced by the antigens. However, antibodies and reactive cells can be identified only on the basis of their reactivity with the immunizing antigen. This rather unsatisfactory situation results in large part from the heterogeneity of cellular and molecular processes that are involved in immune responses as well as the very large number of different kinds of antibodies that can be produced. It is possible to identify and quantify reactions due to rare cells or molecules present at extremely low frequency among other, similar cells and molecules. However, it is difficult to obtain sufficient numbers of specifically reactive cells or antibody molecules to be able to characterize such cells or molecules biochemically or structurally in sufficient detail for independent definition of the basis for their immunological reactivity.

A major advance was made when it was realized that multiple myeloma tumor cells secreted immunoglobulin molecules having the same basic structure as antibody molecules. Since a single kind of immunoglobulin is usually secreted by a given myeloma line, large quantities of a homogeneous antibody-like protein could be obtained for biochemical and structural studies, making it possible to determine the essential features of immunoglobulin composition and struc-

FRANK W. FITCH • Committee on Immunology, Department of Pathology, University of Chicago, Chicago, Illinois 60637.   ANDREW L. GLASEBROOK • Department of Immunology, Swiss Institute for Experimental Cancer Research, Epalinges S./Lausanne, Switzerland CH 1066. Current address for A. L. G.: The Salk Institute, San Diego, California 92138.

ture. Myeloma cells also have facilitated the elegant studies that have characterized the rearrangements of genetic information utilized in immunoglobulin synthesis.

The availability of homogeneous populations of immunoglobulin-producing cells and their products has made it possible to define many of the cellular events and molecules involved in antibody responses in absolute terms without having to resort to operational definitions. Unfortunately, the situation with regard to T-cell responses is not as satisfactory. The participation of T cells in immune responses has been defined mainly in terms of the phenomena that are observed. This is true in large part because homogeneous populations of functional T cells have been unavailable.

However, during the past several years, it has been possible to obtain clonal populations of T cells in quantities that permit analysis of several immunological questions. Several different approaches have been used to obtain such clonal populations: identification or induction of T-cell lymphomas having immunological function, construction of T-cell hybridomas, and derivation of cloned "normal" T cells. Although T-cell lymphomas occasionally retain function, they apparently occur infrequently (Gillis *et al.* 1980b), and the availability of tumors having a given *desired* function is dependent upon chance occurrence. Attempts to induce T lymphomas having a particular function occasionally have been successful (Finn *et al.*, 1979; Ricciardi-Castagnoli *et al.*, 1981). Although T lymphoma cells have limited usefulness for studying cellular interactions, they may be particularly valuable for production of lymphokines (Gillis *et al.*, 1980b; Farrar *et al.*, 1980).

Construction of T-cell hybridomas, using modifications of the fusion technique that has been applied so successfully for obtaining antibody-producing hybridomas, is an alternative approach for obtaining clonal T cells. However, with T-cell hybridomas, the tumor partner may contribute to the observed functional effects in ways that may be difficult to recognize (Pacifico and Capra, 1980; Clark and Capra, 1982). In addition, it should be recognized that identification of particular hybrid cells as the fusion product of two T cells may not always be direct. Some hybridomas formed by fusion of B- and T-cell tumor cell lines have been found to express the Thy-1 antigen of each parent cell (Taussig *et al.*, 1980).

A major limitation is that T-cell hybridomas are susceptible to chromosomal loss, which affects stability of function. Repetitive cloning at frequent intervals may be necessary to maintain functional activity. However, this inherent instability may be exploited in studies attempting to assign a particular phenotypic characteristic to genes present on a given chromosome. Given these limitations, T-cell hybridomas still have been especially useful for analyzing the cytolytic mechanism (Nabholz *et al.*, 1980) and lymphokine secretion (Harwell *et al.*, 1980; Lonai *et al.*, 1981), for production of antigen-specific suppressor factors (Taniguchi and Miller, 1978; Kontiainen *et al.*, 1978; Taussig *et al.*, 1979; Kapp *et al.*, 1980), and for examining properties of the T-cell receptor for antigen (Kappler *et al.*, 1981).

The third approach for obtaining large numbers of uniform functional T lymphocytes is the isolation of clones of "normal" T cells. It is now possible to obtain relatively easily clones of T cells, which can be maintained in culture indefinitely. The essential culture medium component for long-term growth of T lymphocytes is T-cell growth factor (TCGF) (Morgan *et al.*, 1976), more recently designated interleukin 2 (IL 2) (Aarden *et al.*, 1979). Crude conditioned medium from mitogen-stimulated mouse (Watson *et al.*, 1979) or rat (Gillis *et al.*, 1980a) spleen cells, supernatant fluid from secondary mixed leukocyte culture (MLC) (Ryser *et al.* 1978), or supernatant fluid from some T lymphomas (Farrar *et al.* 1980) have been used as sources of IL 2 for deriving and maintaining T-cell clones. Although the relevant biological activity in these different conditioned media has been attributed to IL 2, they all contain other active "factors" as well. Colony-stimulating factor (CSF), interferon, and lymphokines acting on B lymphocytes and macrophages often are also present. These other lymphokines may contribute directly or indirectly to the growth of cloned T cells. For convenience in the subsequent discussion in this chapter, these different preparations used to support proliferation of cloned T cells will be designated IL 2. It should be noted, however, that unless highly purified IL 2 has been used, it is unwarranted to attribute all of the observed effects of a given preparation of conditioned media on T cells to IL 2. In addition, this chapter will deal only with cloned murine T cells, although human T-cell clones also have been derived.

II. Conditions for Cloning T Lymphocytes

Two general techniques have been used to derive T-cell clones, and the technique used may influence the properties of the derived clone. One approach utilizes IL 2 alone. Responding lymphoid cells, often obtained after immunization *in vivo*, are stimulated in culture with the appropriate antigen. They are then subcultured repeatedly at high cell density with IL 2. The frequency of T cells capable of growing in IL 2 alone appears to be low, and usually it is necessary to maintain cells in bulk culture for several months before cloning is possible (Haas *et al.*, 1980). The T cells cultured in IL 2 alone often grow well for about 2 months and then undergo a "crisis" with slowing of the growth rate. When this occurs, the cultures either die or suddenly begin to grow better. The phenotypic characteristics of cells that survive after passage for several months in IL 2 often suggest that they are clonally derived (Haas *et al.*, 1980), but T-cell clones derived and maintained using IL 2 alone may be unstable. Fluctuating levels and patterns of cytolytic activity have been observed with cloned cytolytic T lymphocytes (CTL) obtained in this way (Nabholz *et al.*, 1978). Further, most if not all cloned T cells grown in IL 2 for extended periods have chromosomal abnormalities possibly reflecting a selection and/or generation of a variant that grows in IL 2 alone (Johnson *et al.*, 1982).

The other technique for obtaining cloned T lymphocytes involves repeated stimulation with the appropriate antigen in the presence of "filler" cells and IL 2. For T cells reactive with "conventional" soluble antigens, irradiated syngeneic spleen cells usually are used as a filler cell source. These cells also function as antigen-presenting cells, which are required for T-cell stimulation (Hengartner and Fathman 1980). Filler cells for alloreactive T cells usually consist of irradiated spleen cells bearing the appropriate alloantigens (Glasebrook and Fitch, 1979). In this situation, the stimulating allogeneic spleen cells also are a source of "filler cells." Filler cells/antigen are necessary in order to clone T cells with a high plating efficiency after relatively short exposure to antigen as well as for ease in maintaining cloned T cells in long-term culture (MacDonald *et al.* 1980b; Lutz *et al.*, 1981a). With this technique, alloreactive clones can be derived from primary or secondary MLC with a plating efficiency approaching 100% (MacDonald *et al.* 1980a; Glasebrook *et al.*, 1981b). Adherent cells, probably macrophages, appear to be the essential cell in the filler population. Peritoneal cells and spleen cells depleted of T lymphocytes are fully effective as filler cells (Lutz *et al.*, 1981a). However, it is not clear whether filler cells carry out functions other than presentation of antigen. Cloned T cells maintained in this manner usually are stable and appear to be normal in phenotype and karyotype. The percentage of T-cell clones that can be maintained in long-term culture with antigen/filler cells and IL 2 is very high, and such cells do not appear to undergo a crisis. Filler cells/antigen may function to maintain expression of IL 2 receptors, while cloning and maintenance in IL 2 alone may select for abnormal T cells in which expression of IL 2 receptors is deregulated.

As will be discussed below, several types of cloned T cells can be obtained with this approach. Three different assays have been used to identify antigen-specific reactivity: proliferation of cells after stimulation with antigen, release of lymphokine(s) after stimulation with antigen, or cytolytic activity for target cells bearing the specific antigen. IL 2 may be the primary if not unique signal for T-lymphocyte proliferation, and most cloned T cells die within a short time if IL 2 is not present. Therefore, given the apparent growth requirements for the various kinds of T cell, it may seem to be unnecessary to use IL 2, stimulating antigen, *and* filler cells to maintain all types of clones in long-term culture. Proliferating noncytolytic cells usually can be shown to release IL 2 upon stimulation with antigen, and it would seem to be unnecessary to provide exogenous IL 2 in order to maintain such cells in culture. However, proliferating cloned T cells also can be stimulated to divide by IL 2 alone, and the extent of thymidine incorporation (and presumably cell proliferation) is highly dependent on IL 2 concentration (Glasebrook *et al.*, 1981b). Also, the amount of IL 2 released by such cells after antigen stimulation is related to the concentration of cells in culture (Ely and Fitch, 1983). Thus, at high responding cell density, stimulation with antigen alone may result in production of sufficient IL 2 to achieve the concentration needed for inducing subsequent T-cell proliferation; in this situation, exogenous IL 2 is unnecessary. However, if the density of responding cloned T cells is too low, the concentration of IL 2 released by antigen stimulation may be too low to "rescue" the cloned cells before they die as the result of insufficient IL 2. Thus, some exogenous IL 2 may be needed at low cell density in order to facilitate survival of the cloned cells until sufficient IL 2 for sustained growth is produced.

In the case of CTL, the majority of cloned cells do not produce IL 2 after stimulation with the appropriate alloantigen but are strictly dependent on exogenous IL 2 for growth. Antigenic stimulation, therefore, would seem to be unnecessary for maintaining cloned CTL. However, when cloned CTL are cultured with limiting amounts of IL 2, a synergistic effect is observed when alloantigen is also present (Lutz *et al.*, 1981b). Cloned CTL can produce a variety of lymphokines, including macrophage-activating factor, interferon, and Ia-inducing factor, after antigen stimulation (Glasebrook *et al.*, 1982). These lymphokines, some of which act on macrophages present in the filler population, may indirectly facilitate T-cell proliferation.

Thus, for proliferating, lymphokine-releasing, and cytolytic cloned T cells, the combination of relatively low concentrations of IL 2, antigen, and filler cells appears to provide culture conditions that provide a strong selective force favoring the growth of cells that respond well to the stimulating antigen. This selective pressure probably is useful for maintaining stable characteristics in the cloned cells because there is not selection for the abnormal property of antigen-independent growth. Cloned T cells under optimal conditions divide rapidly, with doubling times frequently in the range of 18–24 hr. Variant cells are certain to develop with prolonged culture. Although variant cells can be useful for certain purposes, unsuspected and unrecognized emergence of variant clones can be troublesome. Recloning every few months and the use of selective culture conditions usually are sufficient for maintaining cloned T lymphocytes having a stable phenotype if IL 2, antigen, and filler cells are used.

The actual cloning can be accomplished by limiting dilution (Glasebrook and Fitch, 1979; MacDonald *et al.*, 1980a), culture in soft agar (Fathman and Hengartner, 1978), or by micromanipulation (Glasebrook 1983; Zagury *et al.*, 1975). A statistical estimate for the likelihood of clonal distribution can be obtained with both limit dilution and soft agar culture methods, but it is not possible to be certain that cells in a given well or colony actually are derived from a single T cell. Repeated cloning by micromanipulation gives the greatest assurance of clonality. If cells display uniform phenotypic characteristics after repetitive cloning, it probably is reasonable to assume that the cells have been clonally derived.

III. Murine T-Cell Clones Reactive with Alloantigen

A. Repertoire of Cytolytic T Cells

Techniques for obtaining clonal growth of CTL have made it possible to analyze the frequency of T cells responding to particular alloantigens, the extent of the cytolytic T cell repertoire, and the range of reactivity of individual T cells. In most experiments designed to estimate the frequency of precursors of CTL (CTL_p), cultures are maintained only for 7 days (Ryser and MacDonald, 1979a,b).

However, it is essential that the culture system be highly efficient in supporting the short-term growth of CTL_p and CTL (MacDonald *et al.*, 1980a,b); optimal conditions include the use of IL2 and stimulating allogeneic spleen cells. These conditions, in which the CTL_p is the only limiting cell, also appear to be optimal for deriving CTL and maintaining them in long-term culture.

Limit dilution analyses generally have confirmed impressions about the relative frequency of CTL_p in various lymphoid cell populations (MacDonald *et al.*, 1980a). In C57BL/6 mice responding to DBA/2 alloantigens, there was a high CTL_p frequency in lymph node (1/68) and peripheral blood (1/180) lymphocytes; the frequency in spleen was lower (1/399), and was lower still among thymocytes (1/1634). The frequency in bone marrow cells (1/2131) probably reflects contamination of bone marrow by peripheral blood (MacDonald *et al.*, 1980a).

However, determination of the clonal frequency using a single type of target cell may not distinguish among different reactivity patterns. For analysis of the extent of the cytolytic T-cell repertoire, it is important to utilize a large array of target cells. For example, early reports suggested that alloreactive cloned CTL had expected patterns of reactivity, lysing only target cells bearing the appropriate alloantigens (Nabholz *et al.*, 1978; Glasebrook and Fitch, 1979). However, as the panel of target cells was expanded, it became clear that CTL clones selected on the basis of cytolytic activity toward target cells from mice of a given haplotype included clones having several different patterns of reactivity. At least seven different patterns of reactivity were observed when nine separate CTL clones derived from secondary C57BL/6 anti-DBA/2 MLC were compared using a panel of 11 different target cells (Glasebrook and Fitch, 1980).

The most discriminating analysis of the repertoire of CTL has been conducted by Sherman (1980, 1982a,b), who has studied the response toward the H-2 alloantigen H-2K^b. This particular antigen was chosen because of the availability of numerous mutant strains that express defined antigenic differences in the H-2K^b molecule (Melief *et al.*, 1977). Cells from these mutant strains can be used to provide the panel of target cells needed to identify CTL clones induced by "wild type" H-2K^b antigen but having different specific reactivities. Extrapolation from results obtained with 43 different clones from seven individual mice led to an estimate of a minimum of 2×10^4 immune T-cell receptor specificities (Sherman, 1980). In later studies, 78 different clones from 28 individual B10.D2 mice sensitized toward B10.A(5R) (H-2K^b) spleen cells were selected on the basis of lytic activity for C57BL/6 (wild-type) target cells. These clones were then assayed on a panel of target cells from seven different H-2K^b mutants; 33 of the 128 possible different receptor specificities were identified (Sherman, 1982a). The repertoire of B10.BR anti-H-2K^b receptor specificities also was highly diverse; 78 different clones from 17 individual mice described a total of 34 different receptor specificities (Sherman, 1982a). However, the frequency of occurrence of some given reactivity patterns seemed not to be distributed randomly. One reactivity pattern (RP 47) appeared in over one-third of B10.D2 mice studied and represented the reactivity of 20% of the anti-H-2K^b-specific clones from this mouse strain. Three reactivity patterns (RP 23, 29, and 87) occurred in CTL clones from B10.BR mice at frequencies of 7.4, 10.4, and 17.9%, respectively; two of these were expressed by over one-third of individual mice (Sherman, 1982a).

The CTL clones from F_1 progeny of these two strains also were diverse in reactivity; 121 different clones from 26 individual mice described 38 reactivity patterns. It is of particular interest, however, that unique specificity patterns were observed. Four reactivity patterns (RP 4, 19, 57, and 60) emerged as uniquely F_1 recurrent specificities (Sherman, 1982a). Analogous results had been obtained in studies of the B-cell repertoire expressed by F_1 hybrid mice (Cancro and Klinman, 1981). The CTL clones derived by Sherman were prepared from mice using responding and stimulating cells from congenic mouse strains having the C57BL/10 genetic background and differing only in the major histocompatibility complex (MHC) region.

Collectively, these data indicate that the antigen receptor of murine cytolytic T lymphocytes is extensive and that MHC-linked genes influence profoundly the frequency of representation of several receptor specificities.

The type of analysis described above usually has been used to determine the extent of the antigen-recognition repertoire for the entire T-cell population. Similar approaches also have been informative in the analysis of the range of reactivity of individual T cells. Sherman (1982c) also has analyzed the specificity of reaction of CTL clones induced in response to antigenic determinants associated with a point mutation in the H-2K^b molecule. In the variant strain B6.C-H-2^{bm11} (bm11), there is a single amino acid substitution at position 77 in the H-2K^b molecule. The cytolytic activity of individual clones from C57BL/6 mouse spleen cells stimulated in MLC with bm11 spleen cells was assayed on target cells from the seven H-2K^b mutant strains. Eighty-three percent of 58 different clones from 11 different mice selected initially for reactivity with bm11 target cells also reacted with target cells from mutant strain bm3, which has amino acid substitutions in positions 77 and 89. The majority of clones (62%) recognized at least one of the other K^b mutants, such as bm8, bm1, and bm9, which are identical to the wild type K^b in position 77 but have amino acid substitutions elsewhere; of these, 24% recognize at least two such H-2K^b mutants. Of particular interest is the finding that about 7% of the clones also reacted with a third-party alloantigen, K^d (Sherman, 1982c). These findings strongly support the hypothesis that conformational alterations in self H-2 antigens can result in immunogenic determinants that do not include the amino acid substitution responsible for the alteration. They also indicate that "cross-reactive" determinants may sometimes be found on allogeneic target cells.

The reactivity patterns of individual T cells also have been studied using cloned CTL directed toward virus-infected or hapten-modified target cells. Such foreign antigenic determinants appear to be recognized by CTL concomitantly with self-alloantigens of the MHC expressed on target cells (Zinkernagel and Doherty, 1979). Some features of this MHC-restricted antigen recognition have been clarified using cloned CTL. The initial description of long-term cultured CTL seemed to indicate that recognition of viral-associated tumor antigens by CTL might not be MHC-restricted (Gillis and Smith, 1977). Two long-term CTL lines, obtained from secondary mixed leukocyte-tumor culture (MLTC), lysed both syngeneic and allogeneic Friend leukemia virus (FLV)-infected target cells. However, one of these long-term cell lines (CTLL-2) was found subsequently to consist of a mixture of cells (Baker *et al.*, 1979). Cloning performed after 14 months of bulk culture in IL 2 yielded clones that had one of four different patterns of cytolytic activity. Some clones preferentially lysed syngeneic FLV-infected tumor target cells, some clones lysed syngeneic FLV-infected tumor target cells as well as allogeneic target cells that did not express FLV-associated antigens, some clones lysed only allogeneic target cells not expressing FLV-associated antigens, and some clones had no lytic activity. The reactivity pattern of the original cell "line" was the sum of those for individual clones (Baker *et al.* 1979). The CTL clones that reacted with syngeneic FLV-infected tumor cells and allogeneic target cells appear to recognize two different antigenic determinants: alloantigen and FLV-associated antigen in the context of self MHC antigen.

Other examples of "dual antigen recognition" by cloned CTL have been described. CTL derived from C57BL/6 lymphoid cells responding to stimulation with Maloney leukemia virus (MoLV)-infected syngeneic cells expressed three reactivity patterns. Some CTL clones were cytolytic only for syngeneic MoLV-derived tumor target cells, some also reacted with allogeneic MoLV-derived tumor target cells, and some were cross-reactive with normal allogeneic cells (A. Weiss *et al.*, 1980). The cytolytic activity of representative clones from each reactivity pattern was inhibited by two different monoclonal anti-H-2D^b antibodies but not by a monoclonal anti-H-2K^b antibody (A. Weiss *et al.*, 1981). For the majority of C57BL/6 CTL clones reactive with MoLV-infected syngeneic target cells, the restriction of the MHC appeared to be in the H-2D^b region; 44 of 51 clones were inhibited by monoclonal anti-H-2D^b antibodies. Regions of the MHC other than H-2D^b or H-2K^b served as restriction elements for three of the remaining seven clones since lytic activity was inhibited by anti-whole H-2^b haplotype antiserum but not by monoclonal anti-H-2D^b or anti-H-2K^b antibodies; restriction elements for the other four clones have not been defined (A. Weiss *et al.*, 1981). Heterogeneity of reactivity patterns also has been observed by Plata (1982) with CTL generated against murine leukemia virus-infected cells. The biological significance of this heterogeneity in receptor repertoire for viral-induced tumor antigens is not clear. It is of interest that five clonal CTL populations isolated from *in vivo* tumors were lytic *only* for MoLV-derived syngeneic target cells (Brunner *et al.*, 1981).

Other examples of cloned CTL that are MHC-restricted in recognition of target cell antigens include those reactive with influenza virus antigen (Lin and Askonas, 1980; Braciale *et al.*, 1981a,b) and with hapten-modified syngeneic cells (Haas *et al.*, 1980; von Boehmer and Haas, 1981). All CTL clones appeared to be restricted in target cell recognition of type A influenza viral antigen by either the H-2K or H-2D region of the appropriate H-2 haplotype (Braciale *et al.*, 1981a). CTL clones of F$_1$ origin were restricted in recognition exclusively to either one or the other of the parental haplotypes (Braciale *et al.*, 1981a); no clones reacting uniquely with F$_1$-infected target cells were observed. These findings are of interest in light of the MHC restriction elements for proliferating, noncytolytic cloned CTL, which are discussed below. "Dual reactivity" also has been observed with virus-reactive CTL. A cloned CTL derived from an (H-2^b × H-2^d) F_1 hybrid mouse exhibited H-2-restricted cytotoxicity for influenza A virus in association with H-$2K^d$ as well as cytotoxicity for H-$2K^k$ alloantigen (Braciale et al., 1981b). The MHC restriction of cytolytic activity for CTL clones reactive with hapten-modified cells often does not appear to be as stringent as that observed with bulk CTL cell populations. Various patterns of reactivity, including cytolytic activity for hapten-modified target cells from several different haplotypes, have been observed with different CTL clones reactive with hapten-modified syngeneic cells (Haas et al., 1980; von Boehmer and Haas, 1981).

Cloned CTL from C57BL/6 female mice that lysed C57BL/6 male target cells (H-Y) also reacted with target cells from male and female mice that bore H-$2D^d$ alloantigen (von Boehmer et al., 1979; von Boehmer and Haas, 1981). These observations have been confirmed in limiting dilution analyses; more than 10% of CTL_p from C57BL/6 female mice that were directed against H-Y target cells also were cytolytic for target cells expressing H-2^d alloantigens (Kanagawa et al., 1982).

Collectively, these results indicate a greater heterogeneity of the antigen-specific CTL repertoire than usually is evident in assays with bulk cell populations. Dual reactivity is frequent and cloned CTL often show unexpected cross-reactivity with apparently unrelated antigens.

B. Alloreactive Proliferating Murine T-Cell Clones

The first alloreactive T-cell clones were derived with cells from strain A mice that had been maintained in vitro by serial restimulation with (C57BL/6 × A) F_1 hybrid spleen cells (Watanabe et al., 1977). One of the reasons for choosing this particular strain combination was the previous observation, made with populations of lymph node cells, which suggested that unique MLC-stimulating determinants existed on cells from F_1 hybrid mice (Fathman and Nabholz, 1977). Proof for such determinants was provided by the observation that some cloned T cells proliferated only when stimulated with F_1 alloantigen. Studies utilizing stimulating cells from congenic and recombinant congenic F_1 mice indicated that the unique stimulating antigenic determinants on F_1 cells were encoded by genes located within the I-A region of the MHC (Fathman and Kimoto, 1981; Fathman and Hengartner, 1979).

Unique F_1 determinants can be produced in this situation since both the α and β chains of the I-A molecular complex are polymorphic, and these particular stimulating determinants appear to be formed as a result of the trans-complementation between I-region gene products of the two parental strains. This situation seems to be different from that involving influenza A virus-specific CTL clones from F_1 mice, which, as noted above, were restricted in recognition exclusively to one of the parental haplotypes; unique F_1 restriction was not observed (Braciale et al., 1981a). In the case of viral-reactive CTL, the restriction elements are specified by either the K or D regions of the MHC; unique F_1 determinants for molecules encoded by genes in these regions are not possible since the β_2-microglobulin component of K and D alloantigen molecular complexes is nonpolymorphic. However, the situation is probably somewhat more complicated than is immediately evident. Cloned T cells that react uniquely with determinants expressed by F_1 stimulating cells appear to include several different specificities since at least three different reactivity patterns can be defined on the basis of inhibition of proliferative responses by anti-Ia antibodies (Beck and Fathman, 1982).

In early studies, CTL clones were found to be dependent on IL 2 for proliferation and did not divide when stimulated with appropriate alloantigen alone. Also, alloreactive proliferating T-cell clones were not cytolytic in either direct or lectin-facilitated cytolytic assays (Glasebrook et al., 1981b). Recent observations, however, indicate that these distinctions in properties are not absolute. The first suggestion that cytolytic T cells might proliferate with alloantigenic stimulation was provided with a T-cell line that had been maintained in culture for 5 years by repetitive stimulation with alloantigen (Dennert and De-Rose, 1976). Proliferation of this cell line, which expressed Lyt-1 but not Lyt-2, was stimulated by Ia^k-positive cells; Ia^k-positive target cells also were lysed by these T cells (Swain et al., 1981). These findings were somewhat suspect when first reported since the T-cell line had not been formally cloned at that time. Widmer and Bach (1981), however, reported that one of seven CTL clones was able to proliferate upon alloantigenic stimulation in the absence of added IL 2. Similar findings have been reported by DiPauli and Opalka (1982), who found that four of seven CTL clones reactive against unknown minor histocopatibility antigens were capable of antigen-dependent proliferation.

Glasebrook (1984) has provided quantitative information about the frequency of helper cell-independent antigen-driven CTL and their properties. His results indicate that such cells are fairly common but also are heterogeneous. In nine independent experiments, a total of 341 short-term CTL clones were derived by micromanipulation after stimulation in vitro or in vivo. Among the total pool of CTL clones derived after stimulation with H-2 and minor loci-incompatible allogeneic spleen cells in vitro, a reproducible frequency of 1/4 CTL clones were observed to proliferate specifically to the stimulating alloantigens in the absence of exogenously added IL 2. However, in vivo or in vitro stimulation with H-2K/D-incompatible allogeneic tumor cells increased the frequency of such antigen-driven CTL clones approximately 2.5-fold to 1/2. In comparison, the frequency of CTL clones able to secrete measurable amounts of IL 2 was always lower, regardless of splenic or tumor cell priming, and constituted a subset among the total pool of antigen-driven CTL. Several representative clones were subcloned and expanded in culture: all demonstrated proliferative and cytolytic specificity for the relevant H-2K/D alloantigens, while IL 2 activity detected in clonal supernatants (antigenic or mitogenic stimulation) was either low or undetectable. All clones analyzed expressed the Lyt-2 marker as judged by flow microfluorometry.

IV. T-Cell Clones Reactive with Soluble Antigens

Recognition of soluble antigen by cloned T cells requires the presence of antigen-presenting cells that bear the appropriate I-region gene products (Fathman *et al.*, 1981). Histocompatibility at the I-A subregion of the MHC for antigen-presenting cells and T cells also was found to be essential for antigen-induced proliferation of cloned T cells reactive with DNP–ovalbumin or with the synthetic random amino acid copolymer GAT (Sredni *et al.*, 1980; Sredni and Schwartz, 1981). GAT-reactive T-cell clones derived from F_1 hybrid mice could be divided into three categories on the basis of the genetic requirements for the antigen-presenting cell: one type responded to antigen only in the presence of F_1 cells, another type responded in the presence of cells from F_1 or from parent "A," and the third type responded in the presence of cells from F_1 or parent "B" (Kimoto and Fathman, 1980; Fathman and Kimoto, 1981). Genetic studies indicated that the relevant unique F_1 hybrid restriction elements for GAT and another synthetic antigen, (TG)-A–L, were formed as a result of *trans*-complementation between gene products encoded by the I-A subregions of the MHC of the two parental strains (Fathman *et al.*, 1981; Kimoto and Fathman, 1981).

The other I-region gene products may also serve as restriction elements for antigen presentation. T-cell clones reacting to antigen only in the presence of cells expressing the molecular complex formed by combinatorial association of an α chain encoded within the I-E subregion and a β chain encoded within the I-A subregion of the MHC have been identified using GL (Sredni *et al.*, 1981) and KLH (Shigeta and Fathman, 1981) as antigens. Indeed, it is possible to derive T-cell clones that recognize individual determinants on a protein molecule and exhibit several patterns of Ia restriction (Infante *et al.*, 1981).

Together, these results indicate that all possible combinations of gene products of the I-A and I-E regions of the MHC can serve as restriction elements for antigen presentation. The importance of different Ia antigens in T-cell stimulation is also shown by the inhibition of proliferative responses of antigen-stimulated cloned T cells by appropriate anti-Ia antibodies (Sredni *et al.*, 1981; Infante *et al.*, 1981; Beck and Fathman, 1982). Results obtained with cells from mutant mice in which the β chain of the $I-A^b$ gene product is altered also supports the importance of Ia antigen in the genetic control of immune responses to soluble antigens (Fathman *et al.*, 1981). Collectively, these data support strongly the concept that Ia antigens that are recognized in association with antigen by helper T cells are the gene products responsible for Ir gene function.

Proliferating alloreactive cells also may exhibit dual reactivity. Webb *et al.* (1981) have reported that a high proportion of cloned T cells selected on the basis of reactivity with Mls determinants also had joint specificity for allo-H-2 determinants. Cloned T cells reactive with soluble antigens also may express dual reactivity. This was first observed with a T-cell clone that proliferated when cultured with DNP–ovalbumin (DNP–OVA) and antigen-presenting cells syngeneic with the T-cell clone at the $I-A^k$ subregion of the MHC. This clone also proliferated after stimulation by cells bearing the $H-2^s$ haplotype. The relevant genetic subregion appeared to be I-A^s; cells from other haplotypes were not stimulatory (Sredni *et al.*, 1980). When this type of analysis was extended to include multiple T-cell clones derived from mice of different haplotypes, two significant findings were evident (Schwartz and Sredni, 1982). First, a high frequency of T-cell colonies (that probably were clonally derived) displayed both antigenic specificity and alloreactivity; from 19 to 44% of colonies obtained from three different mouse strains proliferated when stimulated with cells from at least one of eight independent MHC haplotypes. Second, the distribution of allogeneic specificity in two of the three strains tested was nonrandomly distributed. DNP–OVA-specific colonies from B10.A mice showed a tendency for reactivity to B10.S alloantigens, while antigen-specific colonies from B10.S mice showed a tendency for reactivity to B10.M and B10.B alloantigens. This high frequency of T-cell clones that displayed antigen *and* allogeneic reactivity suggests that all proliferating T cells that recognize nominal antigen must also recognize alloantigen as well.

V. Lymphokine Production by Cloned T Cells

The first indication that cloned T cells might produce lymphokines was provided by the observation that cloned noncytolytic T cells that proliferated in response to alloantigenic stimulation promoted the growth of cytolytic IL 2-dependent T cells (Glasebrook and Fitch 1979). This helper effect was mediated by a soluble factor (Glasebrook and Fitch, 1980), which subsequently has been shown to be IL 2. A variety of other lymphokine activities have been shown to be produced by cloned T cells. "Helper factors" active on B lymphocytes (BCHF) have been assayed in various ways (Schreier and Tees, 1980; Schreier *et al.*, 1980, 1982; Glasebrook *et al.*, 1981a, 1983; Nabel *et al.*, 1981a; Hodes *et al.*, 1981, 1982; Zubler and Glasebrook, 1982). Also produced are colony-stimulating factor (CSF) (Schreier *et al.*, 1980; Ely *et al.*, 1981; Nabel *et al.*, 1981a; Prystowsky *et al.*, 1982), interferon (Prystowsky *et al.*, 1982; Marcucci *et al.*, 1981; McKimm-Breschkin *et al.*, 1982), factor(s) that recruit Ia$^+$ macrophages into the peritoneal cavity and/or induce Ia expression by macrophages *in vitro* (Prystowsky *et al.*, 1982), erythroid burst-promoting activity (Schreier *et al.*, 1980), factor(s) enhancing production of complement components by guinea pig macrophages (Prystowsky *et al.*, 1982a), antigen-specific suppressor factor(s) (Fresno *et al.*, 1981), and factor(s) that induce synthesis of histimine (Dy *et al.*, 1981) and/or stimulate production of proliferation of cloned mast cells (Nabel *et al.*, 1981b).

Although it is not clear how many different molecules account for these multiple lymphokine activities, several terminal molecules must be involved. IL 2 is distinct from CSF and from at least some BCHF since the time course of IL 2 production differs markedly from that for CSF and BCHF (Schreier *et al.*, 1980; Ely *et al.*, 1981), a variant T-cell clone produces CSF and BCHF but not IL 2 (Ely *et al.*, 1981), and IL 2 can be separated physically from CSF and BCHF (Nabel *et al.*, 1981a). Comparison of the array of lymphokine activities produced by parent and variant cloned T cells together with results from time course studies indicate that cloned "helper" T cells produce at least three different biologically active molecules (Prystowsky et al., 1982). This must be regarded as a minimal estimate since it is possible to separate physically two molecules produced by a cloned T cell, each having CSF activity (Prystowsky, 1982b).

Early reports indicated that CTL clones were IL 2-dependent (Nabholz et al., 1978; Baker et al., 1979; Glasebrook and Fitch, 1979), and it was assumed that cloned CTL did not secrete lymphokines. The identification of relatively infrequent CTL clones that produce IL 2 (Widmer and Bach, 1981; Glasebrook et al., 1983) led to a reexamination of this question. It has been found that cloned CTL can produce a varied array of lymphokines, including macrophage-activating factor, Ia-inducing activity, BCHF, and interferon in addition to IL 2 (Glasebrook et al. 1983a,b; Prystowsky et al. 1982; Kelso et al., 1982). Indeed, as increasing numbers of different noncytolytic and cytolytic clones have been studied, it has become clear that several different patterns of lymphokine production can be observed. However, there has not emerged as yet any clear correlation among the nature of the antigen recognized, the phenotypic characteristics of the cloned T cell, and the array or type of lymphokines produced.

The activation of lymphokine secretion by cloned T cells is antigen-specific. However, except for an antigen-specific suppressor factor (Fresno et al., 1981), the lymphokines produced by cloned T cells appear to be immunologically nonspecific in their effects. For example, only the appropriate erythrocytes (RBC) will stimulate release of BCHF by cloned T cells reactive with horse RBC (Schreier and Tees, 1980). However, the antibody response to unrelated sheep RBC antigens is "helped" by horse RBC-stimulated cloned T cells if sheep RBC also are included in the culture. Similar "bystander" effects were observed with (T,G)-A–L-reactive cloned T cells by Hodes et al. (1981) and by Schreier et al. (1982), who studied other antibody responses to other antigens.

Requirements for MHC restriction and for hapten-carrier linkage in B-cell responses depend upon specific experimental conditions. It is possible for a single T-cell clone to provide help that is either carrier-specific or -nonspecific, for which T cell–B cell interaction is either MHC-restricted or -unrestricted, and that results in the activation of either Lyb-5$^-$ or Lyb-5$^+$ B-cell subsets (Hodes et al., 1982). At low antigen concentration, the cloned T helper cells activate primed Lyb-5$^+$ B cells to generate predominately IgG responses. Interactions between cloned T cells and B cells in this pathway is MHC-restricted and help is carrier-specific. At high antigen concentration, the same cloned T helper cells activate primed or unprimed Lyb-5$^+$ B cells to generate predominately IgM responses; interactions between T and B cells in this pathway is not MHC-restricted. The detailed molecular mechanism of these immune responses has not been characterized. However, these findings imply that the different genetic requirements for activating Lyb-5$^-$ and Lyt-5$^+$ B cells relate to differences in the ability of the two B-cell subpopulations to respond to activation signals provided by a single kind of helper T cell rather than to different types of T cells required for activation.

VI. Phenotypic Characteristics of Murine T-Cell Clones

In some situations, apparently simple distinctions about phenotypic characteristics associated with particular T-cell functions have become less rigid on the basis of information provided by cloned functional murine T lymphocytes. For example, Lyt alloantigens have been used to define subsets of T lymphocytes. Generally, helper and antigen-driven proliferating cells are Lyt-1$^+$,2$^-$,3$^-$, while CTL are Lyt-1$^-$,2$^+$,3$^+$ (Cantor and Boyse, 1975), and functional subpopulations of T cells generated in MLC prepared with cells incompatible at the H-2K/D region or the I region have been characterized on the basis of the presence or absence of Lyt-2 antigen (Bach et al., 1977). Although results obtained with most T-cell clones are consistent with these generalizations, there are important exceptions. Helper T cells are generally Lyt-1$^+$ (Glasebrook et al., 1981; Schreier et al., 1980; Nabel et al., 1981), but cloned Mls-reactive helper T cells (Glasebrook and Fitch 1980) and an interferon-producing cloned T cell (Marcucci et al., 1981) lacking Lyt-1 have been reported. Antigen-driven proliferation and IL 2 production has been observed with Lyt-1$^-$,2$^+$ CTL specific for H-K/D alloantigens (Widmer and Bach, 1981; Glasebrook, 1932). In fact, such cells may constitute the majority of CTL clones responding to stimulation with H-2K/D-incompatible tumor cells (Glasebrook, 1983).

Swain et al. (1981) have described a Lyt-1$^+$,2$^-$ antigen-driven proliferating T-cell line reactive with alloantigens encoded by genes of the I-A subregion of the MHC and having both helper and CTL function. In contrast, a Lyt-1$^+$,2$^+$ cloned T cell having similar functions but reactive with alloantigens encoded by genes of the I-C subregion of the MHC has been derived (A. L. Glasebrook, unpublished observations). These observations are consistent with a report that there is heterogeneity in Lyt-2 expression by cells that recognize different I subregions of the MHC; CTL reactive with target cells bearing I-A-subregion encoded products were Lyt-1$^+$,2$^-$, while CTL specific for I-E products were Lyt-1$^+$,2$^+$ (Vidovic et al., 1981). Thus, expression of Lyt surface antigens may relate both to function and to the antigens being recognized.

Cloned T cells also have been useful for characterizing the role of cell surface structures in particular functions. The Lyt-2 molecular complex has been implicated in T-cell-mediated cytolysis, since anti-Lyt-2 antibodies block the cytolytic activity of cloned CTL and Ts cells from MLC (Nakayama et al., 1979; Shinohara and Sachs, 1979; Sarmiento et al., 1980). Three kinds of evidence indicate that the Lyt-2 molecular complex is not involved *directly* in the lytic process: cytolytic activity by cloned CTL is not inhibited with anti-Lyt-2 in a Con A-facilitated assay (Sarmiento et al., 1982); variant clones that do not express cell surface Lyt-2 are lytic in lectin-facilitated assays (Dialynas et al., 1981); CTL clones derived after immunization *in vivo* are heterogeneous with respect to inhibition of cytolytic activity by anti-Lyt-2 antibodies (MacDonald et al., 1981).

Although Lyt-2 does not appear to contribute to receptor antigenic specificity, since the molecule does not exhibit the type of structural heterogeneity that would be required (Sarmiento et al. 1982), Lyt-2 may function to nonspecifically stabilize effector–target cell interactions, possibly via effects on the T-cell receptor (MacDonald *et al.*, 1982b; Springer *et al.* 1982). Pertinent to this are the observations that anti-Lyt-2 can inhibit other noncytolytic functions manifested by Lyt-2$^+$ T cells that are dependent on specific antigenic recognition (i.e., proliferation and lymphokine production), suggesting that Lyt-2 plays a role in antigen recognition (Glasebrook *et al.*, 1983). Heterogeneity of anti-Lyt-2 inhibition at the clonal level may be related to receptor affinity; after *in vitro* stimulation, stabilization with the Lyt-2 molecule is required, but after *in vivo* stimulation, stabilization is not required.

The molecular complex designated 170/100 or LFA-1 also has been implicated in T-cell-mediated cytolysis for similar reasons. Monoclonal antibodies reactive with this complex also inhibit cytolytic activity (Davignon *et al.*, 1981; Pierres *et al.*, 1982; Sarmiento *et al.*, 1982). However, the antigenic determinants recognized by these antibodies are not limited to CTL, and there is no evidence that suggests that this molecular complex is related to the antigen receptor. The 170/100 complex also is not involved directly in the lytic process, since inhibition of cytolysis is overcome in a PHA-facilitated assay (Sarmiento *et al.*, 1982). In contrast, Con A-facilitated lysis *is* inhibited by anti-170/100 antibodies, indicating that the detailed molecular mechanisms of lectin-facilitated lysis differ according to the particular lectin used in the assay.

Alloreactive noncytolytic cloned T cells have been useful for producing "antiidiotypic" antisera in F_1 mice (Infante *et al.*, 1982). These antisera stimulate the proliferation of the appropriate T-cell clones but not other clones even though they bind to irrelevant clones as well as to the specific clones (C. G. Fathman, personal communication). Thus, although these "antiidiotypic" antisera contain antibodies reactive with specific T-cell clones, they also appear to contain antibodies that are cross-reactive with other alloreactive clones. A reasonable candidate for an antibody reactive with the antigen-specific receptor of a cytolytic T-cell clone is a monoclonal antibody raised by immunizing an F_1 mouse with a CTL clone designated L3 (Lancki *et al.*, 1982). This monoclonal antibody binds specifically to and inhibits the cytolytic activity of the CTL clone L3 used for immunization but does not react with or inhibit cytolysis by other CTL clones. Cells reactive with this antibody have not been found among normal lymphoid cells from the strain of origin for the CTL clone L3. However, a small proportion of MLC cells have been found regularly to react with this antibody when the response has been "enriched" genetically for antigen-reactive CTL directed toward H-2D^d alloantigens, the target of CTL clone L3. The amount of antibody bound suggests that there about 10^4 molecules per cell, an estimate consistent with the intensity of staining observed using flow cytofluorometry (Sarmiento *et al.*, 1982).

T-Cell clones have also provided other miscellaneous findings of interest. For example, T-cell-mediated cytolysis has been found to be independent of the growth phase and position in cell cycle, as the result of studies with CTL clones. Cloned cells were sorted using the fluorescence-activated cell sorter according to their position in the cell cycle and then assayed for specific lytic activity (Sekaly *et al.*, 1981). In other studies, differences in the electrophoretic mobility of the Thy-1 antigen were found to be unrelated to specific functions of several cytolytic and noncytolytic clones (Sarmiento *et al.*, 1981).

VII. Functions of Murine T-Cell Clones in Vivo

Several functional activities of cloned T cell have been tested *in vivo*. Only antigen-specific help for B-cell responses has been observed *in vivo*, although, as noted above, "bystander" help for a second antigen can be observed *in vitro* (Schreier and Tees, 1980). It has been possible to reconstitute the response of congenic nude mice to specific antigens by injection of cloned helper T cells (Tees and Schreier, 1980); the magnitude of the response depended upon the number of injected helper cells and could exceed by far the response of normal thymus-bearing litermates.

Delayed-type hypersensitivity reaction (DTH) has been produced when antigen-responsive Lyt-1$^+$,2$^-$ cloned helper T cells were injected subcutaneously along with the specific antigen (Bianchi *et al.*, 1981). Also, an alloreactive, Lyt-1$^+$ helper/cytolytic T-cell clone could mediate DTH when injected locally with the appropriate antigen (S. Weiss and Dennert, 1981). MHC restriction by the I-A subregion of the H-2 complex was observed with cloned helper cells specific for sheep RBC (Bianchi *et al.*, 1981; Schreier *et al.*, 1982). A local DTH reaction also was observed when Lyt-1$^-$,2$^+$ cloned CTL reactive with influenza A virus-infected cells were injected subcutaneously along with purified virus (Lin and Askonas, 1981). However, it has been necessary to inject antigen and cloned T cells together for maximum DTH response. Smaller responses were observed when larger numbers of cloned T cells were injected intravenously and antigen administered subcutaneously (Bianchi *et al.*, 1981), and attempts to elicit DTH responses were unsuccessful after intravenous injection of alloreactive (S. Weiss and Dennert, 1981) or influenza-reactive (Lin and Askonas, 1981) cloned T cells.

In spite of the inability to demonstrate DTH responses after intravenous injection of cloned T cells, sublethally irradiated mice receiving 3×10^6 cloned CTL intravenously survived an intranasal infection with lethal amounts of infective influenza virus (Lin and Askonas, 1981). Virus titers in the lungs also were reduced in mice receiving the cloned CTL. The difficulty in demonstrating DTH after intravenous injection of cloned T cells may relate to altered recirculating and homing patterns of cloned T cells. Several different types of T-cell clones, including antigen-specific, alloreactive, and cytolytic clones, were found to be markedly deficient in their ability to home to peripheral lymphoid tissues (Dailey *et al.*, 1982). This defect appeared to be related to lack of receptors on lymphocytes for the high endothelial venules in lymphoid tissue. Trapping of cloned T cells in the lung was somewhat greater than for normal cells (Dailey *et al.*, 1982), and this may account for the ability of cloned cells to protect against intranasal infection with influenza virus.

CTL have been shown to inhibit tumor growth *in vivo* when injected together with tumor cells as a mixture (Winn-type assay) and to accumulate selectively in grafts and tumors. Allogeneic MLC populations containing CTL have also been shown to function *in vivo* when injected at a site distant from that of tumor inoculation. Tumor elimination and subsequent protection of animals could be shown using positively selected Lyt-2$^+$ cells (containing all the cytolytic activity) but not with negatively selected Lyt-2$^-$ cells (Engers *et al.*, 1982b). In contrast, Lyt-2$^+$ CTL clones have generally been found not to function *in vivo* after intravenous administration, possibly due to altered homing patterns. An alternative explanation, however, may be that cell interactions with other "activated" T-cell subsets (i.e., helper cells) are necessary *in vivo* to promote growth and expansion of CTL clones. Cheever *et al.* (1982) have reported that the efficacy of CTL injected intravenously is increased by repeated administration of IL-2. Engers *et al.* (1982a) have recently reported the first demonstration that cloned CTL injected intravenously can induce rejection of intraperitoneal allogeneic tumor. The striking finding reported in this study was the fact that all Lyt-2$^+$ CTL clones that functioned *in vivo* had been selected originally by screening for autonomous proliferation to alloantigens in the absence of added IL 2. Although a limited number of clones were tested, the implication was that at the clonal level only those CTL clones that manifested "helper cell-like" characteristics were functional *in vivo*.

VIII. Summary

Cloned T lymphocytes already have provided unambiguous answers to several important immunological questions that could not have been addressed using other approaches. The extent of the T-cell repertoire for antigen recognition has been shown to be quite extensive. "Dual" antigen reactivity is common, both with cloned cytolytic T lymphocytes and with proliferating noncytolytic T lymphocytes. Cloned cytolytic T cells may recognize both alloantigen and viral antigens expressed on syngeneic cells. A high proportion of T lymphocytes that proliferate when stimulated with soluble antigen in the presence of syngeneic antigen-presenting cells also have alloreactivity. Indeed, the high frequency of T-cell clones that react with nominal antigens as well as with alloantigen suggests that all antigen-reactive T cells have such dual reactivity. Recognition of soluble antigens requires I-region gene products as well as the nominal antigen, and results with cloned T cells indicate that all possible combinations of I-region gene products can serve as the restriction elements for antigen presentation. Collectively, the data also support the concept that Ia antigens that are recognized in association with nominal antigen by helper T cells are the gene products responsible for Ir gene function.

It is clear from results obtained with cloned T cells that an individual clone can secrete multiple lymphokine activities, that different clones can secrete different arrays of lymphokines, and that different molecules produced by the same clone can be responsible for the same lymphokine activity. Both noncytolytic and cytolytic T lymphocytes can secrete lymphokines. A single T-cell clone can provide help for two independent pathways of B-cell activation.

Cloned T cells also have been useful for characterizing the phenotypic characteristics of different types of T cells. The association of expression of Lyt alloantigens with particular functions seems not to be as stringent as indicated by studies with bulk populations of lymphocytes. Cloned T cells may function *in vivo*, but their effectiveness may be limited by altered recirculating and homing patterns.

Important immunological questions remain unanswered. In spite of vigorous and extensive efforts, the nature of the T-cell receptor for antigen has not yet been determined. However, the use of cloned T cells together with monoclonal antibodies should make it possible to unequivocally identify and characterize that receptor. This information should provide answers to questions about the basis for the dual reactivity and the MHC restrictions observed in T-lymphocyte functions as well.

References

Aarden, L. A., *et al.*, 1979, Revised nomenclature for antigen non-specific T-cell proliferation and helper factors, *J. Immunol.* **123**:2928.

Bach, F. H., Grillot-Courvalin, C., Kupperman, O. J., Sollinger, H. W., Hays, C., Sondel, P. M., and Bach, M. L., 1977, Antigenic requirements for triggering of cytotoxic T lymphocytes, *Immunol. Rev.* **35**:76.

Baker, P. E., Gillis, E., and Smith, K. A., 1979, Monoclonal cytolytic T-cell lines, *J. Exp. Med.* **149**:273.

Beck, B. N., and Fathman, C. G., 1982, Alloreactive T cell clones which recognize hybrid determinants, in: *Isolation, Characterization and Utilization of T Lymphocyte Clones* (C. G. Fathman and F. W. Fitch, eds.), Academic Press, New York, p. 325.

Bianchi, A. T. J., Hooigkaas, H., Benner, R., Tees, R., Nordin, A. A., and Schreier, M. H., 1981, Clones of helper T cells mediate antigen-specific, H-2 restricted DTH, *Nature* **290**:62.

Braciale, T. J., Andrew, M. E., and Braciale, V. L., 1981a, Heterogeneity and specificity of cloned lines of influenza-virus-specific cytotoxic T lymphocytes, *J. Exp. wed.* **153**:910.

Braciale, T. J., Andrew, M. E., and Braciale, V. L., 1981b, Simultaneous expression of H-2-restricted and alloreactive recognition by a cloned line of influenza virus-specific cytolytic T lymphocytes, *J. Exp. Med.* **153**:1371.

Brunner, K. T., MacDonald, H. R., and Cerottini, J.-C., 1981, Quantitation and clonal isolation of cytolytic T lymphocyte precursors selectively infiltrating murine sarcoma virus-induced tumors, *J. Exp. Med.* **154**:362.

Cancro, M. P., and Klinman, N. R., 1981, B cell repertoire ontogeny: Heritable but dissimilar development of parental and F_1 repertoires, *J. Immunol.* **126**:1160.

Cantor, H., and Boyse, E. A., 1975, Functional subclasses of T lymphocytes bearing different Ly antigens. II. Cooperation between subclasses of Ly$^+$ cells in the generation of killer activity, *J. Exp. Med.* **141**:1390.

Cheever, M. A., Greenberg, P. D., Fefer, A., and Gillis, S., 1982, Augmentation of the anti-tumor therapeutic efficacy of long-term cultured T lymphocytes by *in vivo* administration of purified interleukin 2, *J. Exp. Med.* **155**:968.

Clark, A. F., and Capra, J. D., 1982, Ubiquitous nonimmunoglobulin *p*-azobenzene-arsonate-binding molecules from lymphoid cells, *J. Exp. Med.* **155**:611.

Dailey, M. O., Fathman, C. G., Butcher, E. C., Pillemer, E. N., and Weissman, I., 1982, Abnormal migration of T lymphocyte clones, *J. Immunol.* **128**:21.

Davignon, D., Martz, E., Reynolds, T., Kurzinger, K., and Springer, T. A., 1981, Lymphocyte function-associated antigen 1 (LFA-1): A surface antigen distinct from Lyt-2,3 that participates in T lymphocyte-mediated killing, *Proc. Natl. Acad. Sci. USA* **78**:4535.

Dennert, G., and DeRose, M., 1976, Continuously proliferating T killer cells specific for H-2^b target: Selection and characterization, *J. Immunol.* **116**:1601.

Dialynas, D. P., Loken, M. R., Glasebrook, A. L., and Fitch, F. W., 1981, Lyt-2$^-$/Lyt-3$^-$ variants of a cloned cytolytic T cell line lack an antigen receptor functional in cytolysis, *J. Exp. Med.* **153**:595.

DiPauli, R., and Opalka, B., 1982, Antigen-dependent, H-2-restricted cytolytic and monocytolytic T cell lines with specificity for minor histocompatibility antigens, *Eur. J. Immunol.* **12**:365.

Dy, M., Lebel, B., Kamoun, P., and Hamburger, J., 1981, Histamine production during the anti-allograft response, *J. Exp. Med.* **153:**293.

Ely, J. M., and Fitch, F. W., 1983, Alloreactive cloned T cell lines. VI. Comparison of the kinetics of IL 2 release stimulated by alloantigen or lectins, *J. Immunol.* **131:**1274.

Ely, J. M., Prystowsky, M. B., Eisenberg, L., Quintans, J., Goldwasser, E., and Fitch, F. W., 1981, Alloreactive cloned T cell lines. IV. Differential kinetics of IL-2, CSF, and BCSF release by a cloned T amplifier cell and its variant, *J. Immunol.* **127:**2345.

Engers, H. D., Glasebrook, A. L., and Sorenson, G. D., 1982a, Allogeneic tumor rejection induced by intravenous injection of cytolytic T lymphocyte clones, *J. Exp. Med.* **156:**1280–1285.

Engers, H. D., Sorenson, G. D., Terres, G., Horvath, C., and Brunner, K. T., 1982b, Functional activity *in vivo* of effector T cell populations. I. Antitumor activity exhibited by allogeneic mixed leukocyte culture cells. *J. Immunol.* **129:**1292–1298.

Farrar, J. J., Fuller-Farrar, J., Simon, P. L., Hilfiker, M. L., Stadler, B. M., and Farrar, W. L., 1980, Thymoma production of T cell growth factor (Interleukin 2), *J. Immunol.* **125:**2555.

Fathman, C. G., and Hengartner, H., 1978, Clones of alloreactive T-cells, *Nature* **272:**617.

Fathman, C. G., and Hengartner, H., 1979, Crossreactive mixed lymphocyte reaction determinants recognized by cloned alloreactive T cells, *Proc. Natl. Acad. Sci. USA* **76:**5863.

Fathman, C. G., and Kimoto, M., 1981, Studies utilizing murine T cell clones: Ir genes, Ia antigens and MLR stimulating determinants, *Immunol. Rev.* **54:**57.

Fathman, C. G., and Nabholz, M., 1977, *in vitro* secondary MLR. II. Detection of semi-allogeneic (F_1) MLR stimulating determinants, *Eur. J. Immunol.* **7:**370.

Fathman, C. G., Kimoto, M., Melvold, R., and David, C. S., 1981, Reconstitution of Ir genes, Ia antigens and mixed lymphocyte reaction determinants by gene complementation, *Proc. Natl. Acad. Sci. USA* **78:**1853.

Finn, O. J., Boniver, J., and Kaplan, H. S., 1979, Induction, establishment *in vitro* and characterization of functional antigen-specific, carrier-primed murine T-cell lymphomas, *Proc. Natl. Acad. Sci. USA* **76:**4033.

Fresno, M., McVay-Boudreau, L., Nabel, G., and Cantor, H., 1981, Antigen-specific T lymphocyte clones. II. Purification and biological characterization of an antigen-specific suppressive protein synthesized by cloned T cells, *J. Exp. Med.* **153:**1260.

Gillis, S., and Smith, K. A., 1977, Long-term culture of tumour-specific cytotoxic T cells, *Nature* **268:**154.

Gillis, S., Smith, K. A., and Watson, J. D., 1980a, Biochemical and biological characterization of lymphocyte regulatory molecules. II. Purification of a class of rat and human lymphokines, *J. Immunol.* **124:**1954.

Gillis, S., Scheid, M., and Watson, J., 1980b, The biochemical and biological characterization of lymphocyte regulatory molecules. III. The isolation and phenotypic characterization of Interleukin 2 producing T cell lymphomas, *J. Immunol.* **125:**2570.

Glasebrook, A. L., 1984, Cytolytic T lymphocyte clones that proliferate autonomously to specific alloantigenic stimulation. I. Frequency, Interleukin-2 production and Lyt phenotype, *J. Immunol.*, in press.

Glasebrook, A. L., and Fitch, F. W., 1979, T cell lines which cooperate in generation of specific cytolytic activity, *Nature* **278:**171.

Glasebrook, A. L., and Fitch, F. W., 1980, Alloreactive cloned T cell lines. I. Interactions between cloned amplifier and cytolytic T cell lines, *J. Exp. Med.* **151:**876.

Glasebrook, A. L., Quintans, J., Eisenberg, L., and Fitch, F. W., 1981a, Alloreactive cloned T cell lines. II. Polyclonal stimulation of B cells by a cloned helper T cell line, *J. Immunol.* **126:**240.

Glasebrook, A. L., Sarmiento, M., Loken, M. R., Dialynas, D. P., Quintans, J., Eisenberg, L., Lutz, C. T., Wilde, D., and Fitch, F. W., 1981b, Murine T lymphocyte clones with distinct immunological functions, *Immunol. Rev.* **54:**225.

Glasebrook, A. L., Kelso, A., Zubler, R. H., Ely, J. M., Prystowsky, M. C., and Fitch, F. W., 1982, Lymphokine production by cytolytic and noncytolytic alloreactive T cell clones, in: *Isolation, Characterization and Utilization of T Lymphocyte Clones* (C. G. Fathman and F. W. Fitch, eds.), Academic Press, New York, p. 342.

Glasebrook, A. L., Kelso, A., and MacDonald, H. R., 1983, Cytolytic T lymphocyte clones that proliferate autonomously to specific alloantigen stimulation. II. Relationship of the Lyt-2 molecular complex to cytolytic activity, proliferation, and lymphokine secretion, *J. Immunol.* **130:** 1545.

Haas, W., Mathur-Rochat, J., Pohlit, H., Nabholz, M., and von Boehmer, H., 1980, Cytotoxic T cell responses to haptenated cells. III. Isolation and specificity analysis of continuously growing clones, *Eur. J. Immunol.* **10:**828.

Harwell, L., Skidmore, B., Marrack, P., and Kappler, J. W., 1980, Concanavalin A-inducible interleukin-2-producing T cell hybridomas, *J. Exp. Med.* **153:**893.

Hengartner, H., and Fathman, C. G., 1980, Clones of alloreactive T cells. I. A unique homozygous MLR stimulating determinant present on B6 stimulators, *Immunogenetics* **10:**175.

Hodes, R. J., Kimoto, M., Hathcock, K. S., Fathman, C. G., and Singer, A., 1981, Functional helper activity of monoclonal T cell populations: Antigen-specific and H-2 restricted clone T cells provide help for *in vitro* antibody responses to trinitrophenyl-poly-L-(Tyr,Glu)-poly-D,L-(Ala)–poly-L-(Lys), *Proc. Natl. Acad. Sci. USA* **78:**6431.

Hodes, R. J., Asano, Y., Shigeta, M., Hathcock, K. S., Kimoto, M., Fathman, C. G., and Singer, A., 1982, Mechanism of B cell activation by monoclonal T helper cell populations, in: *Isolation, Characterization and Utilization of T Lymphocyte Clones* (C. G. Fathman and F. W. Fitch, eds.), Academic Press, New York, p. 386.

Infante, A. J., Atassi, M. Z., and Fathman, C. G., 1981, T cell clones reactive with sperm whale myoglobin, *J. Exp. Med.* **154:**1342.

Infante, A. J., Infante, P. D., Gillis, S., and Fathman, C. G., 1982, Definition of T cell idiotypes using anti-idiotypic antisera produced by immunization with T cell clones, *J. Exp. Med.* **155:**1100.

Johnson, J. P., Cianfriglia, M., Glasebrook, A. L., and Nabholz, M., 1982, Karyotype evolution of cytolytic T cell lines, in: *Isolation, Characterization and Utilization of T Lymphocyte Clones* (C. G. Fathman and F. W. Fitch, eds.), Academic Press, New York, p. 183.

Kanagawa, O., Louis, J., and Cerottini, J.-C., 1982, Frequency and cross-reactivity of cytolytic T lymphocyte precursors reacting against male alloantigens, *J. Immunol.* **128:**2362.

Kapp, J. A., Arane, B. A., and Clevinger, B. L., 1980, Suppression of antibody and T cell proliferative responses to L-glutamic acid ^{60}–L-alanine^{30}–L-tyrosine^{10} by a specific monoclonal T cell factor, *J. Exp. Med.* **152:**235.

Kappler, J. W., Skidmore, B., White, J., and Marrack, P., 1981, Antigen-inducible H-2 restricted, interleukin-2-producing T cell hybridomas. Lack of independent antigen and H-2 recognition, *J. Exp. Med.* **153:**1198.

Kelso, A., Glasebrook, A. L., Kanagawa, D., and Brunner, K. T., 1982, Production of macrophage activating factor by T lymphocyte clones and correlation with other lymphokine activities, *J. Immunol.* **129:**550–556.

Kimoto, M., and Fathman, C. G., 1980, Antigen reactive T cell clones. I. Transcomplementing hybrid I-A region gene products function effectively, antigen presentation, *J. Exp. Med.* **152:**759.

Kimoto, M., and Fathman, C. G., 1981, Antigen-reactive T cell clones. II. Unique homozygous and (high responder and low responder) F_1 hybrid antigen-presenting determinants detected using poly-L-(Tyr,Glu)-poly-D,L-(Ala)–poly-L-(Lys)-reactive T cell clones, *J. Exp. Med.* **153:**375.

Kontiainen, S., Simpson, E., Bohrer, E., Beverley, P. C. L., Herzenberg, L. A., Fitzpatrick, W. C., Vogt, P., Torano, A., McKenzie, I. F. C., and Feldmann, M., 1978, T-cell lines producing antigen-specific suppressor factor, *Nature* **274:**477.

Lancki, D. W., Lorber, M. I., Loken, M. R., and Fitch, F. W., 1982, A clone specific monoclonal antibody which inhibits T cell mediated cytolysis, *Adv. Exp. Med. Biol.* **146:**557.

Lin, Y.-L., and Askonas, B. A., 1980, Cross-reactivity for different type A influenza viruses of a cloned T-killer cell line, *Nature* **288:**164.

Lin, Y.-L., and Askonas, B. A., 1981, Biological properties of an influenza A virus-specific killer T cell clone, *J. Exp. Med.* **154:**225.

Lonai, P., Puri, J., and Hammerling, G. J., 1981, H-2 restricted antigen binding by a hybridoma clone which produces specific helper factor, *Proc. Natl. Acad. Sci. USA* **78:**549.

Lutz, C. T., Glasebrook, A. L., and Fitch, F. W., 1981a, Alloreactive cloned T cell lines. III. Accessory cell requirements for the growth of cloned cytolytic T lymphocytes, *J. Immunol.* **126:**1404.

Lutz, C. T., Glasebrook, A. L., and Fitch, F. W., 1981b, Alloreactive cloned T cell lines. IV. Interaction of alloantigen and T cell growth factors (TCGF) to stimulate cloned cytolytic T lymphocytes, *J. Immunol.* **127:**391.

MacDonald, H. R., Cerottini, J.-C., Ryser, J.-E., Maryanski, J. L., Taswell, C., Widmer, M. B., and Brunner, K. T., 1980a, Quantitation and cloning of cytolytic T lymphocytes and their precursors, *Immunol. Rev.* **51:**93.

MacDonald, H. R., Maryanski, J. L., and Cerottini, J.-C., 1980b, Cloning of cytolytic T lymphocytes: Requirement for interleukin 2 and irradiated spleen cells, *Behring Inst. Mitt.* **67:**182.

MacDonald, H. R., Thiernesse, N., and Cerottini, J.-C., 1981, Inhibition of T cell-mediated cytolysis by monoclonal antibodies directed against Lyt-2: Heterogeneity of inhibition at the clonal level, *J. Immunol.* **126:**1671.

MacDonald, H. R., Sekaly, R. P., Kanagawa, O., Thiernesse, N., Taswell, C., Cerottini, J.-C., Weiss, A., Glasebrook, A. L., Engers, H. D., Kelso, A., Brunner, K. T., and Bron, C., 1982a, Cytolytic T lymphocyte clones, *Immunobiology* **161:**84.

MacDonald, H. R., Glasebrook, A. L., Bron, C., Kelso, A., and Cerottini, J.-C., 1982b, Clonal heterogeneity in the functional requirement for Lyt-2/3 molecules on cytolytic T lymphocytes (CTL): Possible implications for the affinity of CTL antigen receptors, *Immunol. Rev.* **68:**89–115.

Marcucci, F., Waller, M., Kirchner, H., and Krammer, P., 1981, Production of immune interferon by murine T-cell clones from long-term cultures, *Nature* **291:**79.

McKimm-Breschkin, J. L., Mottram, P. L., Thomas, W. R., and Miller, J. F. A. T., 1982, Antigen-specific production of immune interferon by T cell lines, *J. Exp. Med.* **155:**1204.

Melief, C. J. M., van der Meulen, M. Y., and Postma, P., 1977, CML typing of serological identical H-2 mutants. Distinction of 19 specificities on the cells of four mouse strains carrying zl locus mutations and strain of origin, *Immunogenetics* **5:**43.

Morgan, D. A., Ruscetti, F. W., and Gallo, R. C., 1976, Selective *in vitro* growth of T lymphocytes from normal human bone marrows, *Science* **193:**1007.

Nabel, G., Greenberger, J. S., Sakakeeny, M. A., and Cantor, H., 1981a, Multiple biologic activities of a cloned inducer T-cell population, *Proc. Natl. Acad. Sci. USA* **78:**1157.

Nabel, G., Galli, S. J., Dvorak, A. M., Dvorak, H. F., and Cantor, H., 1981b, Inducer T lymphocytes synthesize a factor that stimulates proliferation of cloned mast cells, *Nature* **291:**332.

Nabholz, M., Engers, H. D., Collavo, D., and North, M., 1978, Cloned T cell lines with specific cytolytic activity, *Curr. Top. Microbiol. Immunol.* **81:**176.

Nabholz, M., Cianfriglia, M., Acuto, O., Conzelmann, A., Haas, W., von Boehmer, H., MacDonald, H. R., Pohlit, H., and Johnson, J. P., 1980, Cytolytically active murine T-cell hybrids, *Nature* **287:**437.

Nakayama, E., Shiku, H., Stockert, E., Oettgen, H. F., and Old, L. J., 1979, Cytotoxic T cells: The Lyt phenotype and blocking of killing activity by Lyt antisera, *Proc. Nat. Acad. Sci. USA* **76:**1977.

Pacifico, A., and Capra, J. D., 1980, T cell hybrids with arsonate specificity. I. Initial characterization of antigen-specific T cell products that bear a cross-reactive idiotype and determinants encoded by the murine major histocompatibility complex, *J. Exp. Med.* **152:**1289.

Pierres, M., Goridis, C., and Golstein, P., 1982, Inhibition of murine T cell-mediated cytolysis and T cell proliferation by a rat monoclonal antibody immunoprecipitating two lymphoid cell surface polypeptides of 94,000 and 180,000 molecular weight, *Eur. J. Immunol.* **12:**60.

Plata, F., 1982, Specificity studies of cytolytic T lymphocytes directed against murine leukemia virus-induced tumors, *J. Exp. Med.* **155:**1050.

Prystowsky, M. B., Ely, J. M., Beller, D. I., Eisenberg, L., Goldman, J., Goldman, M., Goldwasser, E., Ihle, J., Quintans, J., Remold, H., Vogel, S., and Fitch, F. W., 1982, Alloreactive cloned T cell lines. VI. Multiple lymphokine activities secreted by helper and cytolytic cloned T lymphocytes, *J. Immunol.* **129:**2337.

Prystowsky, M. B., Ely, J. M., Vogel, S. N., Goldwasser, E., and Fitch, F. W., 1983, Biochemical enrichment of lymphokines secreted by a cloned helper T lymphocyte, *Fed. Proc.* **42:**2757.

Ricciardi-Castagnoli, P., Doria, G., and Adorini, L., 1981, Production of antigen-specific suppressive T cell factor by radiation leukemia virus-transformed suppressor T cells, *Proc. Natl. Acad. Sci. USA* **78:**3804.

Ryser, J.-E., and MacDonald, H. R., 1979a, Limiting dilution analysis of alloantigen-reactive T lymphocytes. I. Comparison of precursor frequencies for proliferative and cytolytic responses, *J. Immunol.* **122:**1691.

Ryser, J.-E., and MacDonald, H. R., 1979b, Limiting dilution analysis of alloantigen-reactive T lymphocytes. III. Effect of priming on precursor frequencies, *J. Immunol.* **123:**128.

Ryser, J.-E., Cerottini, J.-C., and Brunner, K. T., 1978, Generation of cytolytic T lymphocytes. *in vitro.* IX. Induction of secondary CTL responses in primary long-term MLC by supernatants from secondary MLC, *J. Immunol.* **120:**370.

Sarmiento, M., Glasebrook, A. L., and Fitch, F. W., 1980, IgG or IgM monoclonal antibodies reactive with different determinants on the molecular complex bearing Lyt 2 antigen block T cell-mediated cytolysis in the absence of complement, *J. Immunol.* **125:**2665.

Sarmiento, M., Loken, M. R., and Fitch, F. W., 1981, Structural differences in cell surface T25 polypeptides from thymocytes and cloned T cells, *Hybridoma* **1:**13.

Sarmiento, M., Dialynas, D. P., Lancki, D. W., Wall, K. A., Lorber, M. I., Loken, M. R., and Fitch, F. W., 1982, Cloned T lymphocytes and monoclonal antibodies as probes for cell surface molecules active in T cell-mediated cytolysis, *Immunol. Rev.* **68:**135–169.

Schreier, M. H., and Tees, R., 1980, Clonal induction of helper T cells: Conversion of specific signals into non-specific signals, *Int. Arch. Allergy Appl. Immunol.* **61:**227.

Schreier, M. H., Iscove, N. N., Tees, R., Aarden, L., and von Boehmer, H., 1980, Clones of killer and helper T cells: growth requirements, specificity and retention of function in long-term cultures, *Immunol. Rev.* **51:**315.

Schreier, M. H., Tees, R., Nordin, A. A., Benner, R., Bianchi, A. T. J., and van Zwieten, M. J., 1982, Functional aspects of helper T cell clones, *Immunobiology* **161:**107.

Schwartz, R. H., and Sredni, B., 1982, Alloreactivity of antigen-specific T cell clones, in: *Isolation, Characterization and Utilization of T Lymphocyte Clones* (C. G. Fathman and F. W. Fitch, eds.), Academic Press, New York, p. 375.

Sekaly, R. P., MacDonald, H. R., Zaech, P., Glasebrook, A. L., and Cerottini, J.-C., 1981, Cytolytic T lymphocyte function is independent of growth phase and position in the mitotic cycle, *J. Exp. Med.* **154:**575.

Sherman, L. A., 1980, Dissection of the B10.D2 anti-H-2K^b cytolytic T lymphocyte receptor repertoire, *J. Exp. Med.* **151:**1386.

Sherman, L. A., 1982a, Influence of the major histocompatibility complex on the repertoire of allospecific cytolytic T lymphocytes, *J. Exp. Med.* **155:**380.

Sherman, L. A., 1982b, The specificity repertoire of cytolytic T lymphocytes, in: *Isolation, Characterization and Utilization of T Lymphocyte Clones* (C. G. Fathman and F. W. Fitch, eds.), Academic Press, New York, p. 314.

Sherman, L. A., 1982c, Recognition of conformational determinants on H-2 by cytolytic T lymphocytes, *Nature* **297:**511.

Shigeta, M., and Fathman, C. G., 1981, I region genetic restrictions imposed upon the recognition of KLH by murine T cell clones, *Immunogenetics* **11:**493.

Shinohara, N., and Sachs, D. H., 1979, Mouse alloantibodies capable of blocking cytotoxic T-cell function. I. Relationship between the antigen reactive with blocking antibodies and the Lyt-2 locus, *J. Exp. Med.* **150:**432.

Springer, T. A., Davignon, D., Ho, M.-K., Kurzinger, K., Martz, E., Sanchez-Madrid, F., 1982, LFA-1 and Lyt-2,3 molecules associated with T lymphocyte-mediated killing; Mac-1, and LFA-1 homologue associated with complment receptor function, *Immunol. Rev.* **68:**171–195.

Sredni, B., and Schwartz, R. H., 1981, Antigen-specific proliferating T lymphocyte clones. Methodology, specificity, MHC restriction and alloreactivity, *Immunol. Rev.* **54:**187.

Sredni, B., Tse, H. Y., and Schwartz, R. H., 1980, Direct cloning and extended culture of antigen-specific MHC-restricted, proliferating T lymphocytes, *Nature* **283:**581.

Sredni, B., Matis, L. A., Lerner, E. A., Paul, W. E., and Schwartz, R. H., 1981, Antigen-specific T cell clones restricted to unique F$_1$ major histocompatibility complex determinants. Inhibition of proliferation with a monoclonal anti-Ia antibody, *J. Exp. Med.* **153:**677.

Swain, S. L., Dennert, G., Wormsley, S., and Dutton, R. W., 1981, The Lyt phenotype of a long-term allospecific T cell line. Both helper and killer activites to I-A are mediated by Ly-1 cells, *Eur. J. Immunol.* **11:**175.

Taniguchi, M., and Miller, J. F. A. P., 1978, Specific suppressive factors produced by hybridomas derived from the fusion of enriched suppressor T-cells and a T lymphoma cell line, *J. Exp. Med.* **148:**373.

Taussig, M. J., Corvalan, J. R. F., Binns, R. M., and Holliman, A., 1979, Production of an H-2 related suppressor factor by a hybrid T-cell line, *Nature* **277:**305.

Taussig, M., Holliman, A., and Wright, L. J., 1980, Hybridization between T and B lymphoma cell lines, *Immunology* **39:**57.

Tees, R. N., and Schreier, M. H., 1980, Selective reconstitution of nude mice with long-term cultured and cloned specific helper T cells, *Nature* **283:**780.

Vidovic, D., Juretic, A., Nagy, Z. A., and Klein, J., 1981, Lyt phenotypes of primary cytotoxic T cells generated across the A and E region of the H-2 complex, *Eur. J. Immunol.* **11:**499.

Von Boehmer, H., and Haas, W., 1981, H-2 restricted cytolytic and noncytolytic T cell clones: Isolation specificity and functional analysis, *Immunol. Rev.* **54:**27.

Von Boehmer, H., Hengartner, H., Nabholz, W., Lenhardt, W., Schreier, M. H., and Haas, W., 1979, Fine specificity of a continuous growing killer cell clone specific for H-Y antigen, *Eur. J. Immunol.* **9:**592.

Watanabe, T., Fathman, C. G., and Coutinho, A., 1977, Cloned growth of T cells *in vitro:* Preliminary attempts to a quantitative approach, *Immunol. Rev.* **35:**3.

Watson, J., Gillis, S., Marbrook, J., Mochizuki, D., and Smith, K. A., 1979, Biochemical and biological characterization of lymphocyte regulatory molecules. I. Purification of a class of murine lymphokines, *J. Exp. Med.* **150:**849.

Webb, S. R., Volmar-Kimber, K., Bruce, J., Sprent, J., and Wilson, D. B., 1981, T cell clones with dual specificity for Mls and various major histocompatibility complex determinants, *J. Exp. Med.* **154:**1970.

Weiss, A., Brunner, K. T., MacDonald, H. R., and Cerottini, J.-C., 1980, Antigenic specificity of the cytolytic T lymphocyte response to murine sarcoma virus-induced tumors. III. Characterization of cytolytic T lymphocyte clones specific for Maloney leukemia virus associated cell surface antigens, *J. Exp. Med.* **152:**1225.

Weiss, A., MacDonald, H. R., Cerottini, J.-C., and Brunner, K. T., 1981, Inhibition of cytolytic T lymphocyte clones reactive with Maloney leukemia virus-associated antigen by monoclonal antibodies: A direct approach to the study of H-2 restriction, *J. Immunol.* **126:**482.

Weiss, S., and Dennert, G., 1981, T cell lines active in the delayed-type hypersensitivity reaction (DTH), *J. Immunol.* **126:**2031.

Widmer, M. B., and Bach, F. H., 1981, Antigen driven helper cell-independent cloned cytolytic T lymphocytes, *Nature* **294:**750.

Zagury, D., Bernard, J., Thiemesse, N., Foldman, M., and Berke, G., 1975, Isolation and characterization of individual functionally reactive cytotoxic T lymphocytes. Conjugation, killing, and recycling at the single cell level, *Eur. J. Immunol.* **5:**818.

Zinkernagel, R. M., and Doherty, P. C., 1979, MHC-restricted cytotoxic T cells: Studies on the biological role of polymorphic major transplantation antigens determining T cell restriction specificity, function and responsiveness, *Adv. Immunol.* **27:**51.

Zubler, R. H., and Glasebrook, A. L., 1982, Requirement for three signals in "T-independent" (lipopolysaccharide-induced) as well as in T-dependent B cell responses, *J. Exp. Med.* **155:**666.

Appendix

ADDITIONAL METHODS FOR PRODUCTION AND CHARACTERIZATION OF MONOCLONAL ANTIBODIES AND CONTINUOUS CELL LINES

Introduction

The Appendix of our first book on monoclonal antibodies included the basic methods necessary for the production and characterization of monoclonal antibodies. Those who have produced monoclonal antibodies are aware that this is frequently only the beginning of the work involved. Confirmation or identification of the corresponding antigen may, in fact, take even more effort than the initial immunization, hybridization, and screening. We therefore include here a collection of methods, many of which are used for characterization of the antigens detected with monoclonal antibodies. These include a variety of ways to detect specific antigens after the electrophoretic separation of a mixture of molecules, as well as methods for detecting the reaction of antibodies with specific cells or tissue sections.

Also included are methods for *in vitro* immunization, a fusion method used effectively for human cell lines, a rapid screening assay using immunofiltration, and an ELISA method for determination of monoclonal antibody subclasses.

In addition to somatic cell hybridization, other procedures for producing continuous cell lines have been developed. Descriptions of two of these methods are included: (1) the definition of specific growth requirements, such as for T-cell lines, and (2) production of continuous cell lines by transfection of primary cells with oncogenic DNA.

It is our hope that these methods will be as useful to investigators as were the ones included in our initial volume.

In Vitro Immunization of Mouse Spleen Cells

ZDENKA L. JONAK AND ROGER H. KENNETT

Introduction

Since the success in production of hybridomas depends on the availability of specifically stimulated antibody-secreting lymphocytes, the most efficient protocol for immunization is essential. We have generated activated lymphocytes by *in vitro* stimulation or by combination of *in vivo* immunization followed by *in vitro* restimulation. The *in vitro* immunization can be carried out in serum-free medium or in medium supplemented with fetal bovine serum (FBS). The advantage of this method is avoidance of time-consuming repeated immunizations as well as use of large amounts of purified antigenic material. Although it remains to be confirmed, it is also possible that by limiting or reducing suppression, the *in vitro* immunization protocol may make it possible to obtain responses against antigens that do not readily give a good *in vivo* response. The *in vitro* immunization technique is a modification of the procedure described by Luben and Mohler (1980). A variety of *in vitro* immunization techniques for mouse lymphocytes and the various factors to be considered have been reviewed recently by Reading (1982).

Materials

1. Spleen cells from BALB/c mice at a concentration of 10^7 cells/ml of medium. Prepare as for fusion as described by Kennett *et al.* (1978). Do not lyse red cells prior to *in vitro* stimulation.
2. Peritoneal exudate cells (PEC) at a concentration of 10^5 PEC/10^7 splenic

---

ZDENKA L. JONAK AND ROGER H. KENNETT • Department of Human Genetics, University of Pennsylvania School of Medicine, Philadelphia, Pennsylvania 19104.

lymphocytes. These cells are generated by intraperitoneal injection of 0.5 ml thioglycolate broths (BBL Microbiology Systems) into BALB/c mice 4 days prior to the *in vitro* immunization. Remove from peritoneum by infusion with phosphate-buffered saline (PBS) or by washing the opened peritoneal cavity.

3. Serum-free medium is prepared with the following additions to 500 ml of RPMI 1640 medium: 0.5 ml ITS (Collaborative Research) (2.5 mg insulin, 2.5 mg transferrin, 2.5 μg selenium), 1 μl β-mercaptoethanol, 1 μl ethanolamine (Murakami *et al.*, 1982), plus 5ml of stock glucose solution (25 g/100 ml).
4. Hybridoma medium (HY) supplemented with 10% fetal calf serum (FCS) as described by Kennett (1980).
5. Tissue culture flasks, 25 cm² (Corning).

Procedure

In vitro immunization was carried out utilizing spleen cells from unimmunized BALB/c mice or with cells from mice previously immunized with the antigens.

In vitro immunization culture contained the following:

1. Splenic lymphocytes at a concentration of 10^7 cells/ml of medium.
2. PEC cells at a concentration of 10^5 cells/10^7 splenic lymphocytes.
3. Serum-free medium or HY medium with 10% FCS.
4. Antigen: either human complement C_2 was added at a concentration of 10 μg/5×10^7 spleen cells or, if Reh cells were used as an antigen, they were irradiated at 4500 R and added at a concentration of 10^5 Reh cells/ml of spleen cells.

The *in vitro* immunization was done in plastic 25-cm² flasks for a period of 4 days at 37°C in an atmosphere of 5% CO_2–95% air. The stimulated cells were then treated as previously reported (Kennett *et al.*, 1978, 1980) for hybridoma production, including treatment with ammonium chloride to lyse the red blood cells followed by fusion of spleen cells with SP2/0-Ag14 placmacytoma cell line.

Other Factors to Consider

1. The source of antigen can vary as well as the amount used for immunization (Sethi and Brandis, 1981; Herbst and Braun, 1981; Luben and Mohler, 1979; Luben *et al.*, 1982).
2. In our laboratory, we have now used this procedure successfully for a variety of soluble and particulate antigens, including soluble proteins and glycoproteins, cell surface antigens, and retroviral oncogene products bound to Sepharose beads as an immune complex.

3. To increase the number of cells responding to the antigen, one can manipulate the immunization protocol by using *in vivo* immunization followed by *in vitro* restimulation.

4. On the other hand, the *in vitro* stimulation may provide a means of allowing a response to "conserved antigens," the reaction to which is normally suppressed *in vivo* (Reading, 1982).

References

Herbst, H., and Braun, D. G., 1981, Anti-streptococcal group A antibodies: Production after *in vivo* activation and hybridization of mouse spleen cells, *Ann. Immunol. (Paris)* **132 C**:87–100.

Kennett, R. H., Fusion protocols, 1980, in: *Monoclonal Antibodies. Hybridomas: A New Dimension in Biological Analyses* (R. H. Kennett, T. J. McKearn, and K. B. Bechtol, eds.), Plenum Press, New York, pp. 365–367.

Kennett, R. H., Denis, K. A., Tung, A. S., and Klinman, N. R., 1978, Hybrid plasmacytoma production: Fusions with adult spleen cells, monoclonal spleen fragments, neonatal spleen cells, and human spleen cells, *Curr. Top. Microbiol. Immunol.* **81**:77–94.

Luben, R. A., and Mohler, M. A., 1980, *In vitro* immunization as an adjunct to the production of hybridomas producing antibodies against the lymphokine of osteoclast activating factor, *Mol. Immunol.* **17**:635–639.

Luben, R. A., Brazeau, P., Böhlen, P., and Guillemin, R., 1982, Monoclonal antibodies to hypothalamic growth hormone-releasing factor with picomoles of antigen, *Science* **218**:887–889.

Murakami, H., Masui, H., Sato, G. H., Chow, T. P., and Kano-Sueoka, T., 1982, Growth of hybridoma cells in serum-free medium: Identification of ethanolamine as an essential component, *Proc. Natl. Acad. Sci. USA* **79**:1158–1162.

Reading, C. L., 1982, Theory and methods for immunization in culture and monoclonal antibody production, *J. Immunol. Methods* **53**:261–291.

Sethi, K. K., and Brandis, H., 1981, Generation of hybridoma cell lines producing monoclonal antibodies against *Toxoplasma gondii* or rabies virus following fusion of *in vitro*-immunized spleen cells with myeloma cells, *Ann. Immunol. (Paris)* **132C**:29–41.

Fusion of Nonadherent Human Cell Lines

Kenneth E. Truitt, James W. Larrick, and Andrew Raubitschek

Introduction

Somatic cell hybrids between nonadherent human cell lines have been difficult to produce. Our protocol utilizes specific nontoxic lectins to adhere cells both to themselves and to the plate. The postfusion viability of cells is monitored with two fluorescent dyes, propidium iodide (20 μg/ml) for dead cells, and Hoechst 33258 (50 μg/ml) for live cells (dyes from Calbiochem-Boehring).

Materials

1. Fusion plates. Costar 3506, six-well cluster plates, 35-mm well diameter.
2. HBSS−/+. Hank's balanced saline solution, Ca^{2+}-free, 2 mM $MgSO_4$ (Sigma). Filter-sterilize.
3. PNA, peanut agglutinin (Sigma) stock solution; 100 μg/ml, in HBSS−/+, filter-sterilized. Store at −20°C.
4. PEG fusion mixture. Polyethylene glycol 4000 (BDH), 40% (w/v); dimethylsulfoxide (DMSO), 10% (v/v) in HBSS−/+. After autoclaving the mixture, add poly-L-arginine (Sigma, 70K-150K, filter-sterilized 100× stock solution) to a final concentration of 5 μg/ml. Prior to use, the pH is adjusted to between 7.5 and 8.0 with sterile NaOH solution.
5. Fusion dilution mixture (FDM). Five percent DMSO (v/v) in HBSS−/+. Filter-sterilize.

Kenneth E. Truitt, James W. Larrick, and Andrew Raubitschek • Cetus Immune Research Laboratories, Palo Alto, California 94303.

6. Appropriately stimulated peripheral blood lymphocytes (PBLs). Mitogen- or antigen-induced blasts fuse best.
7. Continuous cell line to be used as fusion partner, drug marked or otherwise prepared for hybrid selection.

Procedures

1. Add 2 ml of HBSS$-/+$ and 50 μl of freshly thawed PNA stock to each fusion well. Allow plates to incubate at 37°C for at least 1 hr prior to fusion.
2. Each fusion well can accommodate 10–20 million cells. If the number of available cells is limited, smaller wells can be used. The optimum fusion ratio appears to be 1 : 1 stimulated PBLs to "immortal" cells. Cell line cultures should be in log phase growth.
3. Wash cells twice in HBSS$-/+$ at room temperature.
4. Resuspend and combine cell populations in HBSS$-/+$ warmed to 37°C. Add 2 ml of the suspension (10–20 million cells) to each pretreated well. For best results, do not remove the PNA coating solution.
5. Centrifuge the cells onto the plate at 400–500$\times g$ for 6 min. Centrifuge must be at room temperature or cells will not adhere.
6. Aspirate supernatant from the monolayer.
7. Add 2 ml of warmed PEG fusion mix, 37°C, down the side of the well. Swirl once or twice.
8. After 1 min, begin dilution with FDM, 37°C. Dilute at a rate of 2 ml/min (0.5 ml every 15 sec). Constantly swirl the plate to ensure optimal mixing. Continue for 3 min (or 6 ml). Now dilute at 4 ml/min until fusion well is full. Gently pipette (up and down) a few milliliters of the solution in the well to facilitate mixing. Aspirate the well.
9. Add FDM, 37°C, to the well at a rate of 2 ml/min for 2 min. Always swirl the plate.
10. Over a period of 15 sec, add 5 ml of 37°C HBSS$-/+$. Swirl. Aspirate.
11. Wash plate two times with 5–10 ml warm HBSS$-/+$.
12. Add 5 ml of normal serum-supplemented media to fusion well. Incubate at 37°C for 18 hr.
13. Remove cells from fusion well by pipetting. Use of a rubber policeman is not recommended. If cells still stick to the plate bottom, incubate in the fusion well for another day.
14. Pellet fused cells, and resuspend in selective media (100 mM hypoxanthine and 8 μg/ml azaserine in the case of HGPRT-negative parent lines).
15. Aliquot into 96-well flat-bottomed microtiter plates (Costar) at 10^5 cells/well. Feeder layer requirement, if any, will vary with cell lines.

Other Actions to Consider

1. Choice of lectins used to precoat the fusion plate may vary with needs of the particular experiment. Con A, PHA, and PNA all adhere cells quite nicely. Optimal coating concentrations may differ with cell types.
2. During fusion, always add solutions down the side of the plate. Avoid disturbing the monolayer.
3. Best mixing results by swirling the plate when it is supported on a flat, horizontal surface.
4. Optimum exposure time of the "straight" PEG fusion mixture may be decreased for more sensitive cell lines.
5. This protocol has successfully produced hybrids with U266, Jurkat, U937, and various lymphoblastoid cell lines.

References

Brahe, C., and Serra, A., 1981, A simple method for fusing human lymphocytes with rodent cells in monolayer by polyethylene glycol, *Somatic Cell Genet.* **7:**109–115.

Davidson, R. L., and Gerald, P. S., 1976, Improved techniques for the induction of mammalian cell hybridization by polyethylene glycol, *Somatic Cell Genet.* **2:**165–176.

Norwood, T. H., Ziegler, C. J., and Martin, G. M., 1976, Dimethyl sulfoxide enhances polyethylene glycol-mediated somatic cell fusion, *Somatic Cell Genet.* **2:**263–270.

O'Malley, K., and Davidson, R. L., 1977, A new dimension in suspension fusion techniques with polyethylene glycol, *Somatic Cell Genet.* **3:**441–448.

Pontecorvo, G., 1975, Production of mammalian somatic cell hybrids by means of polyethylene glycol treatment, *Somatic Cell Genet.* **1:**397–400.

Schneiderman, S., Farber, J. L., and Baserga, R., 1979, A simple method for decreasing the toxicity of polyethylene glycol in mammalian cell hybridization, *Somatic Cell Genet.* **5:**263–269.

Sharon, J., Morrison, S. L., and Kabat, E. A., 1980, Formation of hybridoma clones in soft agarose: Effect of pH and of medium, *Somatic Cell Genet.* **6:**435–441.

Steplewski, Z., Koprowski, H., and Leibovitz, A., 1976, Polyethylene glycol-mediated fusion of human tumor cells with mouse cells, *Somatic Cell Genet.* **2:**559–564.

ELISA for Immunoglobulin Subclass Determination

ANSELMO OTERO AND ROGER H. KENNETT

Introduction

The determination of monoclonal antibody subclass by conventional immunodiffusion frequently requires that hybridoma supernatants be concentrated. We describe here an assay that can be done without concentrating the supernatants and that provides results more rapidly than immunoprecipitation in gels. Using an ELISA technique rather than one based on radioimmunoassay also adds to the rapidity of the assay by making it unnecessary to wait for the counting of multiple radioactive samples.

Materials

1. Ninety-six-well, flat-bottomed polyvinylchloride microtiter plates.
2. Phosphate-buffered saline (PBS), pH 7.2.
3. PBS plus 0.05% (v/v) Tween 80 (PBS–Tween 80).
4. PBS plus 0.1% bovine serum albumin (PBS–BSA).
5. PBS–Tween 80 plus 4% fetal bovine serum (PBS–Tween 80 FBS).
6. Goat anti-mouse immunoglobulin (Cappel). Titer to determine how far this can be diluted for use.
7. Rabbit anti-mouse Ig class-specific or light-chain-specific antisera (Nordic or Miles). These should be tested in the assay against known subclones of monoclonal antibodies to confirm the specificity in the assay and to determine how far they can be diluted for use.

ANSELMO OTERO • National Cancer Center for Scientific Research, Havana, Cuba.   ROGER H. KENNETT • Department of Human Genetics, University of Pennsylvania School of Medicine, Philadelphia, Pennsylvania 19104.

8. Peroxidase-conjugated goat anti-rabbit Ig (Ig fraction, Cappel). Titer to determine how far this can be diluted for use.

9. Substrate reaction mixture, make fresh just before use (10 ml of 0.1 M citrate buffer, pH 4.5, 10 mg orthophenylenediamine, 4 µl 30% H_2O_2).

10. Hybridoma supernatants to be tested. The panel should include known standards and medium controls (i.e., supernatant from nonsecretor plasmacytoma lines, also fresh medium). Centrifuge for 5 min in refrigerated microfuge to remove protein aggregates.

Procedure

1. Add 100 µl of solution of goat anti-mouse Ig to each well. We use a 1 : 800 dilution of goat anti-mouse Ig (Cappel) in PBS; room temperature for 2 hr.

2. Wash wells two times with PBS.

3. Add 150 µl of PBS–BSA; room temperature for 30 mins.

4. Flick the plate to remove PBS–BSA and fill wells with PBS–Tween 80. Flick the plate to remove this solution.

5. Add 100 µl of hybridoma supernatant to wells. Incubate overnight at 4°C. Set up enough wells to test each supernatant with each class-specific antiserum; at least in duplicate.

6. Wash four times with PBS–Tween 80.

7. Add 100 µl of each rabbit anti-mouse Ig subclass-specific antiserum to appropriate wells. We use 1 : 1000 dilution in PBS–Tween 80 FBS of these antisera when obtained for the indicated sources; room temperature for 2 hr.

8. Wash four times with PBS–Tween 80.

9. Add 100 µl of peroxidase-conjugated goat anti-rabbit Ig. We use 1 : 1000 dilution in PBS–Tween 80 FBS; room temperature for 2 hr.

10. Wash six times with PBS–Tween 80.

11. Add 200 µl/well of substrate reaction mixture.

12. Determine +/− reaction by eye or transfer 175 µl from each well to polystyrene plate and read $OD_{450\ nm}$ in microtiter plate reader to determine class of monoclonal immunoglobulin.

Immunofiltration

A Rapid Screening Assay for Detection of Antibodies Directed against Cell Surface Antigens

ELLIOTT K. MAIN, MARY KATE HART, AND DARCY B. WILSON

Introduction

Many currently used assays for the detection of antibody binding to whole cells are cumbersome and time-consuming. Hence, they can be impractical for the rapid screening of large numbers of hybridoma supernatants. The following method involves immobilization of cells on filter paper discs within a modified 96-well plate. Each well serves both as an incubation chamber and a filtration manifold. The entire assay can be run in 2 hr and can be set up for either RIA or ELISA. Obviously, such an assay system can have wide uses beyond hybridoma screening (Cleveland *et al.*, 1979; Handley *et al.*, 1982).

Materials

1. Modified 96-well flat-bottom plates, each well having a central hole and a filter disc. Such plates are available commercially from V and P Enterprises, San Diego, CA, and Millipore Corp., Bedford, MA, or can be

ELLIOTT K. MAIN • Department of Pathology, Divisions of Research Immunology and Laboratory Medicine and of Obstetrics and Gynecology, University of Pennsylvania School of Medicine, Philadelphia, Pennsylvania 19104. MARY KATE HART AND DARCY B. WILSON • Department of Pathology, Divisions of Research Immunology and Laboratory Medicine, University of Pennsylvania School of Medicine, Philadelphia, Pennsylvania 19104.

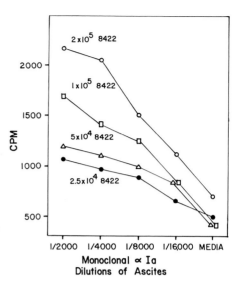

FIGURE 1. Representative radioimmunoassay using an immunofiltration system produced in our laboratory. Monoclonal anti-Ia (ascites) is shown binding to 8422, a human B-cell line, at various target cell numbers. The ordinate units are counts per minute (cpm) of (^{125}I) rabbit anti-mouse F(ab)′$_2$ bound to the target cell following incubation with the first antibody. The abscissa is dilutions of ascites fluid containing antibody. Substituting an irrelevant first antibody (OKT 8 or OKT 3, anti-T-cell antibodies) gives cpm only slightly higher than hybridoma media, 600–750 cpm. For most purposes, we use 2×10^5 cells/well.

easily home-made. Starting with a Costar Cluster 3596, holes are burned into each well with a flamed 27 gauge needle. Filter paper choice may vary depending on the cells to be assayed, but for most uses, Whatman #1 paper will suffice. Discs are cut using a standard ¼-in.-office punch and placed into the wells using a wide-mouth Pasteur pipette attached to a suction bottle. The same suction apparatus is useful for removing the discs for counting at the end of the assay.

2. Vacuum manifold (to apply vacuum to all 96 wells at once): obtainable from either of the sources that produces the filtration plates.
3. Buffers: Phosphate-buffered saline with 1% bovine serum albumin and 0.01% NaN_3 is used for washes; the same buffer with 10% fetal bovine serum is used for incubations (FBS buffer).
4. Iodine-125 rabbit or goat anti-mouse immunoglobulin [anti-F(ab)′$_2$ is preferable].

Procedures

1. Add 50 µl FBS buffer to each well, and allow to incubate 15 min at room temperature. Apply suction.
2. Suspend target cells at 2×10^5/50 µl in FBS buffer and add 50 µl to each test well. Apply suction to immobilize cells to the filter paper. (Before each incubation, be certain that the bottom of the plate is dry to prevent leakage due to capillary action.)

3. To each well, add 50 µl of test supernatant. Incubate for 30 min at room temperature.
4. Add 100 µl of PBS buffer to each well and aspirate; repeat to a total of three washes (each requiring under 30 sec total time).
5. Add 50 µl (^{125}I) anti-mouse Ig (approximately 5×10^4 cpm) to each well and incubate for 30 min at room temperature.
6. Wash three times as in step 4. Dry discs under lamp or in warm room.
7. Harvest discs and count in gamma counter.
8. Results from a representative assay are shown in Figure 1.

References

Cleveland, P. H., Richman, D. D., Oxman, M. N., Wickhan, M. G., Binder, P. S., and Worthen, D. M., 1979, Immobilization of viral antigens on filter paper for a (^{125}I) staphylococcal protein A immunoassay: A rapid and sensitive technique for detection of herpes simplex virus antigens and antiviral antibodies, *J. Immunol. Methods* **29:**369–386.

Handley, H. H., Glassy, M. C., Cleveland, P. H., and Royston, I., 1982, Development of a rapid micro ELISA assay for screening hybridoma supernatants for murine monoclonal antibodies, *J. Immunol. Methods* **54:**291–296.

Binding Inhibition by Cell Extracts

Lois Alterman Lampson

Uses

In this assay, detergent cell extracts are used to inhibit the binding of monoclonal antibodies to glutaraldehyde-fixed target cells. The fixation prevents the target cells from being lysed by the detergent. The assay allows detection of both cell surface and internal antigens in the inhibitor. Thus, it complements quantitative radioimmunoassay against fixed target cells (Morris, 1975), which measures surface antigenicity only. We have used this inhibition assay to quantify the differences in HLA-A,B,C activity in human tissues and cell lines (see Chapter 7) and to compare the retention of antigenic activity after different extraction procedures. The procedure is similar to others in which soluble antigen is used to inhibit binding of antibody to a particulate target (Morris *et al.*, 1975).

Materials

1. Phosphate buffered saline, 0.15 M NaCl, 0.02 M phosphate, pH 7.3 (PBS).
2. Glutaraldehyde (Sigma), diluted to 0.25% in PBS.
3. PBS containing 5% serum (PBS/5% serum). This provides a source of protein to diminish nonspecific binding of the antibody to the other reagents, and any serum source may be used.
4. Nonidet P-40, 1% v/v, in PBS with phenylmethane sulfonyl fluoride at 1 mM. This is the "detergent solution."

Lois Alterman Lampson • Department of Anatomy, University of Pennsylvania School of Medicine, Philadelphia, Pennsylvania 19104.

5. PBS containing 0.5% Nonidet P-40. This is used as the diluent for the inhibition assay.

6. Equipment for radioimmunoassay: Eppendorf pipets, 25 μl microdiluters (Cooke), 25 μl microdroppers (Cooke), Hamilton syringes, plate shaker (Cooke), hot wire apparatus, microtiter plate carriers (Cooke), polyvinyl chloride microtiter plates (U or V wells) (Cooke).

7. ^{125}I labeled rabbit anti-mouse Fab, 30,000–40,000 cpm in 10 μl (diluted into PBS/5% serum). This is the detecting reagent for the radioimmunoassay; other suitable reagents may be used.

Methods

A. Preparation of target cells
   1. Target cells are washed 3 times in PBS, and resuspended to 10^8/ml in PBS.
   2. The cell suspension is mixed with an equal volume of glutaraldehyde solution (materials #2), and incubated at room temperature for 5 min. This fixes the cells.
   3. The fixed cells are washed 3 times in PBS. (Note that the fixation will turn the cells yellow.) The cells may be stored at 4°C in PBS/0.02% NaN$_3$ for several months or longer.
   4. For use in the assay, the cells are washed once in PBS, and resuspended to 2–2.5×10^7/ml in PBS/5% serum.

B. Preparation of inhibitory extracts
   1. Cells to be used as inhibitors are washed 3 times in PBS and resuspended to 2×10^8/ml in PBS. The PBS used for the resuspension should be at 4°C. From this point on, the preparation should be kept at 4°C.
   2. The cell suspension is mixed with an equal volume of detergent solution (materials #4) and incubated for 30 min on ice.
   3. Nuclei and other particulate matter are removed from the extract by centrifugation at 2000 times g for 15 min (at 4°C). Additional material is removed by centrifugation at 25,000 times g for 2 hr. The extract may be stored at −70°C, either before or after the final centrifugation.

C. Preliminary titration of the antibody
   1. Each antibody to be inhibited is titrated against the appropriate target cell in a radioimmunoassay:
   2. Serial 2-fold dilutions of the antibody are made in a microtiter plate, using the microdiluters, and PBS as the diluent.
   3. Ten microliters of the target cell preparation (see step A, above) are added to each well, using the Hamilton syringe.
   4. The plate is incubated for 30 min at room temperature.

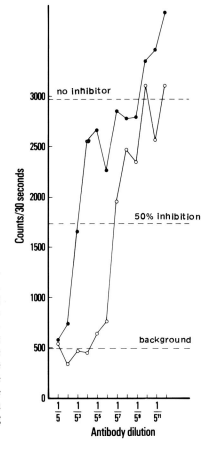

Figure 2. Binding inhibition by detergent extracts. Homogenates of brain (●) or spleen (○), obtained at autopsy, were extracted with NP-40 and used to inhibit the binding of a monoclonal antibody to β_2-microglobulin (L368) to a fixed B-cell target. Binding with no inhibitor and background binding are each the mean of 9–10 values. The volumes of extract required to give 50% inhibition were read from the graph, and the micrograms of protein were calculated, based on the results of a Lowry assay of the starting material. The spleen extract is calculated to be approximately 70 times more efficient than the brain extract, per microgram of extract protein, in inhibiting the antibody.

5. To wash, the cell pellets are loosened by shaking the plate on a vibrator, and the wells are then filled with PBS/5% serum. The plate is then centrifuged, in a carrier, at 250 times g for 8 min. This will pellet the cells, and the supernatant can be removed by flicking the plate. The cell pellets are washed 3 times in this way.

6. After the final wash, the pellets are resuspended (by shaking the plate) in 10 μl of detecting reagent (materials #7) that has been added to each well.

7. After being incubated at room temperature for 2 hr, the plates are washed 4 times in PBS/5% serum, as above.

8. Individual wells are cut from the plate with scissors, or, more conveniently, a hot wire, for gamma counting.

9. The results are plotted as counts/min versus antibody dilution, and an antibody dilution is chosen that is on the shoulder or falling edge of the titration curve, rather than on the plateau. This will ensure that the final assay is most sensitive to inhibition by the extracts.

D. Inhibition assay
   1. Varying volumes of inhibitory extract (for example, 100, 50, and 25 μl), or 25 μl volumes of 2-fold serial dilutions, are added to wells of a microtiter plate. One row is used for each extract. PBS/NP-40 is used as the diluent, and to make each well to the same final volume. One row of wells containing diluent, but not inhibitor, is used to establish baseline binding.
   2. The antibody is diluted, as determined from the preliminary titration, in PBS/5% serum, and 25 μl are delivered to each well with the microdropper.
   3. The extracts have been kept cold during steps 1 and 2, and the plate is incubated at 4°C overnight.
   4. The following morning, 2–2.5×10^5 target cells, (or an equivalent volume of fixed tissue homogenate) is added to each well. After a 30 min incubation at room temperature, the plate is centrifuged to pellet the target cells, and the supernatant is removed by flicking the plate.
   5. The plates are washed, and exposed to detecting reagent, following the RIA procedure in steps C.5–9.
   6. Data is plotted as shown in Figure 2. Relative efficiencies may be expressed in terms of μl of extract, or in terms of μg of extract protein (as determined by Lowry assay).

References

Morris, R. J., 1975, Antigens on mouse and rat lymphocytes recognized by rabbit antiserum against rat brain: The quantitative analysis of a xenogeneic antiserum, *Eur. J. Immunol.* **5**:274–281.

Morris, R. J., Letarte-Muirhead, M., and Williams, A. F., 1975, Analysis in deoxycholate of three antigenic specificities associated with the rat Thy-1 molecule, *Eur. J. Immunol.* **5**:282–285.

Immunoblots and Autoradiography Used to Analyze the Proteins Recognized by Monoclonal Antibodies

CHERYL A. FISHER AND LOIS ALTERMAN LAMPSON

Introduction

Immunoblots complement immunoprecipitation in the characterization of proteins recognized by monoclonal (or conventional) antibodies (Figure 3). Some antigens that cannot be immunoprecipitated easily can be readily visualized on the blots. A second advantage is that the blots indicate which chain(s) of a multichain molecule is being recognized by the antibody. A third is that the starting material is an unlabeled extract. Thus, this procedure is particularly useful for the analysis of molecules or tissues that cannot be radiolabeled conveniently.

The procedure below is essentially that of Towbin *et al.* (1979), as modified by Burnette (1981). To examine the sensitivity and specificity of the assay, we have examined a panel of antibodies to proteins whose structures were already known (Figure 4; Lampson and Fisher, in preparation).

Materials

Background Information

1. The tissue to be analyzed is extracted with detergent (Nonidet P-40) as in Lampson, this Appendix.

CHERYL A. FISHER AND LOIS ALTERMAN LAMPSON • Department of Anatomy, University of Pennsylvania School of Medicine, Philadelphia, Pennsylvania 19104.

Figure 3. Schematic representation of immunoprecipitation compared to immunoblotting.
The figure illustrates the behavior of a monoclonal antibody to a determinant on one chain of
a protein made up of two noncovalently linked
polypeptides. In immunoprecipitation, the antibody is used to precipitate the entire molecule
that bears the determinant from a radioactively
labeled (*) cell extract. The antigen–antibody
complex is then solubilized and denatured in
SDS/2-ME and electrophoresed on an SDS polyacrylamide gel. Because the antibody reacts with
the molecule *before* denaturation, both chains are
precipitated and appear as two radioactive (*)
bands on the gel. In the immunoblots, the (unlabeled) extract is *first* denatured with SDS/2-
ME, and the proteins are separated by
SDS–PAGE and then transferred electrophoretically to nitrocellulose. Then the trans-

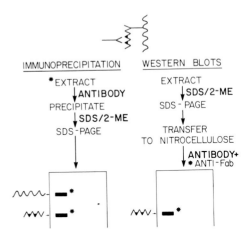

STRATEGIES FOR BIOCHEMICAL ANALYSIS

ferred, separated proteins are exposed to the antibody. Because the two chains have been separated
before exposure to antibody, only the chain that bears the antigenic determinant is detected. When a
radioactive (*) detecting reagent is used, this chain appears as a radioactive (*) band on the nitrocellulose.

2. Slab gels: SDS polyacrylamide gel electrophoresis uses the Laemmli buffer system (Laemmli, 1970).

Transfer

1. Nitrocellulose, 0.2 μm pore size (Schleicher and Schuell).
2. Plastic gloves.
3. Transfer buffer: 25 mM Tris (BioRad), 192 mM glycine (BioRad), 20%
   methanol.
4. Blotter paper (Hoefer).
5. Transfer apparatus (Hoefer).

Radioimmunoassay

1. 5% BSA (Sigma) in Tris-saline.
2. 10 mM Tris-HCl (Baker).
3. 0.9% NaCl.
4. 0.05% Nonidet P-40 in Tris-saline.
5. Detecting reagent: ^{125}I rabbit anti-mouse Fab.
6. 0.1% amido black (Baker) in 30% methanol, 40% glacial acetic acid.

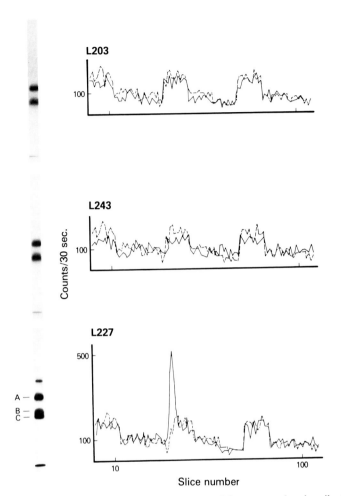

FIGURE 4. Immunoprecipitation and immunoblot analysis of three monoclonal antibodies. L203 and L243 recognize determinants on a two-chain human Ia-like molecule, which is probably formed by both chains of the molecule (Lampson and Levy, 1980; Shackelford *et al.*, 1981). The chains precipitated from a ^{125}I-labeled extract of the human B-cell line Raji are shown in the gel lanes at the left of the figure. L227, which recognizes a second form of human Ia-like molecules, precipitates three specific chains from Raji, which are marked A–C in the figure. Previous studies suggest that the L227 determinant is contained on a single chain, either B or C. To obtain the results shown in the figures at the right, the antibodies were used to label the separated proteins of Raji extracts in immunoblots. The gel lanes were cut into 1-mm slices for gamma counting (solid lines). A lane from the same nitrocellulose sheet which had been exposed to P3/X63 supernatant was used as the control (dashed lines). As expected, neither L203 nor L243 showed any specific peaks, whereas L227 showed a single specific peak. Thus, each of these results is in agreement with the previous characterization of the antibodies by other methods. (The L227 peak is in the expected position for the B–C material, but the weights are too close to distinguish between them in this particular gel.)

Procedures

Transfer

1. The buffer tank is filled with 4 liters of transfer buffer (25 mM Tris, 192 mM glycine, 20% methanol).
2. The tray is filled with about 1 in. of electrode buffer, and the transfer cassette is assembled in the buffer.
3. The Dacron sponge is placed in the bottom half of a transfer cassette in the tray, followed by one sheet of blotter paper. The nitrocellulose is then placed on top of the blotter paper, followed by the gel, two pieces of blotter paper, and the top half of the cassette. (The sponge, the blotter paper, and the nitrocellulose have all been wetted with transfer buffer.) Care must be taken to eliminate any air bubbles that may be trapped under the nitrocellulose and the gel.
4. The cassette is then placed in the transfer chamber with the nitrocellulose facing the anode.
5. A voltage of 15 V/1.5 mm gel is applied for 16–22 hr at room temperature with a heat exchanger in the transfer chamber.

Radioimmunoassay

1. Following transfer, the nitrocellulose is placed in 5% BSA/0.05% NP=40 in Tris-saline and incubated at 40°C for 60 min on a rocker.
2. The nitrocellulose is then incubated with specific antibody diluted in Tris-saline with 5% BSA/0.05% NP-40 and rocked at room temperature for 60 min. Monoclonal antibody-containing culture supernatants are diluted 1/20 and hyperimmune serum is diluted 1/160.
3. The nitrocellulose is washed on a rocker in Tris-saline, then for 5–10 min in two changes of Tris-saline containing 0.05% NP-40, and finally for 5–10 min in two changes of Tris-saline.
4. The nitrocellulose is incubated in Tris-saline with 5% BSA/0.05% NP-40 containing $(2–5) \times 10^5$ cpm/10 μl of ^{125}I rabbit anti-mouse Fab for 60 min at room temperature on a rocker. To reduce the background binding by the detecting reagent, it can be preincubated with an extra piece of nitrocellulose from the transfer. The label is saved after this incubation and is used in the actual assay.
5. The washing procedure in step 3 is repeated.
6. The nitrocellulose is allowed to dry on filter paper and exposed to Kodak X-Omat AR-5 film. Alternatively, the nitrocellulose can be cut into 1-mm slices for gamma counting.

Interpretation

It should be emphasized that immunoblots and immunoprecipitation are complementary and not interchangeable. In some cases, molecules that are not readily immunoprecipitated are easily seen on the blots. In other cases, molecules that can be visualized by immunoprecipitation may not be detected on the blots. This may be because the antigenic determinant is formed by two or more noncovalently linked chains, as is the case for L203 and L243 in Figure 4, or because the determinant has been denatured by the SDS.

Another way in which the two procedures are complementary is illustrated in both Figures 3 and 4. The immunoprecipitation reveals all chains that are associated with the one bearing the antigenic determinant, but does not reveal which chain actually has the determinant. To test this by immunoprecipitation, it would first be necessary to separate the chains. The blots, on the other hand, show only those chains that bear the antigenic determinant. However, they give no information about other chains that might be joined to the antigenic one.

A final point should be made concerning the sensitivity of the blotting technique. When we have used the blots to study antibodies to well-characterized molecules, we have always found the results to be in agreement with the previously established molecular weights and number of the component chains. The blots do not, in general, reveal unexpected chains. In Figure 3, for example, a single expected chain was seen with L227, and no chains were seen with L203 and L243, also as expected. Thus, while the blots can reveal antigens that are not easily seen by other techniques, they are not "too sensitive" to be useful (Lampson and Fisher, in preparation).

References

Burnette, W. N., 1981, "Western blotting": Electrophoretic transfer of proteins from sodium dodecyl sulfate–polyacrylamide gels to unmodified nitrocellulose and radiographic detection with antibody and radioiodinated protein A, *Anal. Biochem.* **112**:195–203.

Laemmli, U. K., 1970, Cleavage of structural proteins during the assembly of the head of bacteriophage T4, *Nature* **227**:680.

Lampson, L., and Fisher, C., Monoclonal antibody analysis of human neuronal proteins: Immunoblot analysis of HLA-A,B,C expression by neuronal cell lines, in preparation.

Lampson, L. A., and Levy, R., 1980, Two forms of Ia-like molecules on a human B cell line, *J. Immunol.* **125**:293–299.

Shackelford, D. A., Lampson, L. A., and Strominger, J. L., 1981, Analysis of HLA-DR antigens by using monoclonal antibodies: Recognition of conformational differences in biosynthetic intermediates, *J. Immunol.* **127**:1403–1410.

Towbin, H., Staehelin, T., and Gordon, J., 1979, Electrophoretic transfer of proteins from polyacrylamide gels to nitrocellulose sheets: Procedure and some applications, *Proc. Natl. Acad. Sci. USA* **76**:4350–4354.

Peroxidase as an Alternative to Radiolabels for Immunoblotting Assays

GERD G. MAUL

Introduction

Pathologists routinely use horseradish peroxidase-labeled probes to identify antigens. However, in most research applications, immunofluorescence or, in the case of immunoblotting assays, radiolabeled antibodies or iodinated protein A are used. Protein A does not bind to all IgG of all species nor to IgM, and the handling of radioactive materials has obvious hazards. The use of other labels in immunoblotting assays is therefore becoming more popular. Procedures with horseradish peroxidase-labeled antibody are described here.

Materials

1. 1% Triton X-100 in water.
2. 4 M urea in 50 mM NaCl, 1 mM Na EDTA, 0.1 mM dithiothreitol (DTT), 10 mM Tris, pH 7.0 (urea buffer).
3. Nitrocellulose sheets (BioRad).
4. Transfer buffer: 25 mM Tris, 192 mM glycine, 20% methanol.
5. 0.1 M phenylmethylsulfonamide (PMSF), 20 mM EDTA (20× PMSF–EDTA).
6. 1% bovine serum albumin (BSA), 1% gelatin, or 1% serum in phosphate-buffered saline (PBS) with 1 × PMSF–EDTA (blocking solution).
7. Self-sealing plastic bags.
8. PBS with or without 0.5% Nonidet P-40 (NP-40).

GERD G. MAUL • The Wistar Institute of Anatomy and Biology, Philadelphia, Pennsylvania 19104.

9. Horseradish peroxidase-coupled anti-mouse Ig or Vector Stain ABC Kit with biotinylated anti-mouse Ig, biotinylated horseradish peroxidase, and avidin.
10. 1 mg/ml diaminobenzidine tetrahydrochloride (DAB) in 0.1 M Tris buffer, pH 7.2.
11. 30% hydrogen peroxide (concentrated stock).
12. 4 M urea or 2% SDS, 25 mM DTT in 0.1 M Tris, pH 7.5.
13. Linbro 96-well plates.
14. 10% Triton X-100, 8 M urea in 0.1 M Tris, pH 7.5.

Procedures

Transfer and Renaturation of Proteins

Separated proteins can be transferred directly from sodium dodecyl sulfate (SDS) gels by the method of Towbin *et al.* (1979), as described in the preceding article (Fisher and Lampson, Appendix, this volume). Many antigenic determinants either survive this procedure or are restored by renaturation of the molecule when SDS is removed during transblot electrophoresis of the protein onto the nitrocellulose. However, some proteins may not renature and thus lack the configuration necessary for antibody binding. In this case, the gel can be washed with 1% Triton X-100 to remove most of the SDS. The Triton is then largely removed by washing with urea buffer (with gentle agitation for 3 hr) (Bowen *et al.*, 1980), which keeps many proteins soluble and allows additional renaturation upon transfer, substantially improving antibody binding.

After protein transfer, the nitrocellulose sheets should be kept wet in the transfer buffer, as drying and rewetting reduces antibody binding to many proteins and eliminates it for some. Storage of transferred proteins on nitrocellulose before immunostaining should be short (not more than 3–5 days) and in the cold, with 1× PMSF–EDTA in transfer buffer.

The nitrocellulose sheet can be blocked 1 hr or overnight with 1% BSA, 1% gelatin, or 1% serum in the buffer used for antibody incubations (PBS). Serum of species other than that used in production of the second antibody should not be used for incubations since low levels of cross-reactivity could lead to some background staining. For our incubations, we use small self-sealing plastic bags and 10 ml of blocking solution per 5 × 10 cm sheet of nitrocellulose with rocking for 1 hr at 37°C or overnight in the cold. The immune serum, the purified immunoglobulins, or the antibody containing culture supernatant can be added directly to the nitrocellulose sheets in plastic bags, although the amount of liquid is kept to 3–5 ml to conserve antibody. Incubation is 1–2 hr at room temperature followed by four washes over 15 min in phosphate-buffered saline (PBS) with or without 0.5% NP40. The detergent is added to reduce background. A clear white background is achieved with some loss of sensitivity.

Affinity-purified peroxidase-labeled antibodies are used in both types of peroxidase assays commercially available. Boehringer-Mannheim manufactures excellent products with either IgG or IgM specificity. These can be used at 1/200–1/1000. If the isotype of the monoclonal antibodies is known, this selection can be used to reduce background; if not, a mixture of anti-IgG and anti-IgM antibodies allows screening for any class of antibodies. The paper is washed with PBS with or without NP40 to remove unbound antibodies and to clear the preparation of any azide or other enzyme-inhibiting substances before the enzyme-coupled antibody is added. Incubation of the nitrocellulose with this second antibody for 1 hr at 37°C or at room temperature is sufficient. Several substrates are available, including the known carcinogen DAB. This is traditionally used and gives excellent results if prepared immediately before use and mixed in equal volumes with 0.02% hydrogen peroxide (made in distilled water), also freshly prepared from concentrated stock. BioRad has a new product which, if used according to the manufacturer's specifications, produces an excellent color reaction (purple). However, it does fade and should be recorded photographically within 1 or 2 days using an appropriate filter. The color development for the horseradish peroxidase-labeled antibody system may proceed for 30 min. It can be stopped at any time if the background between the protein lanes becomes obvious.

Another system available is that from Vector Laboratories (1429 Rollins Road, Burlingame, CA 94010). The Vector Stain ABC Kit was developed for the pathologist to stain slides. Though expensive, it also lends itself to the immunoblotting procedure. It is based on the extremely high affinity of the biotin–avidin interaction. The second antibody (anti-Ig) is biotinylated, and in a third incubation the nitrocellulose sheet is exposed to a freshly prepared avidin–horseradish peroxidase complex. The manufacturer's instructions can be followed as given, though we double all incubation times. The concentration of the biotinylated antibody (the limiting reagent in the kit) can be decreased to one-third, which substantially lowers the cost per sample. The avidin–horseradish peroxidase complex can also be reduced down to one-sixth with excellent results.

An initial dot blotting test is recommended since it allows optimizing antigen solubilization and reagent concentrations without the time-consuming protein separation and transfer procedure, minimizing the number of tests performed. For the initial test, we solubilized samples in 4 M urea, then diluted to 0.1 M urea, and spotted on small nitrocellulose squares in Linbro plates. Many membrane components are not solubilized at that concentration of urea, and other solubilization methods can also be tested. For example, a pellet of cells can be solubilized in a small volume (0.1 ml) of 2% SDS, 25 mM DTT, with or without boiling. Subsequent addition of 0.2 ml of 10% Triton and 8 M urea will help renaturation of the solubilized antigens. After 100-fold dilution in water, the resulting supernatant can be spotted on nitrocellulose squares directly or in small petri dishes. This can then be used as target antigen for initial optimizing of the assay method.

As shown in Figure 5, use of the Vector Stain ABC Kit results in a strong

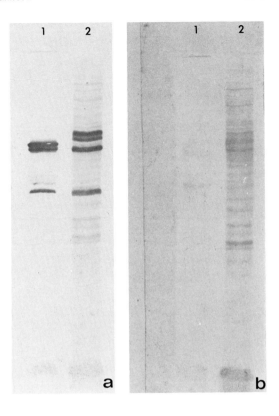

FIGURE 5. Proteins separated by 7–15% SDS–PAGE. Lanes 1, proteins from the rat liver nuclear envelope (NE). Lanes 2, human melanoma cells NE. The monoclonal antibody (IgM) used to stain panel a reacts with the major proteins of the NE. Low background development time was 2 min. Panel b was incubated with a monoclonal antibody that does not bind NE protein; development was 15 min. Background appears over all transferred proteins but not in the areas that contain no proteins. There is also a slight background over areas of the nitrocellulose paper that had not been covered by the gel during electrophoretic transfer.

signal [see Baglia and Maul (1982) for other examples]. The whole nitrocellulose sheet is presented in Figure 5a to show that the area not in contact with the SDS-containing gel shows some background. It may be that there is SDS "washing" of the paper during transblotting or that the gel prevents the deposition of horseradish peroxidase-binding substances from the pressure pad of the sandwich. This is a fortuitous benefit of the gel in the transfer system. Figure 5a shows the assay with a monoclonal antibody of the IgM class. Because of their size, these antibodies give the strongest amplification and therefore the quickest reaction with DAB–H_2O_2 (30 sec to 2 min). The control (Figure 5b) was incubated with the DAB–H_2O_2 until the background became visible. Small dots of nonspecific reaction product seen on the histone band, unlike the specific reaction products, can be removed by slight rubbing. These spots appear where minute pieces of gel have remained stuck to the nitrocellulose sheet.

The sensitivity of the system is such that antigens not visible by Coomassie blue staining (Figure 6a) can still be detected (Figure 6b). We used an antiserum to label clam nuclear envelope (NE) protein and compared its ability to label rat liver NE proteins. Only two protein bands showed cross-species reactivity (Figure 6b, Lane 2). The Coomassie blue-stained gel shows only faint bands, but the immunoperoxidase-stained bands are very prominent and develop within 2 min. This speed of reaction is another advantage of the peroxidase method over the radiolabeled system. The entire assay can be completed in 1 day.

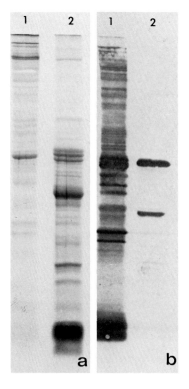

FIGURE 6. Nuclear envelopes (NE) from clam (lanes 1) and rat (lanes 2) separated by SDS–PAGE, blotted, stained with coomassie blue (panel a) or incubated with anti-total clam NE antibodies (panel b). Many bands in the clam sample (panel b, lane 1) react with the antibodies, including several where the band is not apparent by Coomassie blue staining (panel a, lane 1), indicating the sensitivity of the system. The rat NE has only two bands staining (panel b, lane 2) due to cross-reactivity. The high-molecular-weight proteins of the clam NE transfer less readily than those of lower molecular weight and are therefore present on the nitrocellulose sheets in amounts less than those indicated by protein staining of the gel before transfer.

We have experienced difficulties on occasion with background staining of all proteins transferred with no background staining between lanes. The reasons for this finding are unclear as yet, but may be related to excessive amounts of protein bound on the nitrocellulose sheet. Washing with 0.3 M NaCl is helpful. The possibility of product variability has not been excluded.

In conclusion, the peroxidase assay provides the advantages of being more rapid than the autoradiographic system and avoiding the use of radioactive materials. The sensitivity is comparable to that using iodine-labeled second antibodies.

References

Baglia, F. A., and Maul, G. G., 1983, Nuclear RNP release and NTPase activity are inhibited by antibodies directed against one nuclear matrix glycoprotein, *Proc. Natl. Acad. Sci. USA* **82**: 2285–2289.

Bowen, B., Steinberg, J., Laemmli, U. K., and Weintraub, H., 1980, The detection of DNA-binding proteins by protein blotting, *Nucleic Acid Res.* **8**:1–20.

Towbin, H., Straehelin, T., and Gordon, J., 1979, Electrophoretic transfer of proteins from polyacrylamide gels to nitrocellulose sheets: Procedure and some applications, *Proc. Natl. Acad. Sci. USA* **76**:4350–4354.

The Use of Streptavidin in the Detection of Monoclonal Antibodies

Rosemary J. Versteegen and Christine Clark

Introduction

In recent years, widespread interest has developed in the rapid and simple enzyme-linked detection of monoclonal antibodies. Utilization of the avidin–biotin complex has led to increased sensitivity in many immunological and histological detection systems (Bayer and Wilchek, 1979). The development of reagents for an "avidin–biotin"-based ELISA (enzyme-linked immunosorbent assay) has increased the speed and sensitivity of this type of system.

Streptavidin is an avidin analog isolated from culture filtrates of *Streptomyces avidinii* (Chaiet and Wolf, 1964) and is central to the functioning of the Streptavidin HyBRL Screen Kit. Streptavidin exhibits the same biotin-binding capability as egg white avidin. The physical characteristics of the protein, however, are such that nonspecific protein–protein interactions at physiological pH are minimized. The use of streptavidin bridging reagent for hybridoma screening gives rise to a rapid procedure with high sensitivity. Considerably lower background values are obtained than with egg white avidin. Using this methodology, as little as 1 ng of material can be detected in 2 hr.

The reagents developed for this use have also been used to great effect for Western blotting and for immunomicroscopy at both the light and EM levels. Protocols are provided here for both ELISA and Western blot techniques.

Rosemary J. Versteegen and Christine Clark • Bethesda Research Laboratories, Gaithersburg, Maryland 20877.

Materials, Reagents, and Equipment

1. Bovine serum albumin (Calbiochem #126575). This must be free of peroxidase activity.
2. Polyvinylchloride 96-well microtiter plates, flat-bottomed.
3. Multiscan (Flow) or equivalent, to read optical density of microwell contents at 450 nm.
4. Streptavidin HyBRL Screen Kit (BRL #9505 SA). This kit includes:

   a. Biotinylated goat anti-mouse immunoglobulin (BRL #9505A1). The biotinylated antibody is supplied in PBS with 1% BSA containing 0.05% sodium azide. The reagent should be stored at 4°C. This reagent is used at a dilution of 1 : 1000 in PBS with 1% BSA.
   b. Streptavidin bridging reagent (BRL #9505A2). The streptavidin-biotinylated horseradish peroxidase complex is supplied in PBS containing 1% BSA with 0.05% sodium azide. The reagent should be stored at 4°C. This reagent should be freshly diluted 1 : 1000 in PBS containing 1% BSA before use.
   c. o-Phenylenediamine (BRL #9505A3). The o-phenylenediamine is supplied as a crystalline powder. The reagent should be stored at 4°C. o-Phenylenediamine should be dissolved in a fresh solution of 0.1 M citrate buffer, pH 4.5, with 0.012% hydrogen peroxide (H_2O_2) to a concentration of 1 mg/ml. For minimum handling, o-phenylenediamine may be dissolved in the buffer described above (without H_2O_2) to a concentration of 10 mg/ml, aliquoted, and stored at −20°C. This should be warmed to room temperature and diluted 1 : 10 in the citrate buffer with H_2O_2 (0.012%) prior to use.

5. 4-Chloro-1-naphthol (Sigma #C8890). 4-Chloro-1-naphthol is supplied in crystalline form. It should be stored dark. A stock solution of 4-chloro-1-naphthol, 1.5 mg/ml in methanol, can be stored in the dark at 4°C for at least 2 weeks or until it starts to yellow. Prior to use, 1 ml of this stock solution should be diluted with 5 ml of 0.05 M Tris, pH 7.5, 0.2 M NaCl. Immediately before use, 2 μl of 30% H_2O_2 should be added.

Procedures

Preparation of Plates for Hybridoma Screening

1. Coat each well of microtiter plates with the required antigen in a volume of 50 μl using individual preferred protocols. The volumes of reagents used throughout should be adjusted, if necessary, to the volume of antigen solution used when coating the microtiter plate.

2. Wash plate four times with PBS with 0.1% BSA.
3. Add to each well 50 µl of hybridoma supernatant and incubate at room temperature for 1 hr.
4. Wash plate four times with PBS with 0.1% BSA.

Reaction of Hybridoma Supernatant with Biotinylated Second Antibody

1. The biotinylated antibody solution is routinely diluted 1 : 1000 in PBS with 1% BSA. This dilution may vary, depending on the nature of the primary antibody. (*Note:* The biotinylated antibody is stable up to 2–3 days at 4°C after dilution in PBS with 1% BSA.)
2. Add 50 µl of the diluted biotinylated antibody to each well and incubate at room temperature for 1 hr with constant shaking.
3. Wash the plate four times with PBS with 0.1% BSA.

Incubation with Streptavidin Bridging Reagent

1. The streptavidin bridging reagent should be *freshly* diluted 1 : 1000 in PBS with 1% BSA before each use.
2. Add 50 µl of the diluted streptavidin bridging reagent to each well and incubate at room temperature for 30 min with constant shaking.
3. Wash the plate six times with PBS with 0.1% BSA.

Color Development

1. Add 100 µl of o-phenylenediamine solution to each well.
2. Incubate 15–30 min at room temperature with constant shaking in the dark.
3. Monitor the extent of reaction on the plate at 450 nm. If the primary antigen is of a cellular nature, the test supernate should be transferred to a new plate and read at 450 nm.

Result

Wells containing media used for the growth of monoclonal antibody-producing hybridomas will develop a golden yellow color. The existence of a strongly positive reaction will be indicated by an A_{450} of greater than 2.

Western Blot: Enzyme-Linked Detection System

Transfer

1. Transfer proteins to nitrocellulose using standard procedures (Burnette, 1981; Towbin *et al.*, 1979).
2. Block nitrocellulose with 1% BSA in 0.05 M Tris-HCl (pH 7.5), 0.2 M NaCl (TBS), 30 min at room temperature.
3. Discard blocking solution.

Reaction with Primary Antibody

1. Incubate nitrocellulose with antibody solution (antiserum diluted in TBS) for 60 min at room temperature with agitation. As a general rule, 5.0 ml of antibody solution is required per lane. Polyvalent serum can generally be diluted 1 : 1000, while ascites fluid can usually be diluted further. Cell culture medium is used undiluted in this method.
2. Wash two times with TBS for 15 min/wash.

Reaction with Biotinylated Second Antibody

1. Incubate with biotinylated goat α-mouse IgG, diluted around 1 : 250 in TBS. Again, use 5.0 ml of solution per lane for 30 min at room temperature with agitation.
2. Wash two times with TBS for 15 min/wash.

Incubation with Streptavidin Bridging Reagent

1. Incubate with streptavidin–horseradish peroxidase complex diluted in TBS. A working dilution of 1 : 500 will be in the approximate range to give good results but can be optimized for individual systems. Again, use 5.0 ml per lane for 30 min at room temperature with agitation.
2. Wash two times with TBS for 15 min/wash.

Color Development

1. Incubate with substrate solution (4-chloro-1-naphthol) for 15 min at room temperature with agitation (5.0 ml/lane).
2. Rinse in distilled water and dry.

Result

The location of proteins recognized by the monoclonal antibodies of interest will be signaled by the appearance of a purplish-blue band. This is amenable to photography and can be stored in an airtight bag in the dark for some months without fading.

References

Bayer, E. A., and Wilchek, M., 1979, The Use of Avidin–Biotin Complex As a Tool in Molecular Biology, The Weizmann Institute of Science, Department of Biophysics, Rehovot, Israel.

Burnette, W. N., 1981, Western blotting: Electrophoretic transfer of proteins from sodium dodecyl sulfate–polyacrylamide gels to unmodified nitrocellulose and radiographic detection with antibody and radioiodinated protein A, *Anal. Biochem.* **112:**195–203.

Chaiet, L., and Wolf, F. S., 1964, The properties of streptavidin, a biotin binding protein produced by streptomyces, *Arch. Biochem. Biophys.* **106:**1–5.

Towbin, H., Staehelin, T., and Gordon, J., 1979, Electrophoretic transfer of proteins from polyacrylamide gels to nitrocellulose sheets: Procedure and some applications, *Proc. Natl. Acad. Sci. USA* **76:**4350–4354.

Solid Phase Identification and Molecular Weight Determination of Cell Membrane Antigens with Monoclonal Antibodies

Roberto L. Ceriani

Introduction

Molecular weight determinations of antigens identified by monoclonal antibodies are routinely performed by immunoprecipitation methods; however, when these antigens are poorly soluble cell surface proteins, current methodology might prove less valuable. Alternatively, for the determination of molecular weights of cell membrane antigens recognized by monoclonal antibodies, a successful approach is presented which entails the following steps: (1) solubilization of the cell membrane proteins by appropriate means; (2) their electrophoresis in polyacrylamide gel in the presence of detergents; (3) the sequential fragmentation of the gels in desired fractions; (4) the extraction from the gel fractions of the antigen(s) contained by elution; (5) the conjugation of the eluted antigens on a solid phase in appropriate order; and (6) the recognition of the fraction containing the antigen with the radioiodinated monoclonal antibody, or with the aid of a radioiodinated second antibody directed against the monoclonal antibody. The migration coefficient of molecular weight markers run simultaneously is used to determine the molecular weight of the antigen identified.

As an example here, we describe the method for determining the molecular identification and weight determination of an antigen on the membranes of

Roberto L. Ceriani • Children's Hospital Medical Center, Bruce Lyons Memorial Research Laboratory, Oakland, California 94609.

FIGURE 7. Radioactivity profile of components of human milk fat globules (HMFG) identified by monoclonal antibody Mc₃. HMFG was run in a homogeneous 8% polyacrylamide gel, the gel sectioned, and the protein in each fraction bound to solid phase. Antigenic components in fractions were exposed to Mc₃ and binding of the antibody detected by radioiodinated anti-mouse Ig. Bar on top: Coomassie blue stain of HMFG run in 8% polyacrylamide gel electrophoresis. Molecular weight markers: (1) bovine serum albumin dimer,

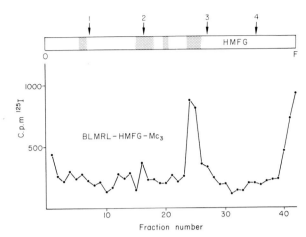

136,000; (2) bovine serum albumin, 68,000; (3) ovalbumin, 45,000; (4) ribonuclease, 13,700. Antigen was prepared as follows: (1) Spin recently obtained human milk in refrigerated centrifuge for 10 min at 5000 × g. Remove cream overlayer, melt at 37°C, resuspend in PBS at 37°C, and centrifuge again. Repeat washes three times. (2) Delipidate HMFG in a negative pressure chemical hood, as described by Ceriani et al. (1977). (3) Dissolve the delipidated HMFG material in cell membrane solubilizing solution (Laemmli, 1970), place solution in ice bath and sonicate with 10-sec bursts for a total time of 1 min, immerse in boiling water for 2 min.

human milk fat globules (Figure 7). This can be adapted to a variety of other antigens present in complex moieties that can be separated on sodium dodecyl sulfate polyacrylamide gel electrophoresis (PAGE).

Materials

1. Cell membrane preparation, whole-cell homogenate of a cell line or tissue containing antigen(s), or other complex mixtures of proteins.
2. Slab gel electrophoresis device, prefably able to run 10–12 lanes and with a run length of 12–14 cm, with corresponding power source.
3. Cell membrane solubilizing solution: 5% mercaptoethanol, 2% sodium dodecyl sulfate, 10% glycerol, and 0.1% bromophenol blue in 0.0625 M Tris buffer, pH 6.8.
4. Scalpel and sharp blade or any adjustable gel-slicing device cutting sections from 1 to 3 mm.
5. Plastic 3.5-ml tubes, Sarstedt (Federal Republic of Germany).
6. Microtiter plates, Dynatech Labs, polyvinylchloride 12.7 × 9.5 cm, 96 conical wells.
7. Bovine serum albumin (BSA), Sigma.
8. Buffered methylated BSA (Met-BSA); 0.01% Met-BSA + 0.3% Triton X-100 + 0.05% Na azide in PBS. Prepared as described by Fraenkel-Conrat, (1957).

9. Dry incubator at 37°C.
10. Phosphate-buffered saline (PBS); 176 ml of 0.05 M KH_2PO_4, 608 ml of 0.05 M Na_2HPO_4, 8 g of NaCl up to 1000 ml in distilled H_2O, pH 7.4.
11. Buffered glutaraldehyde; 0.25% glutaraldehyde in PBS.
12. Buffered glycine; 0.5% glycine in PBS.
13. Anti-mouse immunoglobulin made in sheep, goat, or rabbit.
14. Monoclonal antibody (either from cell culture medium or ascites).
15. Molecular marker kit, Pharmacia.

Procedures

Antigenic Separation and Elution

1. Load 50 μg of solubilized protein per slot on the slab gel according to Laemmli (1970). Prepare at least five lanes.
2. In additional lanes, add molecular markers.
3. Run at volts and amps at room temperature until bromophenol blue front is 1 cm from end of slab.
4. Remove slab, cut out lanes longitudinally from origin to front, fix one for routine coomassie blue staining (Fairbanks *et al.*, 1971).
5. Cut one lane in transverse fashion in consecutive fragments of 1-mm width and place these fragments in consecutive numbered plastic tubes (in the order they were in the gel) containing 0.5 ml of running buffer. Comigrating fragments of contiguous lanes can be put in same tubes; however, resolution could be affected. Lanes not employed at this point can be frozen at −80°C sealed in Parafilm.
6. With a glass rod for each fragment, pulverize gel in each tube and cover with Parafilm.
7. Let stand at room temperature for 48 hr.

Solid Phase Preparation

1. Add 50 μl of Met-BSA per microtiter well. Prepare several plates.
2. Dry overnight at 37°C.
3. Add 200 μl of PBS per well and let stand 30 min at room temperature. Aspirate and repeat once. Plates can be stored dry at this stage at room temperature for at least 6 months.
4. Add 50 μl of buffered glutaraldehyde per well and let stand at room temperature for 1 hr.
5. Wash twice with 200 μl of PBS. Plates can be stored dry at this stage for at least 6 months.
6. Add 5–50 μl from each fraction of gel eluates above to Met-BSA-coated, glutaraldehyde-treated plates, agitate horizontally in rotating agitator for

1 hr, then dry overnight at 37°C. With small volumes, 5–30 µl, it is preferable to dissolve the eluate to a larger volume so as to have a larger surface of contact of the eluate to the coated microtiter plate.

7. Wash twice with 200 µl PBS.
8. Add 200 µl of buffered glycine per well and let stand for 1 hr at room temperature.
9. Wash once with 200 µl PBS.

Molecular Weight Determination

1. Add 200 µl of PBS to microtiter wells, let stand 10 min, aspirate.
2. Add dilution of monoclonal antibody, 50 µl per microwell, to every microtiter well containing the eluates of the sequential fragments of the gel.
3. Cover microtiter well openings with translucent tape.
4. Rotate horizontally in gyratory agitor at room temperature overnight.
5. Remove tape, wash microtiter wells five times with 200 µl of PBS.
6. Add 200×10^3 cpm of ^{125}I-labeled anti-mouse immunoglobulin labeled by the chloramine-T method (Sasaki $et\ al.$, 1981) per microtiter well, cover again with translucent tape, and rotate horizontally in gyratory agitator for 3 hr at room temperature.
7. Wash five times with 200 µl PBS.
8. Cut out microtiter wells from matrix and count for radioactivity.
9. Plot radioactivity counts obtained versus fraction number.
10. Compare to already destained coomassie blue staining of comigrated gel.
11. Plot the slope of migration coefficients of standard marker proteins on graph of cpm versus fraction number, and obtain molecular weight of antigen.

ACKNOWLEDGMENTS

This work was supported by NIH Grant No. CA 20286 and Biomedical Research Grant No. RRO 5467 from DHEW.

References

Ceriani, R. L., Thompson, K. E., Peterson, J. A., and Abraham, S., 1977, Surface differentiation antigens of human mammary epithelial cells carried by the human milk fat globule, $Proc.\ Natl.\ Acad.\ Sci.\ USA$ **74**:582–586.

Fairbanks, G., Steck, T. L., and Wallach, D. F. H., 1971, Electrophoretic analysis of the major polypeptides of the human erythrocyte membrane. $Biochemistry$ **10**:2606–2617.

Fraenkel-Conrat, H., 1957, Methods of investigating the essential groups of enzyme activity, in: $Methods\ of\ Enzymology$, Volume IV, Academic Press, New York, p. 254.

Laemmli, U. K., 1970, Cleavage of structural proteins during the assembly of the head of phage T4, *Nature* **227**:680–685.

Sasaki, M., Peterson, J. A., and Ceriani, R. L., 1981, Quantitation of human mammary epithelial antigens in cells cultured from normal and cancerous breast tissues, *In Vitro* **17**:150–158.

Antigen Localization in Tissue Sections

Kathleen B. Bechtol

Introduction

Information about the development of antigen expression and the cell type and subcellular localization of antigens can be gained by immunostaining of tissue sections for light or electron microscopy. The use of tissue sections conserves information inherent in the histological and cytological organization of the sample, be it normal tissue or tumor biopsy. The technique is sufficiently sensitive to recognize individual tumor cells dispersed in a normal tissue and different cell types present in low frequency within a complex tissue. This approach tends to be most successful for describing antigens present in high local concentration. Indeed, many antigens present in small total amounts, but highly localized in their distribution, are more easily detected by this method than by radioimmunoassay or ELISA.

Materials for Paraffin Sections

Bouin's fixative, Paraplast wax, xylene, ethanol, phosphate-buffered saline (PBS), 0.5 M NaCl, Wheaton staining dishes with slide racks.

Purified monoclonal antibody in buffer (pH 7–8), antibody-containing culture supernatant or ascites fluid, or immune serum.

Horseradish peroxidase-coupled anti-mouse Ig (for mouse monoclonal antibody) in NKH buffer (8.5 g NaCl, 0.4 g KCl, 3.57 g HEPES, 1 g gelatin per liter, pH 7.3), 3′,3′-diaminobenzidine tetrahydrochloride monohydrate (DAB, Aldrich Chemical Co.; *Caution:* known carcinogen), H_2O_2, light microscope.

Kathleen B. Bechtol • The Wistar Institute of Anatomy and Biology, Philadelphia, Pennsylvania 19104.

Procedures

Fix a small tissue chunk (up to 6 mm by 4 mm) in ice-cold Bouin's fixative. For encapsulated tissues such as testis, the capsule must be torn to allow access of the fixative to the tissue. After 2 hr, wash the tissue chunk once with ice-cold 70% ethanol, transfer to ice-cold 70% ethanol for 2 hr, then 95% ethanol in a tighly capped container in the refrigerator overnight. This produces light Bouin's fixation as a function of depth from the tissue surface, followed by alcohol fixation. With mouse testis, this has given good light microscopic morphology with good antigen preservation in many cases.

Continue the standard dehydration procedure, keeping tissue and solvents ice-cold until just before wax embedding. Warm the xylene-infiltrated tissue chunk to room temperature and infiltrate with several changes of 56°C Paraplast. Tissue embedded in blocks can be stored for up to 2 weeks, 1 month, or in some cases years, depending on the stability of the antigen (e.g., Atkinson *et al.*, 1982). While the morphology of the section may be fixed, not all antigenic moieties will survive for long periods, presumably due to slow degradation by moisture, oxidants, etc. Sections can be spread on a 44°C water bath briefly and dried on the slide at 37°C for up to 1 hr. Slides can be stained immediately or, in many cases, can be stored in the refrigerator, preferably with dryrite, for several weeks or more (depending again on the stability of the antigenic determinant).

Before immunostaining, the paraffin is removed from sections by three 15-sec baths in ice-cold xylene, followed by two 15-sec washes in ice-cold 95% ethanol, two 15-sec washes in ice-cold PBS, and one 15-min wash in cold PBS. All of the short washes are with gentle agitation (Sainte-Marie, 1962). The slide is dried with a paper towel, except for the area immediately surrounding the tissue section, thus creating a surface-tension well in which to localize the added antibody.

One hundred milliliters of first antibody is added to each section and incubated in a humid chamber for 1 hr on ice. Negative control for this step is incubation of a section with an equal concentration of another antibody of the same class, but not binding to the tissue or binding to an antigen with different distribution within the tissue. A section incubated with buffer but no first antibody will show cells reacting directly with the labeling reagents (e.g., Ig-positive cells, erythrocytes with endogenous peroxidase activity). Before addition of the labeled anti-Ig, the sections are washed at room temperature in racks dipped into Wheaton staining dishes: 5 min each in PBS, 0.5 M NaCl, and PBS. The slides are again dried around the sections and 100 ml of labeled anti-Ig in NKH buffer is added and incubated 45 min on ice in a humid chamber. For Kirkeguaard-Perry (Gaithersburg, MD) peroxidase-coupled, affinity-purified goat anti-mouse IgG(H + L), a $\frac{1}{8}$ dilution gives sensitive staining and low background.

After removal of the unbound anti-Ig by the series of PBS–NaCl–PBS washes described above and drying around each section, the slides are developed by adding for 10 min at room temperature one drop of 0.05% DAB in 0.05 M Tris-HCl, 0.13 M NaCl, pH 7.6, with 10 μl of 30% H_2O_2 added per 25 ml of DAB solution. The DAB should be dissolved at room temperature no more than

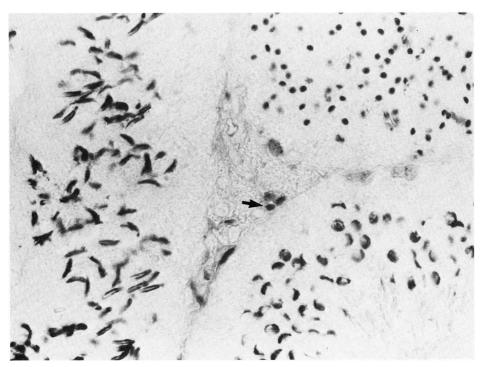

FIGURE 8. Cross section through a portion of three adjacent tubules in mouse testis indirectly immunoperoxidase-stained with an IgG1 monoclonal antibody to an acrosomal antigen and peroxidase-coupled, affinity-purified anti-mouse Ig, developed with DAB and OsO$_4$. Each of the tubules contains cells in different stages of spermatogenesis. In the upper right are early round spermatids with a small (button-shaped) acrosomal cap. The lower right tubule contains late round spermatids with larger, beany-shaped developing acrosomes, and the left-hand tubule contains elongating spermatids whose heads have cycle-shaped acrosomes. Note also the erythrocytes with endogenous peroxidase activity in capillaries in the intertubular space (arrow). Five-micrometer section.

15 min before use, and peroxidase should be added immediately before the solution is added to the slide. Wash off the unreacted DAB by flooding the slide with NKH buffer five times. The product of the DAB–peroxide radical reaction is osmiophilic, and the density of staining can be enhanced by treating at this point with 1.33% OsO$_4$ in PBS for 20 min in the dark in the refrigerator. The slides are then washed by flooding five times with NKH buffer. Dry around the section and add a drop of 50% glycerine in NKH buffer with 0.1% gluteraldehyde, add a cover slip, and observe and photograph the results. An example is shown in Figure 8.

Variations on the Procedure

Fixatives other than Bouin's can be used. The choice will depend on the tissue source and the sensitivity of the antigenic determinant to various fixatives.

Alternatives include the following: buffered picric acid–formaldehyde (PAF; Stefanini *et al.*, 1967), 1% formalin in ethanol, or 0.2% gluteraldehyde in aqueous buffer. Following fixation with gluteraldehyde, free aldehyde groups must be blocked with amino acids or amine-containing buffer (e.g., 0.05 M triethanolamine, glycine, or Tris buffer). When the antigenic determinant fails to survive fixation or embedding or when rapidly prepared sections are desired, the staining procedure can be carried out on frozen sections.

There are alternative chromogens to DAB for development of the peroxidase immunostaining. These include 4-chloro-1-naphthol (Hawkes *et al.*, 1982) and benzidine derivatives. The quality of results obtained with these chromogens is thought to depend in part on the water used. It may therefore be advantageous to test several in one's own situation.

The immunoperoxidase labeling can be made more sensitive, if necessary, by using the peroxidase–antiperoxidase method (PAP method; Sternberger, 1979). For localization of mouse monoclonal antibodies, mouse antibodies to horseradish peroxidase that are of the same class as the monoclonal antibody or that cross-react with it at the level of the cross-bridging anti-mouse Ig are needed (Dr. M. Willingham, NIH, personal communication). The peroxidase–antiperoxidase (PAP) complex is then bound to the monoclonal antibody on the tissue section by anti-mouse Ig, which forms a bridge between the two mouse antibodies. A modification of the PAP method that does not require mouse antiperoxidase is to use mouse monoclonal antibody as above, but followed by rabbit anti-mouse Ig and then add rabbit antiperoxidase PAP complexes and cross-bridge with anti-rabbit Ig (Hancock *et al.*, 1982).

Fluorescein- or rhodamine-coupled anti-Ig offers an alternative to the peroxidase-coupled second reagent. After immunofluorescent staining, the cover slip should be added with pH 8.2 buffer to enhance fluorescence emission (Lennette, 1978). The results are then observed in a dark-field fluorescent microscope. Fluorescent staining may be more sensitive in detecting antigens present on long, narrow structures, such as tubules, filament, and flagella, than is peroxidase staining. The bright line of immunofluorescence is more easily distinguished than is the slightly darker or thicker rod produced by deposition of the peroxide product on top of an already visible line. In contrast, on larger or more complex structures, peroxidase staining may be more sensitive than fluorescence. Stain localization can be more easily distinguished in a narrow focal plane of peroxidase-stained sections where there is no interfering bright haze from the staining in adjacent regions and focal planes. In addition, peroxidase offers the advantage that the stain does not fade and provides a permanent record of the results.

Plastic Sections for Light and Electron Microscopy

Tissues embedded in plastic (e.g., araldite, epon, Spurr's) can be immunostained following etching of the sections in 10% H_2O_2 for 10 min to reexpose the tissue. Several water-permeable plastics (e.g., JB4, methacrylate), which do not require etching before staining, are also available. If the antigen fails to survive either type of plastic embedding and thin sections are desired, the tissue can be embedded in wax initially, and 5 μm sections mounted on plastic cover slips can be immunostained as usual. The stained sections can then be reembedded (this time in plastic) and resectioned to 1 μm for light microscopy or thinner for electron microscopy. The morphology in the resulting sections is not as good as with direct plastic embedding, but in combination with immunostaining is often sufficient to provide adequate definition of antigen localization. For electron microscopy, the anti-Ig can be labeled with horseradish peroxidase, ferritin, virus particles, or colloidal gold (e.g., De Mey *et al.,* 1981).

Conclusion

Immunostaining of sections is both a sensitive method for screening new hybridomas and a powerful descriptive tool for determining antigen localization (i.e., the distribution of the antigen in a given cell and the *in situ* detection of antigen-positive cells).

References

Atkinson, B. F., Ernst, C. S., Herlyn, M., Steplewski, Z., Sears, H. F., and Koprowski, H., 1982, Gastrointestinal cancer-associated antigen in immunoperoxidase assay, *Cancer Res.* **42:**4820–4823.

De Mey, J., Moeremans, M., Geuens, G., Nuydens, R., and De Brabander, M., 1981, High resolution light and electron microscopic localization of tubulin with the IGS (immunogold staining) method, *Cell Biol. Int. Rep.* **5:**889–899.

Hancock, W. W., Becker, G. J., and Atkins, R. C., 1982, A comparison of fixatives and immunohistochemical techniques for use with monoclonal antibodies to cell surface antigens, *Am. Soc. Clin. Pathol.* **78:**825–831.

Hawkes, R., Niday, E., and Gordon, J., 1982, A dot-immunobinding assay for monoclonal and other antibodies. *Anal. Biochem.* **119:**142–147.

Lennette, D. A., 1978, An improved mounting medium for immunofluorescence microscopy, *Am. J. Clin. Pathol.* **69:**147.

Sainte-Marie, G., 1962, A paraffin embedding technique for studies employing immunofluorescence. *J. Histochem. Cytochem.* **10:**250–256.

Stefanini, M., De Martino, C., and Zamboni, L., 1967, Fixation of ejaculated spermatozoa for electron microscopy, *Nature* **216:**173–174.

Sternberger, L. A., 1979, *Immunocytochemistry*, Wiley, New York, pp. 104–169.

Microscopic Analysis of Monoclonal Antibody Binding to Agarose-Embedded Cell Lines

LOIS ALTERMAN LAMPSON, JAMES P. WHELAN, AND CAROL J. LAWTON

Introduction

The unlabeled antibody, peroxidase–antiperoxidase (PAP) method (Sternberger, 1979) is an immunocytochemical technique that has been widely used for both conventional and monoclonal antibodies. In this variation, cells from tissue culture are lightly fixed with glutaraldehyde, embedded in agarose, and then cut into 50-μm vibratome sections. The sections are placed in separate wells of a 96-well Linbro plate and then exposed to the staining reagents in the plate. Finally, the cells are mounted on slides for microscopy.

This procedure permits the rapid screening of large numbers of antibodies, while avoiding the difficulties that may be encountered when mounted sections are stained (such as the loss of sections from the slides). Because the cells are cut open, internal as well as cell surface antigens are directly exposed to the antibodies (Figure 9). We have used this procedure to examine human cell lines fixed directly from culture or after they have been stored (fixed), and also to examine bone marrow biopsies. We have also used this procedure to stain sections of cat retina that had been embedded in albumin (Lampson, Chapter 7, this volume).

LOIS ALTERMAN LAMPSON, JAMES P. WHELAN, AND CAROL J. LAWTON • Department of Anatomy, University of Pennsylvania School of Medicine, Philadelphia, Pennsylvania 19104.

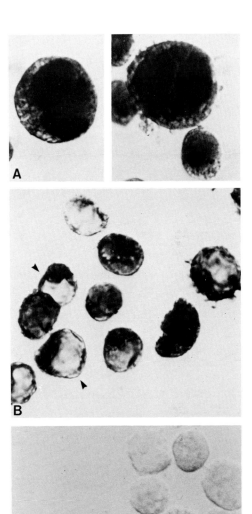

FIGURE 9. Binding of antineural antibodies to IMR-5. Monoclonal antibodies were used to label the human neuroblastoma-derived cell line IMR-5, as described in the text. (A) Antibody A257 stains both cytoplasm and nuclei. (B) Antibody A359 stains the cytoplasm and cell membrane (not easily seen here), but spares the nuclei (arrows). (C) Spent culture medium containing the myeloma protein MOPC21 was used as the negative control. This is an illustration of the way in which we have used this technique to help determine the subcellular localization of antineural antibodies. Monoclonal antibody A257 (part A) clearly stains both cytoplasm and nuclei. It does not bind to lightly fixed whole cells in radioimmunoassay, suggesting that it does not stain the outer membrane. In contrast, monoclonal antibody A359 (part B) does bind strongly to fixed whole cells in radioimmunoassay, suggesting that it does bind to the outer membrane. The microscopic analysis gives the additional information that the antibody stains the cytoplasm but not the nucleus. Although it need not always be so, the behavior of these antibodies against the cell line is consistent with the staining seen in normal neural tissue (L. Lampson and P. Sterling, unpublished). Further examples are shown in Lampson, Chapter 7, this volume.

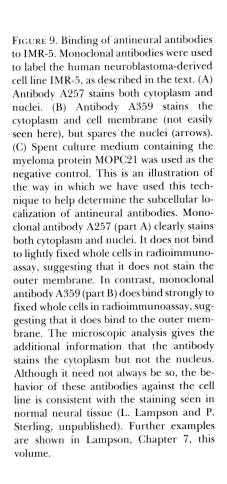

Embedding Cells in Agarose

Materials

1. Agarose powder (BioRad), 4% (w/v) in distilled water.
2. Cells to be embedded (at least 10^6, fixed in 0.1% glutaraldehyde for 5 min at room temperature) (Lampson *et al.*, 1977), maintained in 0.02% sodium azide in phosphate-buffered saline (PBS) (0.0026 M KH_2PO_4, 0.0104 M K_2HPO_4, 0.15 M NaCl) at 4°C.
3. Eppendorf microtest tubes, 1.5 ml (Brinkman).
4. Ice bath.
5. Water bath maintained at 60°C.

Procedures

1. The 4% agar can be melted in a boiling water bath. Once melted, the agar should be kept at 60°C on a hot plate (agar solidifies at 42°C).
2. Centrifuge the fixed cells ($250 \times g$, 8 min) and remove all of the buffer. Gently tap the tube to loosen the pellet.
3. Pipette approximately 0.3 ml of agar into an Eppendorf microtest tube, close the cap, and place the tube in the 60°C water bath. Repeat for as many tubes as necessary. (The pipetting of agar may be facilitated by first filling the pipette for a moment with 60°C H_2O.)

   Note: To avoid heat damage to the cells, steps 4–6 should be performed quickly.

4. Remove one of the agar-filled microtest tubes from the 60°C water bath and hold it at room temperature for 30–45 sec.
5. With a clean Pasteur pipette, draw up approximately 25 μl of the cells, insert into the agar, and release the cells.
6. Stir the agar/cell suspension with a wooden applicator stick to disperse the cells, close the cap of the microtest tube, and plunge it into the ice bath.
7. Repeat steps 4–6 for each tube.
8. After allowing sufficient time for solidification (5–10 min), the agar blocks may be removed from the microtest tube for sectioning by slicing off the bottom tip of the tube with a razor blade and then pushing the block out with a wooden applicator stick.
9. If sectioning is not to take place immediately, the microtest tube should be left uncut and filled with 0.02% NaN_3/PBS. This can be kept at 4°C until ready for use. (We have obtained good results with agar blocks that have been stored for as long as 4 months.)

PAP Staining

The following procedure, which may be used for staining 40- to 60-μm-thick sections of tissue or agar blocks, is an adaptation of Sternberger's method (Sternberger, 1979).

Materials

1. Ninety-six-well, flat-bottom Linbro plate, well capacity of 0.35 ml (Flow Laboratories).
2. Goat anti-mouse Ig "bridge" antibody. This procedure pertains to antibody of mouse origin. If antibody of a different origin is to be utilized, appropriate changes of "bridge" and PAP should be made.
3. Mouse peroxidase–antiperoxidase (PAP) (Sternberger–Meyer, "Clono-PAP").
4. Antibody to be tested (monoclonal antibodies in culture supernatant, serum or ascites, or conventional polyclonal serum may be used).
5. Phosphate-buffered saline (PBS), pH 7.3.
6. Three percent normal goat serum (NGS) in PBS.
7. One percent NGS in PBS.
8. Diaminobenzidine tetrahydrochloride (DAB) (Aldrich).
9. Thirty percent hydrogen peroxide solution.
10. Mechanical rocker.
11. 0.05 M Tris buffer, pH 7.6.

Procedure

1. Place one section of tissue in each well of the Linbro plate. Each well should contain PBS, pH 7.3. (A 0.25% Triton X-100/PBS solution may be substituted for PBS in this step and for all subsequent washes; the detergent is useful when better penetration of the antibody is desired if tissue, rather than an embedded cell suspension, is being stained.)
2. After sectioning is complete, remove the PBS from each well and add 100 μl of 3% NGS. Gently rock the plate for 30 min at room temperature. This reduces nonspecific binding in later steps.
3. Remove the 3% NGS from each well and add 50 μl of the test antibody. The antibody may be diluted in 1% NGS. (Typically, monoclonal antibodies in spent culture medium are used at 1/3–1/30, while serum or ascites may be diluted to 1/10,000 without a significant loss of staining. Optimal dilutions should be determined for each antibody.) Incubate for 48 hr at 4°C.
4. Remove the antibody and wash each section three times by filling each well with PBS and then removing the PBS after 2 min.
5. Add 50 μl of goat anti-mouse Ig "bridge" antibody diluted in PBS. (The

"bridge" antibody should be titrated beforehand. Normally, we employed a 1/11 dilution.)

6. Remove the "bridge" and wash each section three times in PBS.
7. Add 50 µl of "Clono-PAP" diluted 1/200 in 1% NGS/PBS to each well. Incubate 30 min at room temperature.
8. Remove the PAP solution and wash each section three times in PBS.
9. Add 100 µl of a solution containing 0.05% DAB and 0.001% H_2O_2 in the 0.05 M Tris buffer to each well. Incubation time should be determined empirically. We have used incubation times of up to 2 hr without any significant background staining problems. Prepare the DAB/H_2O_2 solution as described below. Note that this solution must be prepared immediately before use. Also note that DAB is a carcinogen and should be handled in a fume hood.

   a. Add 5 mg of DAB to 10 ml of 0.05 M Tris. Note that the free-base form of the DAB must be used.
   b. Add 10 µl of 30% hydrogen peroxide to 3 ml of distilled water.
   c. Add 0.30 ml of the hydrogen peroxide solution to the DAB solution.

10. Remove the DAB solution and wash each section three times in PBS.
11. Sections may be mounted in glycerin and coverslips sealed with Permount. Slides are examined with differential interference contrast (Normarski) optics.

References

Lampson, L. A., Royston, I., and Levy, R., 1977, Homogeneous antibodies directed against human cell surface antigens: I. The mouse spleen fragment culture response to T and B cell lines derived from the same individual. *J. Supramol. Struct.* **6**:441.
Sternberger, L. A., 1979, *Immunocytochemistry,* 2nd ed., Wiley, New York.

Derivation of T-Cell Clones

ANDREW L. GLASEBROOK AND FRANK W. FITCH

Materials

Medium

Dulbecco's modified Eagle's medium (DMEM), high-glucose formulation (4500 mg/liter), with the following additives (Cerottini *et al.,* 1974) (RPMI 1640 or Iscove's modification of DMEM also have been used by some investigators):

1. L-Glutamine, 216 mg/liter (added weekly).
2. L-Asparagine, 36 mg/liter.
3. L-Arginine, 116 mg/liter.
4. Folic acid, 6 mg/liter; 5×10^{-5} M 2-mercaptoethanol.
5. 10 mM morpholinopropanesulfonic acid or 25 mM HEPES.
6. Penicillin, 100 μg/ml.
7. Streptomycin 100 units/ml.

Serum

Fetal calf serum (heat-inactivated at 56°C for 45 min and decanted to avoid transfer of precipitate) is used in all cultures. Concentration is 2% in mixed leukocyte cultures and in maintenance cultures for clones unless otherwise indicated.

Mixed Leukocyte Culture Supernatant Fluid (MLC SF)

Secondary MLC SF generally is used to maintain cloned T cells. Primary MLC are prepared by mixing 25×10^6 C57BL/6 responding spleen cells with an

ANDREW L. GLASEBROOK • Department of Immunology, Swiss Institute for Experimental Cancer Research, Epalinges S./Lausanne, Switzerland CH 1006. FRANK W. FITCH • Committee on Immunology, Department of Pathology, University of Chicago, Chicago, Illinois 60637. Current address for A. L. G.: The Salk Institute, San Diego, California 92138.

equal number of irradiated (1400 rad) DBA/2 stimulating spleen cells in 20 ml culture medium in plastic culture flasks (Falcon #3013). Flasks are incubated upright at 37°C in a humidified atmosphere for 14 days. Secondary MLC are established by culturing $3.5–5 \times 10^6$ viable primary MLC cells with 25×10^6 irradiated DBA/2 stimulating spleen cells in 20 ml medium. Culture supernatant is collected 48 hr later, centrifuged at $3000 \times g$ for 5 min, and stored at $-20°C$. The MLC SF can be filtered, but there may be some loss of activity with some types of filters.

Concanavalin A-Induced Supernatant Fluid (Con A SF)

Lewis rat spleen cells are cultured at a density of 1.25×10^6 cells/ml culture medium (without MOPS or HEPES) in the presence of 2.5 μg/ml concanavalin A. Culture supernatant is collected 48 hr later and processed as described for MLC SF. The Con A SF can be absorbed with Sephadex G-25 (0.2 g/100 ml SF) to remove Con A.

EL-4 Supernatant Fluid (EL-4 SF)

Some sublines of EL-4 mouse lymphoma cells can be stimulated with phorbol myristate acetate (PMA) to produce very high levels of IL 2. One microgram of PMA is added to 10^8 EL-4 cells in 100 ml of medium. Culture supernatant is collected 48 hr later and centrifuged. PMA is removed by adsorption with charcoal (Farrar *et al.*, 1980).

Culture Plates, Flasks, and Miscellaneous Supplies

96-well plates, Costar (#3596); 24-well plates, Linbro (#76-033-05) or Costar (#3524); 50-ml tissue culture flasks, Falcon (#3013); 60×15 mm tissue culture dishes, Falcon (#3002); 10-cm plastic petri dishes, Falcon (#1005); micro hematocrit tubes, plain, Becton and Dickinson (#1021); Bacto agar (Difco Laboratories).

Preparation and Initial Culture of Cells

It is possible to obtain alloreactive clones from unstimulated spleen or lymph node cells, but the frequency of clones is much higher if the responding cells are stimulated first with alloantigen in mixed leukocyte culture. If unstimulated lymphoid cells are used, several hundred cells must be added to each microwell. With secondary MLC cells obtained as described above, 0.1–1 cell is added to each microwell (Glasebrook and Fitch, 1980).

To obtain T-cell clones reactive with soluble antigens, mice are immunized with appropriate amounts (usually 100 μg) of antigen, emulsified in complete Freund's adjuvant, subcutaneously at the base of the tail (Corradin *et al.*, 1977). The draining inguinal and paraaortic lymph nodes are removed 7 days later, and cultures are established using 5×10^6 cells per macrowell in 1.5 ml of medium containing 100–400 μg/ml antigen. After 4 days of culture with antigen, cells are transferred to macrowells containing only irradiated syngeneic cells, and this cycle of passage alternating antigen stimulation with culture on syngeneic cells is repeated several times before cloning (Fathman and Hengartner, 1978; Kimoto and Fathman, 1980). It probably is possible to clone directly from initial bulk cultures, although repetitive stimulation with antigen may increase the frequency of antigen-reactive cells.

Cloning of T cells

At Limiting Dilution (Glasebrook and Fitch, 1980)

T-cell populations to be cloned are suspended in either MLC SF or Con A SF at the appropriate density. In the case of cells previously stimulated *in vitro*, cell concentration usually is adjusted to 1–10 cells/ml, and 100 μl (0.1–1 cell) is added to each microwell of a 96-well culture plate containing 10^6 irradiated (1400 rad) spleen cells in 0.1 ml of medium containing 20% FCS. The appropriate allogeneic stimulating cells are used to obtain alloreactive cloned T cells; syngeneic cells and antigen (100–400 μg/ml) are used to obtain antigen-reactive T cells. The plate is incubated in a humidified atmosphere at 37°C, and 50 μl of medium with 11% FCS and 50 μl of SF are added after 4 days of incubation. Clusters of cells are evident in cloning wells after 7–10 days of culture. Screening for cytolytic activity is performed directly with an aliquot of cells from microwells using a sensitive micro-^{51}Cr-release assay (Engers and Fitch, 1979).

In Soft Agar (Fathman and Hengartner, 1978)

Twenty-four hours after initiation of restimulated allogeneic MLC, 3×10^4 to 1×10^6 cells are resuspended in 1 ml of their MLC culture supernatant fluid and mixed with 2 ml of 0.5% agar in MLC SF. For antigen-reactive cells, 2×10^5 cells are restimulated with soluble antigen (100–400 μg/ml) and 5×10^6 syngeneic irradiated spleen cells in macrowells (24-well plate) in 2 ml of medium. After culture for 24 hr, the entire mixture from a macrowell is mixed with 0.05% agar (1–2 v/v). The cell mixture in agar is spread over a supporting layer of 0.5% agar (15 ml in a 10-cm plastic petri dish, Falcon # 1005). Colonies become visible within 7 days. Individual colonies are picked using a drawn-out Pasteur pipette and transferred to microwells containing 1×10^6 irradiated syngeneic cells and antigen in 200 μl of medium. Cells can be recloned by limit dilution or in soft agar containing 10% Con A SF.

By Micromanipulation (Glasebrook 1984)

Approximately 10^4 cells to be cloned are transferred to a 60 × 15 mm tissue culture dish (Falcon #3002) containing 3 ml of culture medium. Cells are allowed to settle for 45 min and single cells are isolated with a drawn-out capillary pipette (Becton-Dickinson #1021) using an inverted microscope at 200× magnification. A single isolated cell is then transferred to a culture dish containing culture medium and repeatedly expelled and aspirated to ensure the presence of only a single cell. The cell is then transferred to a microwell containing 10^6 irradiated (1400 rad) allogeneic spleen cells (or syngeneic spleen cells and soluble antigen), 50% MLC SF, or Con A SF (or 3% EL-4 SF), and 10% FCS in a final volume of 200 μl.

Maintenance of Cloned T Cells

Both cytolytic and noncytolytic alloreactive cloned T cells are maintained routinely by culture with irradiated allogeneic spleen cells and either MLC SF or EL-4 SF. From $1.6 × 10^4$ to $3.2 × 10^4$ cloned T cells in 100 μl of medium are added to macrowells of a 24-well plate which contains $6 × 10^6$ irradiated (1400 rad) allogeneic spleen cells in 1 ml of medium and 0.5 ml of MLC SF (or 0.5 ml of EL-4 SF diluted 1 : 15). Although peak numbers of cells usually are observed 5 days after transfer, cloned T cells are transferred at 7-day intervals. Cells transferred at shorter intervals have not been found to grow as well.

Antigen-reactive cloned T cells may be maintained by transfer every 7–14 days. From 10^4 to 10^5 cloned T cells are cultured with $10 × 10^6$ irradiated syngeneic spleen cells, the optimal concentration of antigen, and 10% Con A SF (or 33% MLC SF or 2% EL-4 SF) in a final volume of 2 ml in macrowells of a 24-well tray. Transfer to syngeneic cells alone after 4 days will avoid possible presence of antigen if cells are to be used in assays of antigen-specific B-cell help.

Storage of T-Cell Clones

Cloned T cells may be stored frozen by suspending cells obtained 4–5 days after initiation of maintenance culture in 1 ml of medium containing 10% FCS and 10% dimethylsulfoxide at 4°C. After transfer to freezing vials, cells are stored overnight in a −70°C freezer. Cloned cells survive freezing better if stored in liquid nitrogen. Cells are recovered by thawing rapidly in a 37°C water bath with gentle shaking. Cells are centrifuged, resuspended in medium, and restimulated with allogeneic spleen cells (or syngeneic spleen cells and antigen) and MLC SF.

References

Cerottini, J. C., Engers, H. D., MacDonald, H. R., and Brunner, K. T., 1974, Generation of cytotoxic T lymphocytes *1p12in vitro*. I. Response of normal and immune spleen cells in mixed leukocyte cultures, *J. Exp. Med.* **140:**703–717.

Corradin, G., Etlinger, H. M., and Chiller, J. M., 1977, Lymphocyte specificity to protein antigens. I. Characterization of the antigen-induced *in vitro* T-cell-dependent proliferative response with lymph node cells from primed mice, *J. Immunol.* **119:**1048–1053.

Engers, H. D., and Fitch, F. W., 1979, An estimate of the minimal frequency of cytolytic T lymphocyte effector cells generated in allogeneic reactions, *J. Immunol. Methods* **25:**13–20.

Farrar, J. J., Fuller-Farrar, J., Simon, P. L., Hilfiker, M. L., Stadler, B. M. and Farrar, W. L., 1980, Thymoma production of T cell growth factor (Interleukin 2), *J. Immunol.* **125:**2555–2558.

Fathman, C. G., and Hengartner, H., 1978, Clones of alloreactive T cells, *Nature* **272:**617–618.

Glasebrook, A. L., 1984, Cytolytic T lymphocyte clones that proliferate autonomously to specific alloantigenic stimulation. I. Frequency, Interleukin-2 production and Lyt phenotype, *J. Immunol.*, in press.

Glasebrook, A. L., and Fitch, F. W., 1980, Alloreactive cloned T-cell lines. I. Interactions between cloned amolifier and cytolytic T-cell lines, *J. Exp. Med.* **151:**876–895.

Kimoto, M., and Fathman, C. G., 1980, Antigen reactive T-cell clones. I. Transcomplementing hybrid I-A region gene products function effectively in antigen presentation, *J. Exp. Med.* **152:**759–770.

Methods for Transfection of Human DNA into Primary Mouse Lymphocytes and NIH/3T3 Mouse Fibroblasts

ZDENKA L. JONAK AND ROGER H. KENNETT

Introduction

With the purpose of developing a system for further analysis of oncogenic sequence(s), we have developed methods for transfer of genetic information from human tumor cell line Reh (Venuat *et al.*, 1981; Goutner *et al.*, 1977) into two different recipient cells. Transfection by calcium phosphate–DNA coprecipitate has been used in many laboratories. In cases reported previously, the recipient cells used for transfection of oncogenic DNA sequences were exclusively cultured fibroblast cell lines, such as NIH/3T3 (Kucherlapati, 1982; Weinberg, 1981; Lane *et al.*, 1982). Due to the observation by many investigators that NIH/3T3 may not be a true representative of a "normal cell," we chose primary mouse spleen cells as another source of recipient cells for DNA transfection. Our data (Jonak *et al.*, 1983) indicate that we are able to transfect both types of cells, fibroblasts and lymphocytes, with DNA from the same human tumor cell line. This system offers many opportunities for analysis, isolation, and comparison of oncogenic DNA sequence(s), as well as the ability to study the gene product(s) of these sequences(s). This technique has, in addition, the advantage of allowing one to immortalize primary cells, such as mouse lymphocytes, and potentially a variety of other cell types. In the case of the immortalized primary lymphocytes, we have demonstrated that they produce monoclonal immunoglobulin (Jonak *et al.*, 1984). This technique, therefore, has the potential to be expanded to make possible the production of a variety of cell-specific products.

ZDENKA L. JONAK AND ROGER H. KENNETT • Department of Human Genetics, University of Pennsylvania School of Medicine, Philadelphia, Pennsylvania 19104.

Materials

Cells and Cell Lines

1. The Reh cell line (acute lymphocytic leukemia) has been well characterized and described in the literature (Venuat *et al.*, 1981; Goutner *et al.*, 1977). These cells were grown in RPMI 1640 medium with 10% fetal bovine serum (FBS).
2. NIH/3T3 cells were grown in Dulbecco's minimal essential medium (DMEM) with high glucose plus 10% FBS.
3. Lymphocytes: Mouse lymphocytes were used for transfection after *in vivo* stimulation with a subcutaneous injection of 10^6 Reh cells 3 weeks prior to the transfection. The primed lymphocytes were removed from the spleen and treated as reported for hybridoma production (Kennett *et al.*, 1978; Kennett, 1980a).

DNA Preparation

1. Lysis solution: 0.1 M Tris, pH 7.9, 0.1 M NaCl, 0.05 M EDTA, 0.5% SDS.
2. Proteinase K: final concentration 50 μg/ml.
3. Chloroform–isoamyl alcohol (24 : 1).
4. Pancreatic RNase: final concentration 50 μg/ml.
5. TEN buffer: 0.01 M Tris, pH 7.5, 0.01 M NaCl, 0.001 M EDTA.
6. Redistilled phenol.
7. 95–100% alcohol.

Calcium Phosphate–DNA Coprecipitation

1. 10× salt solution: 1.37 M NaCl, 0.05 M KCl, 0.007 M Na_2HPO_4, 0.06 M dextrose.
2. Solution A: 19 ml sterile H_2O, 5 ml 10× salt solution, 1 ml of 1 M HEPES buffer, pH 7.0.
3. Solution B: 1 ml of 2 M $CaCl_2$, 3 ml H_2O.

Media and Solutions for Transfection

1. HY medium (Kennett, 1980a) with or without serum.
2. TY medium is prepared by making the following additions to 500 ml of HY medium: 1 ml ITS (Collaborative Research) (5 mg insulin, 5 mg transferrin, and 5 μg selenium), 2 μl β-mercaptoethanol, 2 μl ethanolamine, and 20% FBS.
3. T-RPMI medium is prepared by adding to 500 ml of RPMI 1640: 1 ml

ITS (5 mg insulin, 5 mg transferrin, 5 µg selenium), 2 µl ethanolamine, 150 mg glutamine, gentamicin (10 µg/ml), 20% (v/v) FBS.
4. Conditioned medium A: TY or T-RPMI medium incubated with mouse spleen cells at a concentration of 10^4/ml for 8–10 days.
5. Conditioned medium B: Equal volumes of TY medium and HY medium which was conditioned by mid-log (6 × 10^5/ml) growth of the plasmacytoma line Sp$_2$/0-Ag14 were mixed and filtered through a 0.2-µm filter.
6. PEG mixture: 35% polyethylene glycol 1000, 5% DMSO prepared in medium without serum.

Procedures

Protocol for Preparation of DNA

DNA for transfections or for Southern blot analysis was prepared by harvesting the cells and washing them three times in Dulbecco's Ca- and Mg-free phosphate-buffered saline. The cells (10^8) were suspended in 1 ml of 0.1 M Tris, 0.1 M NaCl, 0.05 M EDTA, and 1% NP40, and vortexed gently. An equal volume of lysis solution (proteinase K added just prior to use) was added, followed by incubation at 37°C for 2 hr. The preparation was extracted with one-half volume of redistilled phenol plus one-half volume of chloroform–isoamyl alcohol. The aqueous phase was reextracted with an equal volume of chloroform–isoamyl alcohol, and after addition of 0.1 volume of 5 M sodium chloride and 2.5 volumes of cold alcohol, the precipitated DNA was dissolved in a small volume of TEN buffer and dialyzed against the same buffer overnight. The preparation was incubated with pancreatic RNase for 45 min at 37°C. Proteinase K was then added and incubation continued for an additional 60 min. The DNA was reextracted as described above dissolved in a small volume of TEN, and dialyzed against the same buffer. Optical density was measured at A_{260} and A_{280}. The 260/280 ratio should be between 1.6 and 1.9. Prior to use in transfection, the DNA was sterilized by ethanol precipitation and resuspended in sterile TEN (500 µg/ml) or directly in solution A.

Protocol for Preparation of DNA Coprecipitate

The DNA coprecipitate used for transfection was prepared as described in published reports (Graham and van der Eb, 1973). Briefly: Per 20 µg of DNA, add 75 µl of solution A. Mix gently and add dropwise an equal amount (75 µl) of solution B while air is being bubbled through the DNA solution. Vortex this mixture for 5 sec at maximal agitation and allow the precipitate to form for 45–60 min at room temperature.

Method for Transfection of Mouse Lymphocytes

A single cell suspension of stimulated mouse lymphocytes was prepared. The red blood cells were lysed by ammonium chloride (10 min on ice), and the cells were washed by centrifugation. Cells were suspended in HY medium without serum (2 ml per 5×10^7 cells). Thirty micrograms of DNA precipitate was added and the mixture was incubated at 37°C for 2 hr. After centrifugation at 1000 rpm for 10 min, the supernatant was aspirated and the cells were gently resuspended in PEG mixture and centrifuged at 1000 rpm for 5 min. Five milliliters of HY medium without serum was added to the mixture and was followed by addition of another 5 ml of the same medium with 10% FBS. The suspension was centrifuged for 10 min at 1000 rpm. Cells were suspended in 15 ml of TY medium and distributed dropwise into three 96-well microplates. Fresh medium was added once a week. After approximately 14–20 days, the transformed lymphocytes appeared as clumps of cells slightly larger in size compared to nontransformed lymphocytes. These cells were passaged to additional wells in the same size plates and then to wells of a 24-well plate before being passaged to flasks. Alternatively, T-RPMI medium was used for growth of some transfectants. In early experiments, conditioned medium B was used. Recently, it has been found that conditioned medium A is more effective. This medium was used preferentially for cloning of the transfectants in semisolid agarose [technique described for hybridomas (Kennett, 1980b)].

Method for Transfection of NIH/3T3 Cells

NIH/3T3 cells were seeded in 60-mm petri dishes 18–24 hr prior to the transfection, which was done when the cells achieved 70–80% confluency. After removing all the medium and washing with HY without serum, the calcium phosphate–DNA coprecipitate (15 μg of DNA/plate of 5×10^5 cells) was added along with 1 ml of HY medium without serum. Cells were incubated for 4 hr at 37°C (5% CO_2). The medium was then removed and 1 ml of PEG solution was added for 3 min. Cells were washed with medium without serum and three times in HY medium with serum. HY medium with 10% FBS was then added. After 24 hr, the cells were divided into three 100-mm plates. The cells were fed with fresh HY with 10% FBS every 4 days, and 7–20 days later were scored for transformed foci. Transfectants were cloned in semisolid agarose as described previously for hybridomas (Kennett, 1980b).

References

Graham, F. L., and van der Eb, A. J., 1973, *Virology* **52**:456–467.

Goutner, A., Choquet, C., Venaut, A. M., Kayibanda, B., Pico, J. L., Rosenfeld, C., and Greaves, M. F., 1977, *Nature* **267**:841–843.

Jonak, Z. L., Braman, V., and Kennett, R. H., 1984, *Hybridoma*, in press.

Kennett, R. H., 1980a, in: *Monoclonal Antibodies. Hybridomas: A New Dimension in Biological Analyses* (R. H. Kennett, T. J. McKearn, and K. B. Bechtol, eds.), Plenum Press, New York, pp. 365–367.

Kennett, R. H., 1982b, in: *Monoclonal Antibodies. Hybridomas: A New Dimension in Biological Analyses* (R. H. Kennett, T. J. McKearn, and K. B. Bechtol, eds.), Plenum Press, New York, pp. 372–373.

Kennett, R. H., Denis, K. A., Tung, A. S., and Klinman, N. R., 1978, *Curr. Top. Microbiol. Immunol.* **81:**77–94.

Kucherlapati, R., 1982, in: *Advances in Cell Culture* (K. Maramorosch, ed.), Academic Press, New York, pp. 69–98.

Lane, M., Sainten, A., and Cooper, G. M., 1982, *Cell* **28:**873–880.

Venuat, A., Testu, M. and Rosenfeld,C., 1981, *Cytogenet. Cell Genet.* **3:**327–334.

Weinberg, R. A., 1981, *Biochim. Biophys. Acta* **651:**25–35.

Cell Lines for Hybridoma Formation and References to Other Methods

Introduction

Several of the plasmacytoma cell lines and a variety of hybridomas are currently available from the American Type Culture Collection, 12301 Parklawn Drive, Rockville, Maryland 20852. A smaller collection is also available at the Institute for Medical Research, Copewood Street, Camden, New Jersey.

References are given for publications that include detailed descriptions of methods used in the production and application of monoclonal antibodies.

Mouse Plasmacytomas

P3/X63-Ag8: the original hybridoma parental cell (κ_1, γ_1)

Kohler, G., and Milstein, C., 1975, Continuous cultures of fused cells secreting antibody of pre-defined specificity, *Nature* **256**:495–497.

P3/NS1/1-Ag4-1: nonsecretor variant of P3/X63-Ag8 (κ chain is secreted in hybridomas)

Kohler, G., and Milstein, C., 1976, Derivation of specific antibody producing tissue cultured tumor cell lines by cell fusion, *Eur. J. Immunol.* **6**:511–519.

MCP11-45.6.TG1.7 (κ, γ_{2b})

Margolies, D. N., Koehl, W. M., and Scharff, M. D., 1976, Somatic cell hybridization of mouse myeloma cells, *Cell* **8**: 405–415.

Sp2/0-Ag14: a nonproducer derived from a P3/X63-Ag8 hybridoma

Shulman, M., Wilde, C. D., and Kohler, G., 1978, A better cell line for making hybridomas secreting specific antibodies, *Nature* **276:**269–270.

S194/5.XXO.BU.1: a nonproducer

Trowbridge, I. S., 1978, Interspecies spleen–myeloma hybrid producing monoclonal antibodies against mouse lymphocyte surface glycoprotein, T200, *J. Exp. Med.* **148:**313–323.

Rat Plasmacytomas

210.RCY3-Ag.1.2.3: (κ) derived from a LOU rat

Galfre, G., Milstein, C., and Wright, B., 1979, Rat × rat hybrid myelomas and a monoclonal anti-Fd portion of mouse IgG, *Nature* **277:**131–133.

IR983F

Bazin, H., 1982, Production of rat monoclonal antibodies with the LOU rat non-secreting IR983F myeloma cell line in: *Protides of the Biological Fluids 29th Colloquium, 1981* (H. Peeters, ed.), Pergamon Press, New York, pp. 615–618.

Human Cell Lines

See references to the various human cell lines used in Buck *et al.,* Chapter 11, this volume.

References to Other Methods

Hunnell, J. G. R. (ed.), 1982, *Monoclonal Hybridoma Antibodies: Techniques and Applications,* CRC Press, Boca Raton, Florida.
Kohler, G. (ed.), 1980, *Hybridoma Techniques,* Cold Spring Harbor Laboratory, Cold Spring Harbor, New York.
Langone, J. J., and van Vunakis, H. (eds.), 1983, *Monoclonal Antibodies and General Immunoassay Methods, Methods in Enzymology,* Volume 92, Part E, Academic Press, New York.

Index